ILLUSTRATED ANATOMY of the HEAD and NECK

SECOND EDITION

ILLUSTRATED ANATOMY of the HEAD and NECK

MARGARET J. FEHRENBACH, RDH, MS
Dental Hygienist, Educational Consultant,
*   and Oral Biologist*
Private Practice, Seattle, Washington
Adjunct Faculty, Marquette University
Milwaukee, Wisconsin

SUSAN W. HERRING, PhD
Anatomist and Researcher
Professor of Orthodontics, School of Dentistry
Adjunct Professor of Biological Structure, School of Medicine
University of Washington,
Seattle, Washington

Illustrated by
PAT THOMAS, CMI
Certified Medical Illustrator, AMI
Oak Park, Illinois

W.B. SAUNDERS COMPANY
A Harcourt Health Sciences Company
Philadelphia ■ London ■ New York ■ St Louis ■ Sydney ■ Toronto

W.B. SAUNDERS COMPANY
A Harcourt Health Sciences Company

The Curtis Center
Independence Square West
Philadelphia, Pennsylvania 19106

Library of Congress Cataloging-in-Publication Data

Fehrenbach, Margaret J.
Illustrated anatomy of the head and neck / Margaret J. Fehrenbach, Susan W. Herring:
illustrated by Pat Thomas—2nd ed.

p. cm.

Includes bibliographical references and index.

ISBN 0–7216–9363–6

1. Head—Anatomy, 2. Neck—Anatomy. I. Herring, Susan W. II. Title.
[DNLM: 1. Head—anatomy & histology—Programmed Instruction. 2. Neck—anatomy
& histology—Programmed Instruction.   WE 18.2 F296i 2002]

QM535 .F44 2002   611′.91—dc21   2001049539

Publishing Director: Andrew Allen
Acquisition Editor: Shirley Kuhn
Project Manager: Agnes Hunt Byrne
Production Manager: Peter Faber
Illustration Specialist: Lisa Lambert
Book Designer: Gene Harris

ILLUSTRATED ANATOMY OF THE HEAD AND NECK   ISBN 0–7216–9363–6

Printed in the United States of America.

Last digit is the print number: 9   8   7   6   5   4   3   2   1

Reviewers

JOSEPH E. BAUGHMAN, DDS
Lanier Technical Institute
Oakwood, Georgia

CAROL A. BIBB, PhD, DDS
University of California, Los Angeles, School of Dentistry
West Los Angeles College Department of Dental Hygiene
Los Angeles, California

JOHN W. CAMPBELL, PhD, MS, MBA, BS, CCC-SLP
University of Oklahoma Health Sciences Center
Department of Veterans Affairs Medical Center
Oklahoma City, Oklahoma

NANCY CUTTIC, BSDH, MEd
Harcum College
Bryn Mawr, Pennsylvania

JANICE P. DeWALD, BSDH, DDS, MS
Baylor College of Dentistry
The Texas A & M University System
Health Science Center
Dallas, Texas

SARAH ANN TURNER, RDH, MAE
Hawkeye Community College
Waterloo, Iowa

Preface

OVERVIEW

To meet the needs of today's dental professional, this textbook on head and neck anatomy has more than the basic information on the topic. Special emphasis is placed on the specific anatomy of the temporomandibular joint in order to allow the dental professional to understand the disorders associated with this joint. The textbook also includes a chapter on the anatomical basis of local anesthesia for pain control. Another chapter explains the routes of the spread of dental infection.

The authors and illustrator of this textbook have tried to make it easy to understand, as well as interesting to read. We hope that it challenges the reader to incorporate the information presented into clinical situations.

FEATURES

Each chapter topic has been chosen to be relevant to the present needs of the dental professional and to build on former topics. Each chapter begins with an outline of subjects covered, learning objectives, and a list of key words with a pronunciation guide. This pronunciation guide is based on *Dorland's Medical Dictionary*, 29th edition, W.B. Saunders Company, Philadelphia. The chapters continue with an organized text and pronunciation guide for each anatomical structure, original illustrations where possible, and clinical photographs where applicable. The anatomical terms follow those outlined in the internationally approved official body of anatomical nomenclature, *Nomina Anatomica*, 6th edition, Churchill Livingstone, New York.

Further study of the subject has been made easier with tables that summarize information, identification exercises, and review questions and activities for each chapter. A bibliography, answers to each chapter's review questions, a glossary of key words and anatomical terms, and an index are at the end of the textbook. Within each chapter, there may be references to other chapters so that the reader can review or investigate interesting interrelated subjects.

NEW EDITION

With the new edition, there is an increase in the number of identification exercises, and review questions and activities. Additionally, references to clinical situations have been further emphasized throughout the textbook. The important anatomy-related chapters on the temporamandibular joint, local anesthesia, and spread of dental infection have been revised. The chapter on the nervous system has also been revised to include information on the central nervous system. Finally, within the added *Appendix* there are *Head and Neck Anatomy Review Cases* with initial narrative, related photographs, and associated review questions and answers. In addition, there is a table outlining the procedure for *Conducting an Extraoral and Intraoral Examination*. The associated *Slide Series* has also been updated.

MARGARET J. FEHRENBACH

SUSAN W. HERRING

Acknowledgments

The authors would like to thank photographer Jim Clark, University of Washington, Seattle, who provided many of the skull photographs.

We would also like to thank Doreen Naughton, RDH, BS, Dental Hygiene Health Services, Seattle, and Dental Public Health Sciences Department, University of Washington Dental School, Seattle, for her clinical expertise on the local anesthesia chapter. We also thank Mary Bath-Balogh, BA, BS, MS, Faculty, Biological and Health Sciences, Pierce College, Tacoma, Washington, for her assistance on the chapter on the nervous system, as well as Heidi Schlei, RDH, MS, Instructor, Dental Hygiene Program, Waukesha County Technical College, Pewaukee, Wisconsin. Finally, we would like to thank our editor, Shirley Kuhn, and the staff of the W.B. Saunders Company for making the new edition possible.

MARGARET J. FEHRENBACH

SUSAN W. HERRING

Contents

Introduction

CHAPTER OUTLINE

This chapter discusses the following topics:

I. Clinical Applications
II. Anatomical Nomenclature
III. Normal Anatomical Variation

LEARNING OBJECTIVES

After studying this chapter, the reader should be able to:

1. Define and pronounce all the key words and anatomical terms in this chapter.
2. Discuss the clinical applications of the study of head and neck anatomy by dental professionals.
3. Apply the correct anatomical nomenclature during the study of head and neck anatomy.
4. Discuss normal anatomical variation and how it applies to different structures of the head and neck.
5. Correctly complete the review questions and activities for this chapter.

KEY WORDS

Anterior (an-**tere**-ee-or) Front of an area of the body.

Apex (**ay**-peks) Pointed end of a conical structure.

Contralateral (kon-trah-**lat**-er-il) Structures on the opposite side of the body.

Deep (deep) Structures located inward, away from the body surface.

Distal (**dis**-tl) Area that is farther away from the median plane of the body.

Dorsal (**dor**-sal) Back of an area of the body.

External (eks-**tern**-il) Outer side of the wall of a hollow structure.

Frontal plane (**frunt**-il) Plane created by an imaginary line that divides the body at any level into anterior and posterior parts.

Frontal section (**frunt**-il) Section of the body through any frontal plane.

Horizontal plane (hor-i-**zon**-tal) Plane created by an imaginary line that divides the body at any level into superior and inferior parts.

Inferior (in-**fere**-ee-or) Area that faces away from the head and toward the feet of the body.

Internal (in-**tern**-il) Inner side of the wall of a hollow structure.

Ipsilateral (ip-see-**lat**-er-il) Structures on the same side of the body.

Lateral (**lat**-er-il) Area that is farther away from the median plane of the body or structure.

Medial (**me**-dee-il) Area that is closer to the median plane of the body or structure.

Median (**me**-dee-an) Structure at the median plane.

Median plane (**me**-dee-an) Plane created by an imaginary line dividing the body into right and left halves.

Midsagittal section (mid-**saj**-i-tl) Section of the body through the median plane.

Posterior (pos-**tere**-ee-or) Back of an area of the body.

Proximal (**prok**-si-mil) Area closer to the median plane of the body.

Sagittal plane (**saj**-i-tl) Any plane of the body created by an imaginary plane parallel to the median plane.

Superficial (soo-per-**fish**-al) Structures located toward the surface of the body.

(continued)

Superior (soo-**pere**-ee-or) Area that faces toward the head of the body, away from the feet.

Transverse section (**trans**-vers) Section of the body through any horizontal plane.

Ventral (**ven**-tral) Front of an area of the body.

CLINICAL APPLICATIONS

The dental professional must have a thorough knowledge of head and neck anatomy when performing patient examination procedures, both extraoral and intraoral (Figure 1–1). The knowledge of normal anatomy will help determine if any abnormalities or lesions exist and possibly indicate the etiology and amount of involvement. This knowledge will also provide a basis for the description of the lesion and its location for record-keeping purposes.

Head and neck anatomy is also useful when performing dental radiology procedures. Landmarks are used by the dental professional in the placement of the films, and knowledge of anatomy is important in the mounting and analysis of the films.

A patient may also present features of a temporomandibular joint disorder. A dental professional must have knowledge of the normal anatomy of the joint in order to understand the various disorders associated with it.

More specifically, the administration of local anesthesia is based on landmarks of the head and neck. The knowledge of anatomy will facilitate treatment planning of local anesthesia by the dental professional for the reduction of pain during various dental procedures. This knowledge will also allow for the correct placement of the syringe, potentially avoiding complications.

During the examination of the patient, the dental professional may also note the presence of a dental infection. It is important to know the source of the infection as well as the areas it could spread to by way of certain anatomical features of the head and neck. Knowledge of the anatomy will supply the background for understanding the spread of dental infection.

FIGURE 1–1 ■ Extraoral, as well as intraoral, examination of the patient is based on knowledge of head and neck anatomy.

ANATOMICAL NOMENCLATURE

Before beginning the study of head and neck anatomy, the dental professional may need to review the basic *anatomical nomenclature* (an-ah-**tom**-ik-al **no**-men-kla-cher), which is the system of names of anatomical structures. This review will allow for the easy application of these terms to the head and neck area.

The nomenclature of anatomy is based on the body's being in *anatomical position* (Figure 1–2). In anatomical position, the body is standing erect. The arms are at the sides with the palms and toes directed forward and the eyes looking forward. This position is assumed even when the body may be supine (on the back) or prone (on the front).

FIGURE 1–2 ■ Body in anatomical position.

When studying the body in anatomical position, certain terms are used to refer to areas in relationship to other areas (Figure 1–3). The front of an area in relationship to the entire body is its *anterior* (an-**tere**-ee-or) portion. The back of an area is its *posterior* (pos-**tere**-ee-or) portion. The *ventral* (**ven**-tral) portion is directed toward the anterior and is the opposite of the *dorsal* (**dor**-sal) portion when considering the entire body.

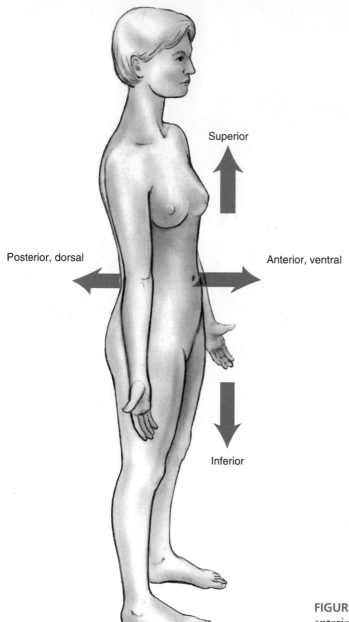

Superior

Posterior, dorsal

Anterior, ventral

Inferior

FIGURE 1–3 ■ Body in anatomical position with the anterior (or ventral), posterior (or dorsal), superior, and inferior areas noted.

Other terms can be used to refer to areas in relationship to other areas of the body (Figure 1–3). An area that faces toward the head and away from the feet is its *superior* (soo-**pere**-ee-or) portion. An area that faces away from the head and toward the feet is its *inferior* (in-**fere**-ee-or) portion. As an example, the face is on the anterior side of the head, and the hair is superior and posterior to the

face. The *apex* (**ay**-peks) or tip is the pointed end of a conical structure, such as the tongue's apex or tip.

The body in anatomical position can be divided by planes or flat surfaces (Figure 1–4). The *median plane* (**me**-dee-an) or midsagittal plane is created by an imaginary line dividing the body into right and left halves. On the surface of the body, these

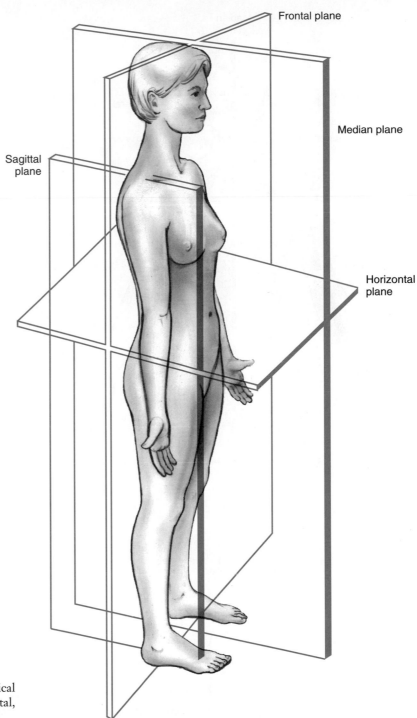

Frontal plane

Median plane

Sagittal plane

Horizontal plane

FIGURE 1–4 ■ Body in anatomical position with the median, sagittal, horizontal, and frontal planes noted.

halves are generally symmetrical in structure, yet the same symmetry does not apply to all internal structures.

Other planes can be created by different imaginary lines (Figure 1–4). A *sagittal plane* (**saj**-i-tl) is any plane created by an imaginary plane parallel to the median plane. A *frontal plane* (**frunt**-il) or coronal plane is created by an imaginary line dividing the body at any level into anterior and posterior parts. A *horizontal plane* (hor-i-**zon**-tal)

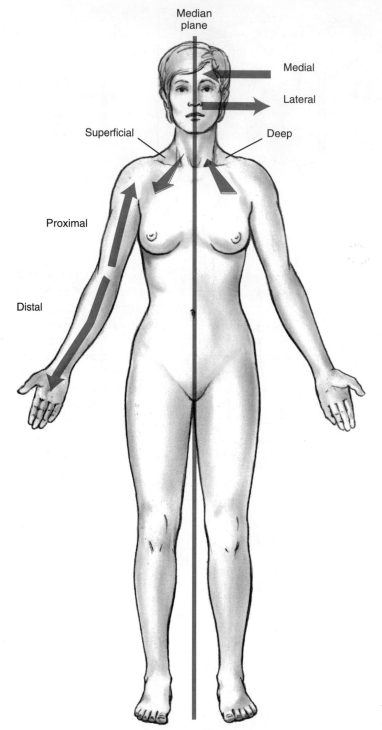

FIGURE 1–5 ■ Body in anatomical position with the medial (or proximal), lateral (or distal), and superficial (or deep) areas noted.

is created by an imaginary line dividing the body at any level into superior and inferior parts and is perpendicular to the median plane.

Portions of the body in anatomical position can also be described in relationship to these planes (Figure 1–5). A structure located at the median plane, for example the nose, is considered *median* (**me**-dee-an). An area closer to the median plane of the body or structure is considered *medial* (**me**-dee-il). An area farther from the median plane of the body or structure is considered *lateral* (**lat**-er-il). For example, the eyes are medial to the ears, and the ears are lateral to the eyes.

Terms can be used to describe the relationship of portions of the body in anatomical position (Figure 1–5). An area closer to the median plane is considered by anatomists *proximal* (**prok**-si-mal), and an area farther from the median plane is *distal* (**dis**-tl). For example, in the upper limb, the shoulder is proximal, and the fingers are distal.

Additional terms can be used to describe relationships between structures. Structures on the same side of the body are considered *ipsilateral* (ip-see-**lat**-er-il). Structures on the opposite side of the body are considered *contralateral* (kon-trah-**lat**-er-il). For example, the right leg is ipsilateral to the right arm but contralateral to the left arm.

Certain terms can be used to give information about the depth of a structure in relationship to the surface of the body (Figure 1–5). The structures located toward the surface of the body are *superficial* (soo-per-**fish**-al). The structures located inward, away from the body surface, are *deep* (deep). For example, the skin is superficial, and the bones are deep.

Terms also can be used to give information about location in hollow structures such as the braincase of the skull. The inner side of the wall of a hollow structure is referred to as *internal* (in-**tern**-il). The outer side of the wall of a hollow structure is *external* (eks-**tern**-il).

The body or portions of it in anatomical position can also be cut or divided into sections along various planes in order to study the specific anatomy of a region (Figure 1–6). The *midsagittal section* (mid-**saj**-i-tl) or median section is a cut through the median plane. The *frontal section* (**frunt**-il) or coronal section is a cut through any frontal plane. The *transverse section* (**trans**-vers) or horizontal section is a cut through a horizontal plane.

▓ NORMAL ANATOMICAL VARIATION

When studying anatomy, the dental professional must understand that there can be anatomical variation of head and neck structures that is still within normal limits. The number of bones and muscles in the head and neck is usually constant, but specific details of these structures can vary from patient to patient. Bones may have different sizes of processes. Muscles may differ in size and details of their attachments. Joints, vessels, nerves, glands, lymph nodes, and fascial planes and spaces of an individual can vary in size, location, and even presence. The most common variations of the head and neck that affect dental treatment are discussed in this text.

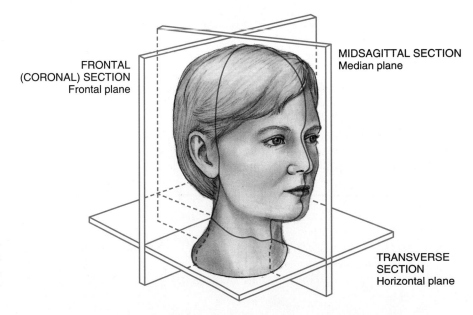

FRONTAL (CORONAL) SECTION
Frontal plane

MIDSAGITTAL SECTION
Median plane

TRANSVERSE SECTION
Horizontal plane

FIGURE 1–6 ■ Head and neck in anatomical position showing the midsagittal, transverse, and frontal sections.

REVIEW QUESTIONS

1. Which of the following planes *divides* the body in anatomical position into right and left halves?
   A. Horizontal plane
   B. Median plane
   C. Coronal plane
   D. Frontal plane

2. Which of the following is used to describe an area of the body that is farther from the median plane?
   A. Proximal
   B. Lateral
   C. Medial
   D. Ipsilateral
   E. Contralateral

3. Structures on the *same* side of the body are considered:
   A. Proximal
   B. Lateral
   C. Medial
   D. Ipsilateral
   E. Contralateral

4. An area of the body in anatomical position that faces toward the head is considered:
   A. Inferior
   B. Superior
   C. Proximal
   D. Distal
   E. Dorsal

5. Through which plane of the body in anatomical position is a midsagittal section taken?
   A. Horizontal plane
   B. Median plane
   C. Coronal plane
   D. Frontal plane

6. Which of the following statements concerning anatomical position is correct?
   A. Body is erect with eyes looking forward.
   B. Arms are at sides with palms directed backward.
   C. Arms are behind the head with toes directed forward.
   D. Body is supine with eyes closed.

7. Which of the following sections is a horizontal section?
   A. Midsagittal section
   B. Transverse section
   C. Frontal section
   D. Median section

8. Structures that are located inward, away from the body surface, are considered:
   A. Distal
   B. Superficial
   C. Deep
   D. Contralateral
   E. External

9. Which plane divides any part of the body into anterior and posterior parts?
   A. Sagittal plane
   B. Horizontal plane
   C. Frontal plane
   D. Median plane

10. Which of the following is a correct statement concerning human anatomy?
    A. The apex of a conical structure is the flat base.
    B. The two halves of the body are completely symmetrical.
    C. The external surface is the inner wall of hollow structure.
    D. Joints, vessels, nerves, glands, and nodes vary in size.

REVIEW ACTIVITIES

1. Stand in anatomical position in front of a long mirror.

2. Standing in anatomical position in front of a long mirror, describe parts of your body using the correct anatomical nomenclature, such as medial and lateral.

3. Standing in anatomical position in front of a long mirror, use a long ruler to show the different planes, such as horizontal and frontal.

Surface Anatomy

CHAPTER OUTLINE

This chapter discusses the following topics:

I. Surface Anatomy
II. Regions of the Head
   A. Frontal Region
   B. Parietal and Occipital Regions
   C. Temporal Region
   D. Orbital Region
   E. Nasal Region
   F. Infraorbital, Zygomatic, and Buccal Regions
   G. Oral Region
   H. Mental Region
III. Regions of the Neck

LEARNING OBJECTIVES

After studying this chapter, the reader should be able to:

1. Define and pronounce all the key words and anatomical terms in this chapter.
2. Discuss the anatomical considerations for patient examination and dental radiology of the head and neck region.
3. Locate and identify the regions and associated surface landmarks of the head and neck on a diagram and a patient.
4. Correctly complete the review questions and activities for this chapter.
5. Integrate the knowledge of surface anatomy into the clinical practice of patient examination and dental radiology of the head and neck regions.

KEY WORDS

Buccal (**buk**-al) Structures closest to the inner cheek.

Facial (**fay**-shal) Structures closest to the facial surface.

Labial (**lay**-be-al) Structures closest to the lips.

Lingual (**ling**-gwal) Structures closest to the tongue.

Palatal (**pal**-ah-tal) Structures closest to the palate.

SURFACE ANATOMY

The dental professional must be thoroughly familiar with the surface anatomy of the head and neck in order to examine patients. (See Appendix, page 339, for the procedure table for Performing an Extraoral and Intraoral Examination.) The features of the surface provide essential landmarks for many of the deeper anatomical structures. Thus the examination of these accessible surface features by visualization and palpation can give information about the health of deeper tissues. Any changes in these surface features need to be recorded by the dental professional.

Many of the radiographs taken by the dental professional also use surface landmarks. Portions of the eye, nose, and ear are used for this purpose. This use of landmarks allows for easy film placement and consistency in taking radiographs.

A certain amount of variation in surface features is within a normal range. However, a change in a surface feature in a given person may signal a condition of clinical significance. Thus it is not the variations among individuals that should be noted but the changes in a particular individual.

The study of anatomy of the head and neck begins with the division of the surface into regions.

Within each region are certain surface landmarks. Practice finding these landmarks in each region on yourself to improve the skills of examination.

REGIONS OF THE HEAD

The **regions of the head** include the frontal, parietal, occipital, temporal, orbital, nasal, infraorbital, zygomatic, buccal, oral, and mental regions (Figure 2-1). These regions are all noted during an overall evaluation of the face, head, and neck. During an extraoral examination, the patient is seated upright and relaxed, and the symmetry and coloration of the surface is noted.

The superficial to deep relationships of the head are relatively simple over most of its posterior and superior surfaces but are more difficult in the region

of the face. The underlying bony structure of the head is covered in Chapter 3. The underlying muscles of the head are covered in Chapter 4. The underlying glandular tissue, such as the salivary and lacrimal glands and thyroid gland, is covered in Chapter 7. Lymph nodes that are located throughout the tissues of the head are covered in Chapter 10.

FRONTAL REGION

The **frontal region (frunt**-il) of the head includes the forehead and the area above the eyes (Figure 2–2). Just under each eyebrow is the **supraorbital ridge** (soo-prah-**or**-bit-al) or superciliary ridge. The smooth elevated area between the eyebrows is the **glabella** (glah-**bell**-ah), which tends to be flat in children and adult females and to form a rounded

FIGURE 2–1 ■ Regions of the head: frontal, parietal, occipital, temporal, orbital, nasal, infraorbital, zygomatic, buccal, oral, and mental.

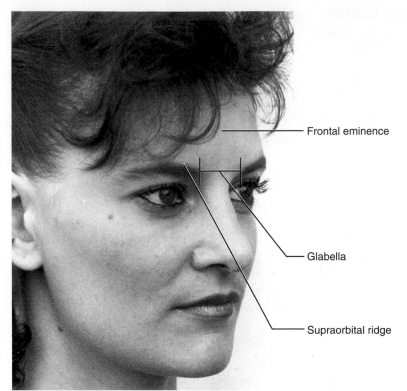

Frontal eminence

Glabella

Supraorbital ridge

FIGURE 2–2 ■ Frontal view of the head with the landmarks of the frontal region noted.

prominence in adult males. The prominence of the forehead, the **frontal eminence** (**frunt**-il **em**-i-nins), is also evident. The frontal eminence is typically more pronounced in children and adult females, and the supraorbital ridge is more prominent in adult males. Standing near the patient, the forehead is visually inspected and bilaterally palpated during an extraoral examination.

PARIETAL AND OCCIPITAL REGIONS

The **parietal region** (pah-**ri**-it-al) and **occipital region** (ok-**sip**-it-al) of the head are covered by the scalp. The **scalp** consists of layers of soft tissue overlying the bones of the braincase. Large areas of the scalp may be covered by hair. It is still important to try to survey these areas during an extraoral examination since many lesions may be hidden visually from the clinician, as well as the patient. During an extraoral examination, standing near the patient, visually inspect the entire scalp by moving the hair, especially around the hairline, starting from one ear and proceeding to the other ear (Figure 2–3).

FIGURE 2–3 ■ Visual inspection of the entire scalp.

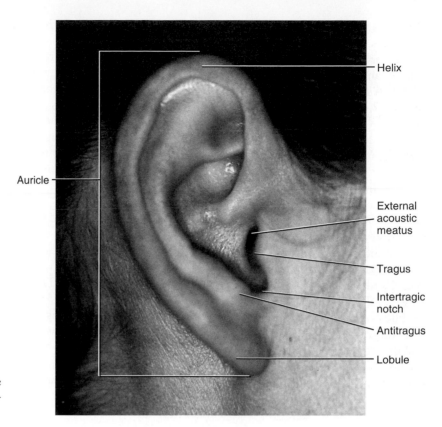

Auricle

Helix

External acoustic meatus

Tragus

Intertragic notch

Antitragus

Lobule

FIGURE 2–4 ■ Lateral view of the external ear and its landmarks within the temporal region noted.

TEMPORAL REGION

Within the **temporal region** (**tem**-poh-ral) of the head, the external ear is a prominent feature (Figure 2–4). The external ear is composed of an **auricle** (**aw**-ri-kl) or oval flap of the ear and the **external acoustic meatus** (ah-**koos**-tik me-**ate**-us). The auricle collects sound waves. The external acoustic meatus is a tube through which sound waves are transmitted to the middle ear within the skull.

The superior and posterior free margin of the auricle is the **helix** (**heel**-iks), which ends inferiorly at the **lobule** (**lob**-yule), the fleshy protuberance of the earlobe (Figure 2–4). The upper apex of the helix is typically level with the eyebrows and the glabella, and the lobule is approximately at the level of the apex of the nose.

The part of the auricle anterior to the external acoustic meatus is a smaller flap of tissue called the **tragus** (**tra**-gus) (Figure 2–4). The tragus, as well as the rest of the auricle, is flexible when palpated due to its underlying cartilage. The other flap of tissue opposite the tragus is the **antitragus** (an-tie-**tra**-gus). Between the tragus and antitragus is a deep notch, the **intertragic notch** (in-ter-**tra**-gic). The external

acoustic meatus and tragus are important landmarks to use when taking extraoral radiographs and performing local anesthesia on a patient. During an extraoral examination, the external ear is visually inspected and palpated (Figure 2–5).

FIGURE 2–5 ■ Palpation of the external ear.

ORBITAL REGION

In the **orbital region (or**-bit-al) of the head, the eyeball and all its supporting structures are contained in the bony socket called the **orbit (or**-bit) (Figure 2–6). The eyes are usually near the midpoint of the vertical height of the head. The width of each eye is typically the same as the distance between the eyes. On the eyeball is the white area or **sclera (skler**-ah) with its central area of coloration, the circular **iris (eye**-ris). The opening in the center of the iris is the **pupil (pew**-pil), which changes size as the iris responds to changing light conditions.

Two movable **eyelids,** upper and lower, cover and protect each eyeball (Figure 2–6). Behind each upper eyelid and within the orbit is the **lacrimal gland (lak**-ri-mal), which produces lacrimal fluid or tears.

The **conjunctiva** (kon-junk-**ti**-vah) is the delicate and thin membrane lining the inside of the eyelids and the front of the eyeball. The outer corner where the upper and lower eyelids meet is called the **lateral canthus** (plural, **canthi**) (**kan**-this, **kan**-thy) or outer canthus. The inner angle of the eye is called the **medial canthus** or inner canthus. These canthi are important landmarks to use when taking extraoral radiographs. During an extraoral examination, the orbital region, including the eyes, is examined by standing near the patient and visually inspecting the eyes and their movements and responses.

NASAL REGION

The main feature of the **nasal region (nay**-zil) of the head is the external nose (Figure 2–7). The **root of the nose** is located between the eyes. Inferior to the glabella is a midpoint landmark of the nasal region that corresponds to the junction between the underlying bones, the **nasion (nay**-ze-on). Inferior to the nasion is the bony structure that forms the **bridge of the nose.** The tip or **apex of the nose** is flexible when palpated since it is formed from cartilage.

Inferior to the apex on each side of the nose is a nostril or **naris** (plural, **nares**) (**nay**-ris, **nay**-rees) (Figure 2–7). The nares are separated by the midline **nasal septum (nay**-zil **sep**-tum). The nares are bounded laterally by winglike cartilaginous structures, the **ala** (plural, **alae**) (**a**-lah, **a**-lay) of the nose. The width between the alae should be about the same width as one eye or the space between the eyes. The nasion and the alae of the nose are important landmarks to use when taking extraoral radiographs. During an extraoral examination, the external nose is visually inspected and palpated (Figure 2–8). Standing near the patient, visually inspect and use bilateral palpation for the nasal region, starting at the root of the nose and proceeding to its apex.

INFRAORBITAL, ZYGOMATIC, AND BUCCAL REGIONS

The infraorbital, zygomatic, and buccal regions of the head are all located on the facial aspect (Figure 2–9). The **infraorbital region** (in-frah-**or**-bit-al) of the head is located inferior to the orbital region and lateral to the nasal region. Farther laterally is the **zygomatic region** (zy-go-**mat**-ik), which overlies the cheek bone, the **zygomatic arch.**

Upper eyelid

Medial canthus

Lower eyelid

Outline of orbit

Lacrimal gland (deep)

Pupil

Lateral canthus

Sclera (covered by conjunctiva)

Iris

FIGURE 2–6 ■ Frontal view of the left eye with the landmarks of the orbital region noted.

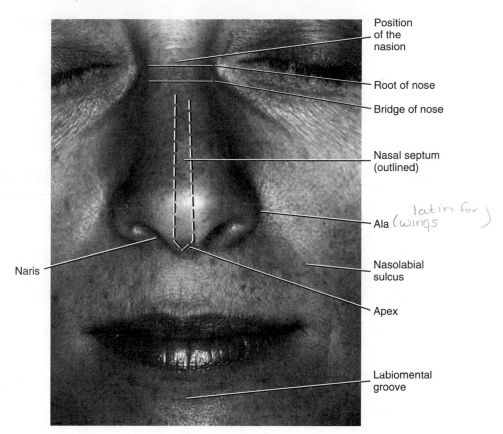

Position
of the
nasion

Root of nose

Bridge of nose

Nasal septum
(outlined)

Ala (*latin for*
wings)

Naris

Nasolabial
sulcus

Apex

Labiomental
groove

FIGURE 2–7 ■ Frontal view of the face with the landmarks of the nasal region noted.

The zygomatic arch extends from just below the lateral margin of the eye toward the upper part of the ear.

Inferior to the zygomatic arch, and just anterior to the ear, is the **temporomandibular joint** (tem-poh-ro-man-**dib**-you-lar) (Figure 2–9). This is where the upper skull forms a joint with the lower jaw. The movements of the joint can be felt when one opens and closes the mouth or moves the lower jaw to the right or left. One way to feel the lower jaw moving at the temporomandibular joint is to place a finger into the outer portion of the external acoustic meatus.

The **buccal region** (**buk**-al) of the head is composed of the soft tissues of the cheek (Figure 2–9). The **cheek** forms the side of the face and is a broad area of the face between the nose, mouth, and ear. Most of the upper cheek is fleshy, mainly formed by a mass of fat and muscles. One of these is the strong **masseter muscle** (**mass**-et-er), which is felt when a patient clenches the teeth together. The sharp angle of the lower jaw inferior to the ear's lobule is termed the **angle of the mandible.** During an extraoral examination, the dental professional stands near the patient, and visually inspects and palpates bilaterally the infraorbital, zygomatic, and buccal regions as well as the temporomandibular joint (see Figures 5–7 and 5–8).

FIGURE 2–8 ■ Palpation of the external nose.

FIGURE 2–9 ■ Landmarks of the zygomatic and buccal regions noted.

ORAL REGION

The **oral region** of the head has many structures within it, such as the lips, oral cavity, palate, tongue, floor of the mouth, and portions of the throat. The lips are the gateway of the oral region, and each lip's **vermilion zone** (ver-**mil**-yon) has a darker appearance than the surrounding skin (Figure 2–10). The lips are outlined from the surrounding skin by a transition zone, the **vermilion border.** The width of the lips at rest should be about the same distance as that between the irises of the eyes.

On the midline of the upper lip, extending downward from the nasal septum, is a vertical groove called the **philtrum** (**fil**-trum) (Figure 2–10). The philtrum terminates in a thicker area or **tubercle of the upper lip** (**too**-ber-kl). The upper and lower lips meet at each corner of the mouth or **labial commissure** (**kom**-i-shoor). The groove running upward between the labial commissure and the ala of the nose is called the **nasolabial sulcus**

FIGURE 2–10 ■ Frontal view of the lips within the oral region.

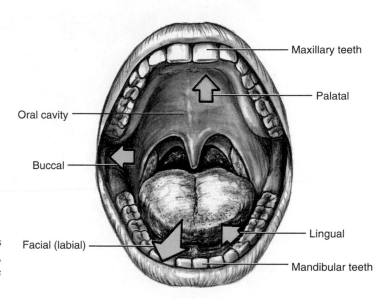

Oral cavity

Buccal

Maxillary teeth

Palatal

Lingual

Mandibular teeth

Facial (labial)

FIGURE 2–11 ■ The oral cavity and jaws with the designation of the terms lingual, palatal, buccal, facial, and labial within the oral cavity.

(nay-zo-**lay**-be-al **sul**-kus) (see Figure 2–7). The lower lip extends to the horizontal **labiomental groove** (lay-bee-o-**ment**-il), which separates the lower lip from the chin in the mental region. The lips are bidigitally palpated during an intraoral examination, as well as visually inspected in a systematic manner, from one commissure to the other.

Oral Cavity

The inside of the mouth is known as the **oral cavity.** The jaws are within the oral cavity and deep to the lips (Figure 2–11). Underlying the upper lip is the upper jaw or **maxilla** (mak-**sil**-ah). The bone underlying the lower lip is the lower jaw or **mandible** (**man**-di-bl).

Many areas in the oral cavity are termed or identified by their relationship to the tongue, palate, cheek, facial surface, or lips (Figure 2–11). Those structures closest to the tongue are termed *lingual* (**ling**-gwal). Those structures closest to the palate are termed *palatal* (**pal**-ah-tal). Those structures closest to the facial surface or lips are termed *facial* (**fay**-shal) or *labial* (**lay**-be-al). Those structures closest to the inner cheek are also considered *buccal* (**buk**-al).

The oral cavity is lined by a mucous membrane or **mucosa** (mu-**ko**-sah) (Figure 2–12). The inner portions of the lips are lined by a pink and thick **labial mucosa.** The labial mucosa is continuous with the equally pink and thick **buccal mucosa** that lines the inner cheek.

The buccal mucosa covers a dense pad of inner tissue, the **buccal fat pad.** To visually examine the labial mucosa, ask the patient to open the mouth slightly. Pull the lips away from the teeth. Then gently pull the buccal mucosa slightly away from the teeth so as to palpate bidigitally, using circular compression.

Further landmarks can be noted in the oral cavity (Figure 2–12). On the inner portion of the buccal mucosa, just opposite the maxillary second molar, is a small elevation of tissue called the **parotid papilla** (pah-**rot**-id pah-**pil**-ah), which contains the duct opening from the parotid salivary gland. An elevation on the posterior aspects of the maxilla is the **maxillary tuberosity** (mak-sil-lare-ee too-beh-**ros**-i-tee).

The upper and lower spaces between the cheeks, lips, and gums are the maxillary and mandibular **vestibules** (**ves**-ti-bules) (Figure 2–12). Deep within each vestibule, the pink and thick labial or buccal mucosa meets the redder and thinner **alveolar mucosa** (al-**ve**-o-lar) at the **mucobuccal fold** (mu-**ko**-buk-al). The **labial frenum** (**free**-num) or frenulum is a fold of tissue located at the midline between the labial mucosa and the alveolar mucosa of the maxilla and mandible (Figure 2–13).

Teeth of the oral cavity are located within the upper and lower jaws of the oral cavity (Figure 2–13). The teeth of the maxilla are the **maxillary teeth** (**mak**-sil-lare-ee), and the teeth of the mandible are the **mandibular teeth** (man-**dib**-

FIGURE 2–12 ■ View of the buccal and labial mucosa of the oral cavity with landmarks noted.

you-lar). The maxillary anterior teeth should overlap the mandibular anterior teeth, and posteriorly, the maxillary buccal cusps should overlap the mandibular buccal cusps. Both dental arches in the adult have permanent teeth that include the **incisors** (in-**sigh**-zers), **canines** (**kay**-nines), **premolars** (pre-**mol**-ers), and **molars** (**mol**-ers).

Surrounding the maxillary and mandibular teeth are the gums or **gingiva** (jin-**ji**-vah), composed of a firm, pink mucosa (Figures 2–13 and 2–14). The gingiva that tightly adheres to the bone around the roots of the teeth is the **attached gingiva.** The attached gingiva may have areas of pigmentation. The line of demarcation between the firmer

and pinker attached gingiva and the movable and redder alveolar mucosa is the scallop-shaped **mucogingival junction** (mu-ko-**jin**-ji-val).

At the gingival margin of each tooth is the nonattached or **marginal gingiva** (**mar**-ji-nal) (Figure 2–14). The inner surface of the marginal gingiva faces a space or **sulcus** (plural, **sulci**) (**sul**-kus, **sul**-ky). The gingiva between the teeth is an extension of attached gingiva and is called the **interdental gingiva** (in-ter-**den**-tal) or interdental papilla. During an intraoral examination, the buccal and labial mucosae are retracted enough to visually inspect the vestibular area. The gingiva is also visually examined and palpated using digital compression.

FIGURE 2–13 ■ Frontal view of the oral cavity with its landmarks noted.

— Alveolar mucosa

— Mucogingival junction

— Attached gingiva

— Marginal gingiva

— Interdental gingiva

— Sulcus (inside)

FIGURE 2–14 ■ Close-up view of the gingiva and its associated landmarks.

Palate

The roof of the mouth or **palate** (**pal**-it) has two portions—an anterior portion and a posterior portion (Figure 2–15). The firmer anterior portion is called the **hard palate.** A midline ridge of tissue on the hard palate is the **median palatine raphe** (**pal**-ah-tine **ra**-fe). A small bulge of tissue at the most anterior portion of the hard palate, lingual to the anterior teeth, is the **incisive papilla** (in-**sy**-ziv pah-**pil**-ah). Directly posterior to this papilla are **palatine rugae**

(**pal**-ah-tine **ru**-ge), which are firm, irregular ridges of tissue.

The looser posterior portion of the palate is called the **soft palate** (see Figures 2–15 and 2–21). A midline muscular structure, the **uvula of the palate** (**u**-vu-lah), hangs from the posterior margin of the soft palate. The **pterygomandibular fold** (teh-ri-go-man-**dib**-yule-lar) is a fold of tissue that extends from the junction of hard and soft palates down to the mandible, just behind the most distal mandibular

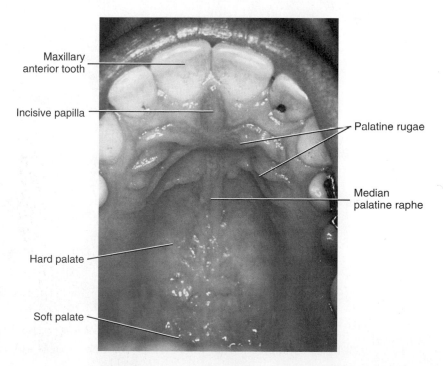

Maxillary anterior tooth

Incisive papilla

Palatine rugae

Median palatine raphe

Hard palate

Soft palate

FIGURE 2–15 ■ View of the palate with its landmarks noted.

tooth, and stretches when the patient opens the mouth wider. This fold covers a deeper fibrous structure and separates the cheek from the throat. Just distal to the last tooth of the mandible is a dense pad of tissue, the **retromolar pad** (re-tro-**moh**-ler). During an intraoral examination, the palate is viewed using a mouth mirror to intensify the light source. The tongue is extended in order to observe the soft palate. The mouth mirror is gently placed (mirror side down) on the middle of the tongue and the patient asked to say "ah." As this is done, the uvula is visually observed. Then the hard and soft palates are compressed with the first or second finger of one hand. Avoid circular compression on the soft palate to avoid initiating the gag reflex.

Tongue

The **tongue** is a prominent feature of the oral region (Figure 2–16). The posterior one third is the **base of the tongue** or pharyngeal portion. The base of the tongue attaches to the floor of the mouth. The base of the tongue does not lie within the oral cavity but within the oral part of the throat. The anterior two thirds of the tongue is termed the **body of the tongue** or oral portion and lies within the oral cavity. The tip of the tongue is the **apex of the tongue.** Certain surfaces of the tongue have small elevated structures of specialized mucosa

called **lingual papillae** (pah-**pil**-ay), some of which are associated with taste buds.

The side or **lateral surface of the tongue** is noted for its vertical ridges of lingual papillae called **foliate lingual papillae** (**fo**-le-ate), some of which contain taste buds. These lingual papillae are more prominent in children.

The top surface or **dorsal surface of the tongue** (Figure 2–17) has a midline depression, the **median lingual sulcus,** corresponding to the position of a midline fibrous structure deeper in the tongue. In the tongue, dorsal and posterior are not equivalent terms, nor are ventral and anterior the same. Instead, they are four different locations. This is because the tongue of humans still has the same orientation as the tongue of four-footed animals, in which anterior and posterior mean toward the nose and tail, respectively, and dorsal and ventral refer to the back and belly, respectively. Upright posture is the reason that dorsal and posterior have become synonyms in the rest of the body.

The dorsal surface of the tongue also has many lingual papillae (Figure 2–17). The slender, thread-like lingual papillae are the **filiform lingual papillae** (**fil-i**-form), which give the dorsal surface its velvety texture. The red mushroom-shaped dots are called **fungiform lingual papillae** (**fun**-ji-form). These lingual papillae are more numerous on the apex and contain taste buds.

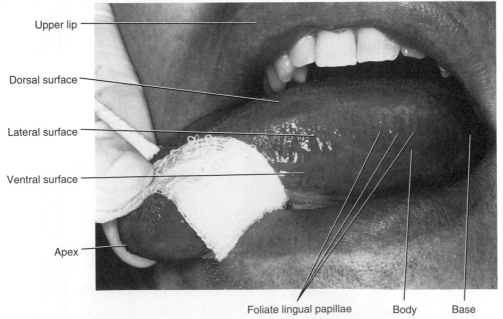

Upper lip

Dorsal surface

Lateral surface

Ventral surface

Apex

Foliate lingual papillae   Body   Base

FIGURE 2–16 ■ Examination of the lateral view of the tongue with its portions and landmarks noted.

FIGURE 2–17 ■ Dorsal view of the tongue with its landmarks noted.

Farther posteriorly on the dorsal surface of the tongue and more difficult to see clinically is a V-shaped groove, the **sulcus terminalis** (**ter**-mi-nal-is) (Figure 2–17). The sulcus terminalis separates the base from the body of the tongue. Where the sulcus terminalis points backward toward the throat is a small pitlike depression called the **foramen cecum** (for-**ay**-men **se**-kum). The **circumvallate lingual papillae** (serk-um-**val**-ate), which are 10 to 14 in number, line up along the anterior side of the sulcus terminalis on the body. These large mushroom-shaped lingual papillae have taste buds. Even farther posteriorly on the dorsal surface of the tongue base is an irregular mass of tonsillar tissue, the **lingual tonsil** (**ton**-sil).

The underside or ventral surface of the tongue is noted for its visible large blood vessels, the deep **lingual veins** (vanes), that run close to the surface (Figure 2–18). Lateral to each deep lingual vein is the **plica fimbriata** (plural, **plicae fimbriatae**) (**pli**-kah fim-bree-**ay**-tah, **pli**-kay fim-bree-**ay**-tay), a fold with fringelike projections. Again, the term used for the underside of the tongue, ventral, referred to four-footed animals in anatomical position.

To examine the dorsal and lateral surfaces of the tongue, a gauze square is wrapped around the anterior one third of the tongue to obtain a firm grasp while the patient gently extends it (see Figure 2–16). If the patient is forced to extend the tongue too far, the gag reflex is triggered. The dorsal sur-

face is palpated digitally. The tongue is turned slightly on its side to inspect its base and lateral borders and is bidigitally palpated. To examine the ventral surface, have the patient lift the tongue; inspect and digitally palpate the surface.

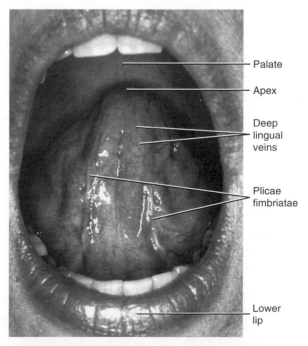

FIGURE 2–18 ■ Ventral surface of the tongue with its landmarks noted.

Sublingual caruncle

Lingual frenum

Sublingual fold

Lower anterior teeth

FIGURE 2–19 ■ View of the floor of the mouth with its landmarks noted.

Floor of the Mouth

The floor of the mouth is located inferior to the ventral surface of the tongue (Figure 2–19). The **lingual frenum** (**free**-num) or frenulum is a midline fold of tissue between the ventral surface of the tongue and the floor of the mouth.

There is also a ridge of tissue on each side of the floor of the mouth, the **sublingual fold** (sub-**ling**-gwal) or plica sublingualis. Together these folds are arranged in a V-shaped configuration from the lingual frenum to the base of the tongue (Figure 2–19). The sublingual folds contain duct openings from the sublingual salivary gland. The small papilla or **sublingual caruncle** (sub-**ling**-gwal **kar**-unk-el) at the anterior end of each

sublingual fold contains the duct openings from both the submandibular and sublingual salivary glands.

Use the mouth mirror to facilitate lighting and direct observation of the floor of the mouth. While the patient lifts the tongue to the palate, observe the mucosa of the floor of the mouth and check the lingual frenum. Bimanually palpate the sublingual area by placing the right index finger intraorally and the fingertips of the left hand extraorally under the chin to feel the tissue between your two hands.

Pharynx

The oral cavity also provides the entrance into the throat or **pharynx** (**far**-inks). The pharynx is

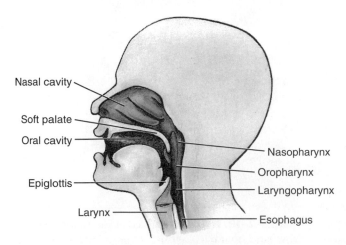

Nasal cavity
Soft palate
Oral cavity
Epiglottis
Larynx
Nasopharynx
Oropharynx
Laryngopharynx
Esophagus

FIGURE 2–20 ■ Midsagittal section of the head and neck illustrating portions of the pharynx.

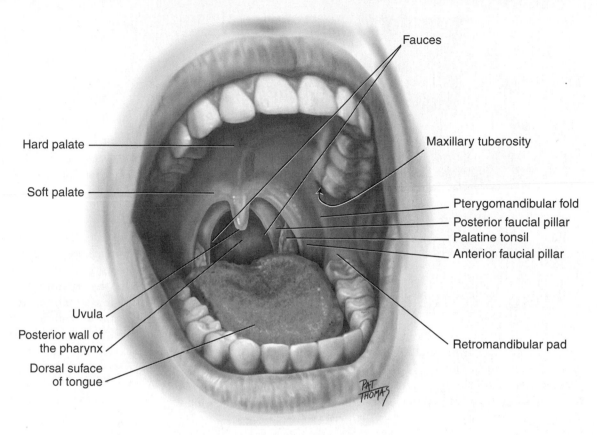

Hard palate

Soft palate

Uvula

Posterior wall of
the pharynx

Dorsal suface
of tongue

Fauces

Maxillary tuberosity

Pterygomandibular fold
Posterior faucial pillar
Palatine tonsil
Anterior faucial pillar

Retromandibular pad

FIGURE 2–21 ■ Oral view of the oropharynx and oral cavity.

a muscular tube that serves both the respiratory and digestive systems. There are three portions to the pharynx: the nasopharynx, the oropharynx, and the laryngopharynx (Figure 2–20). Portions of the nasopharynx and oropharynx are visible in an intraoral examination when examining the palatal area with the patient saying "ah." The **laryngopharynx** (lah-ring-gah-**far**-inks) is more inferior, close to the laryngeal opening, and thus is not visible in an intraoral examination.

The portion of the pharynx that is superior to the level of the soft palate is the **nasopharynx** (nay-zo-**far**-inks). The nasopharynx is continuous with the nasal cavity. The portion of the pharynx that is between the soft palate and the opening of the larynx is the **oropharynx** (or-o-**far**-inks). (Figure 2–21).

The opening from the oral region into the oropharynx is the **fauces** (**faw**-seez) or the faucial isthmus (Figure 2–21). The fauces are formed laterally by the **anterior faucial pillar** (**faw**-shawl **pil**-er) and the **posterior faucial pillar.** Older terms for these structures that border the fauces are the tonsil-

lar pillars or palatal arches. Tonsillar tissue, the **palatine tonsils** (**pal**-ah-tine **ton**-sils), is located between these pillars or folds of tissue created by underlying muscles. The palatine tonsils are the tonsillar tissue that patients call their 'tonsils.'

MENTAL REGION

The chin is the major feature of the **mental region** (**ment**-il) of the head (Figure 2–22). The prominence of the chin is called the **mental protuberance** (pro-**too**-ber-ins). The mental protuberance is often more pronounced in adult males but can also be visualized and palpated bilaterally in adult females. The **labiomental groove** (lay-bee-o-**ment**-il), a horizontal groove between the lower lip and the chin mentioned in the description of the oral region, should be approximately midway between the apex of the nose and the chin and level with the angle of the mandible. Also present on the chin in some individuals is a

Labiomental groove

Mental protuberance

FIGURE 2–22 ■ Frontal view of the head showing the mental region with its landmarks noted.

midline depression or dimple that marks the underlying bony fusion of the lower jaw.

▓ REGIONS OF THE NECK

The neck extends from the skull and mandible down to the clavicles and sternum. The **regions of the neck** can be divided into different cervical triangles based on the large bones and muscles in the area (Figure 2–23). Chapters 3 and 4 further describe these bones and muscles, respectively. Structures deep to the surface of these cervical triangles are also discussed in other chapters.

The large strap muscle, the **sternocleidomastoid muscle** (stir-no-kli-do-**mass**-toid), divides each side of the neck diagonally into an **anterior cervical triangle** (ser-vi-kal) and **posterior cervical triangle** (Figure 2–23). The anterior region of the neck corresponds to the two anterior cervical triangles, which are separated by a midline. The lateral region of the neck, posterior to the sternocleidomastoid

Sternocleidomastoid muscle

Posterior cervical triangle

Hyoid bone

Anterior cervical triangle

Thyroid cartilage

subclavian

FIGURE 2–23 ■ Regions of the neck: the anterior cervical triangle and posterior cervical triangle.

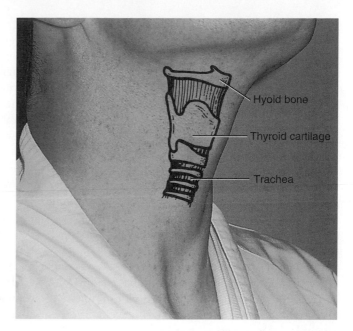

FIGURE 2–24 ■ Lateral view of the anterior cervical triangle of the neck highlighting its skeletal landmarks.

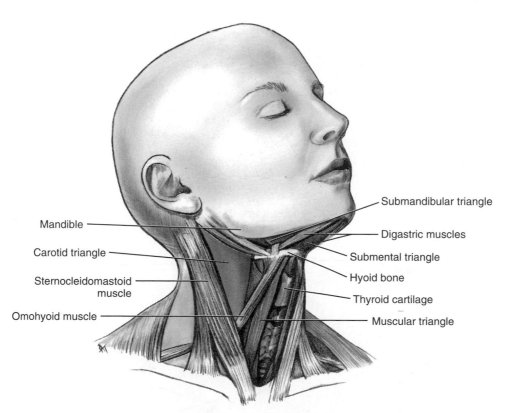

FIGURE 2–25 ■ Divisions of the anterior cervical triangle: submandibular, submental, carotid, and muscular.

muscle, is considered the posterior cervical triangle on each side.

At the anterior midline, the prominence of the larynx, the **thyroid cartilage** (**thy**-roid), is visible as the "Adam's apple," especially in adult males (Figure 2–24). The vocal cords or ligaments are attached to the posterior surface of the thyroid cartilage.

The **hyoid bone** (**hi**-oid) is also found in the anterior midline, superior to the thyroid cartilage (Figure 2–24). Many muscles attach to the hyoid bone. The hyoid bone can be effectively palpated by feeling below and medial to the angles of the mandible. Do not confuse the hyoid bone with the inferiorly placed thyroid cartilage when palpating the neck.

The anterior cervical triangle can be further subdivided into smaller triangular regions by muscles in the area that are not as prominent as the sternocleidomastoid muscle (Figure 2–25). For example, the superior portion of each anterior cervical triangle is demarcated by portions of the digastric muscle (both bellies) and the mandible, forming a **submandibular triangle** (sub-man-**dib**-you-lar). The inferior portion of each anterior cervical triangle is further subdivided by the omohyoid muscle into a carotid triangle (kah-**rot**-id) above and a muscular triangle below. A midline **submental triangle** (sub-**men**-tal) is also formed by portions of the digastric muscle (right and left anterior belly) and the hyoid bone. These triangles are discussed further in Chapter 4.

Each posterior cervical triangle can also be further subdivided into smaller triangular regions by muscles in the area (Figure 2–26). The omohyoid muscle divides the posterior cervical triangle into the **occipital triangle** (ok-**sip**-it-al) above and the **subclavian triangle** (sub-**klay**-vee-an) below on each side. These triangles are discussed further in Chapter 4.

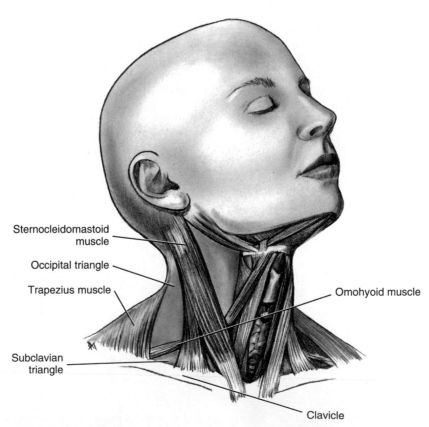

Sternocleidomastoid muscle

Occipital triangle

Trapezius muscle

Omohyoid muscle

Subclavian triangle

Clavicle

FIGURE 2–26 ■ Divisions of the posterior cervical triangle: occipital and subclavian.

REVIEW QUESTIONS

1. Those structures in the oral region that are closest to the tongue are called:
   A. Buccal
   B. Facial
   C. Lingual
   D. Pharyngeal
   E. Palatal

2. Which of the following terms is used to describe the smooth elevated area between the eyebrows in the frontal region?
   A. Supraorbital ridge
   B. Medial canthus
   C. Glabella
   D. Alae
   E. Auricle

3. In which region of the head and neck is the tragus located?
   A. Frontal region
   B. Nasal region
   C. Temporal region
   D. Anterior cervical triangle
   E. Submandibular triangle

4. The tissue at the junction between the labial or buccal mucosa and the alveolar mucosa is the:
   A. Mucogingival junction
   B. Mucobuccal fold
   C. Vermilion border
   D. Labial frenum
   E. Labiomental groove

5. Into which cervical triangles does the sternocleidomastoid muscle divide the neck?
   A. Superior and inferior
   B. Medial and lateral
   C. Anterior and posterior
   D. Proximal and distal

6. The parietal and occipital regions are covered by the:
   A. Temporal region
   B. Layers of scalp
   C. Eyelids
   D. External acoustic meatus

7. Which of the following statements concerning the location of the medial canthus is correct when comparing it to the lateral canthus?
   A. Nearer to the nose
   B. Nearer to the ear
   C. Where upper and lower eyelid meet
   D. Where upper and lower lip meet

8. Which of the following structures extends from just below the lateral margin of the eye toward the ear?
   A. Pterygomandibular fold
   B. Zygomatic arch
   C. Sulcus terminalis
   D. Sternocleidomastoid muscle

9. The opening from the oral region into the oropharynx is the:
   A. Fauces
   B. Palatine tonsils
   C. Pterygomandibular fold
   D. Nasopharynx

10. Which of the following terms is given to the small papilla at the anterior end of each sublingual fold?
    A. Lingual frenum
    B. Plica fimbriata
    C. Foliate papillae
    D. Sublingual caruncle
    E. Incisive papilla

REVIEW ACTIVITIES

1. Standing in front of a mirror that shows your head and neck area, point out the regions of the head and neck, such as the frontal and temporal regions.

2. Standing in front of a mirror that shows your head and neck area, point out the surface features of each region, such as the supraorbital ridge and glabella.

3. Using a hand mirror and lying in a dental chair or on a couch under good lighting, point out the terms used to describe the oral cavity, such as lingual and palatal.

4. Using a hand mirror and lying in a dental chair or on a couch under good lighting, point out the surface landmarks in the oral cavity, using a dental probe or tongue depressor, such as labial and buccal mucosa.

5. Point out the surface landmarks in the oral cavity to your patient (or peer) as the person lies in a dental chair under good lighting; use a dental probe or tongue depressor so the person can see the landmarks in a hand mirror.

Bones

3

LEARNING OBJECTIVES

After studying this chapter, the reader should be able to:

1. Define and pronounce all the key words and anatomical terms in this chapter.
2. Locate and identify the bones of the head and neck and their landmarks on a diagram, a skull, and a patient.
3. Describe in detail the various parts and landmarks of the maxilla and mandible.
4. Discuss certain abnormalities of bone.
5. Correctly complete the identification exercises and review questions and activities for this chapter.
6. Integrate the knowledge about the bones into the overall study of the head and neck anatomy.

KEY WORDS

Aperture (**ap**-er-cher) Opening or orifice in bone.

Arch (arch) Prominent bridgelike bony structure.

Articulation (ar-tik-you-**lay**-shin) Area where the bones are joined to each other.

Bones (bones) Mineralized structures of the body that protect internal soft tissues and serve as the biomechanical basis for movement.

Canal (kah-**nal**) Opening in bone that is long, narrow, and tubelike.

Condyle (**kon**-dyl) Oval bony prominence typically found at articulations.

Cornu (**kor**-nu) Small hornlike prominence.

Crest (krest) Roughened border or ridge on the bone surface.

Eminence (**em**-i-nins) Tubercle or rounded elevation on a bony surface.

Epicondyle (ep-ee-**kon**-dyl) Small prominence that is located above or upon a condyle.

Fissure (**fish**-er) Opening in bone that is narrow and cleftlike.

Foramen/foramina (for-**ay**-men, for-**am**-i-nah) Short windowlike opening in bone.

Fossa/fossae (**fos**-ah, **fos**-ay) Depression on a bony surface.

Head (hed) Rounded surface projecting from a bone by a neck.

Incisura (in-si-**su**-rah) Indentation or notch at the edge of the bone.

Line (line) Straight small ridge of bone.

Meatus (me-**ate**-us) Opening or canal in the bone.

Notch (noch) Indentation at the edge of a bone.

Ostium/ostia (**os**-tee-um, **os**-tee-ah) Small opening in bone.

Perforation (per-fo-**ray**-shun) Abnormal hole in a hollow organ, such as in the wall of a sinus.

(continued)

■ **KEY WORDS** *(continued)*

Plate (plate) Flat structure of bone.

Process (**pros**-es) General term for any prominence on a bony surface.

Spine (spine) Abrupt small prominence of bone.

Sulcus/sulci (**sul**-kus, **sul**-ky) Shallow depression or groove such as that on the bony surface or that between the tooth and the inner surface of the marginal gingiva.

Suture (**su**-cher) Generally immovable articulation in which bones are joined by fibrous tissue.

Tubercle (**too**-ber-kl) Eminence or small rounded elevation on the bony surface.

Tuberosity (too-beh-**ros**-i-tee) Large, often rough, prominence on the surface of bone.

■ SKELETAL SYSTEM

The *bones* (bones) of the skeletal system are mineralized structures in the body. Bones protect the internal soft tissues. Bones also serve as the biomechanical basis for movement of the body along with muscles, tendons, and ligaments. Bones are also a consideration in the spread of dental infection (see Chapter 12 for more information).

The prominences and depressions on the bony surface are landmarks for the attachments of associated muscles, tendons, and ligaments. The openings in the bone are also landmarks where various nerves and blood vessels enter or exit. Areas of the bones can also be demarcated that are not prominences or depressions such as a *plate* (plate), which is a flat bony structure.

BONY PROMINENCES

A general term for any prominence on a bony surface is a *process* (**pros**-es). One specific type of prominence located on the bony surface is a *condyle* (**kon**-dyl), a relatively large, convex prominence usually involved in joints. A rounded surface projecting from a bone by a neck is a *head* (hed). Another large, often rough prominence is a *tuberosity* (too-beh-**ros**-i-tee). Tuberosities are typically attachment areas for muscles or tendons.

An *arch* (arch) is shaped like a bridge with a bowlike outline. A *cornu* (**kor**-nu) is a hornlike prominence.

Other prominences of the bone include epicondyles, tubercles, crests, lines, and spines. These primarily serve as muscle and ligament attachments. An *epicondyle* (ep-ee-**kon**-dyl) is a prominence above or upon a condyle. A *tubercle* (**too**-ber-kl) or *eminence* (**em**-i-nins) is a rounded elevation on the bony surface. A *crest* (krest) is a prominent, often roughened border or ridge. A *line* (line) is a straight small ridge. An abrupt prominence of the bone that may be a blunt or sharply pointed projection is a *spine* (spine).

BONY DEPRESSIONS

One type of depression on the bony surface is an *incisura* (in-si-**su**-rah) or *notch* (noch), an indentation at the edge of the bone. Another depression on a bony surface is a *sulcus* (plural, *sulci*) (**sul**-kus, **sul**-ky), which is a shallow depression or groove that usually marks the course of an artery or nerve. A generally deeper depression on a bony surface is a *fossa* (plural, *fossae*) (**fos**-ah, **fos**-ay). Fossae can be parts of joints, be attachment areas for muscles, or have other functions.

BONY OPENINGS

The bone can have openings such as a foramen or canal. A *foramen* (plural, *foramina*) (for-**ay**-men, for-**am**-i-nah) is a short windowlike opening in the bone. A *canal* (kah-**nal**) is a longer, narrow tubelike opening in the bone. A *meatus* (me-**ate**-us) is a type of canal. Another opening in a bone is a *fissure* (**fish**-er), which is a narrow cleftlike opening. A small opening, especially as an entrance into a hollow organ or canal, is an *ostium* (plural, *ostia*) (**os**-tee-um, **os**-tee-ah). Another opening or orifice is an *aperture* (**ap**-er-cher).

SKELETAL ARTICULATIONS

An *articulation* (ar-tik-you-**lay**-shin) is an area of the skeleton where the bones are joined to each other. An articulation of the bones can be either a movable or an immovable type of joint. A *suture* (**su**-cher) is the union of bones joined by fibrous tissue. Sutures appear on the dry skull as jagged lines. Sutures are considered to be generally immovable but may provide mechanical protection from the force of a blow by moving very slightly to absorb the force. Sutures are the most flexible in infants. Much of the early growth of the skull occurs at the sutural edges of the cranial bones.

BONES OF THE HEAD AND NECK

The bones of the head and neck serve as a base during palpation of the soft tissues in the area. The bones also serve as markers when identifying the location of soft tissue lesions. These bones are also examined externally during a head and neck examination by a dental professional since they may be affected by a disease process. A dental professional must not only locate each of the head and neck bones but also recognize any abnormalities in the bony surface structure (discussed later in this chapter).

In order to recognize any bony abnormalities, the dental professional must know the normal anatomy of the bones of the head and neck. The knowledge of the normal anatomy includes locating the surface bony prominences, depressions, and articulations. It also includes knowing the openings in these bones and the blood vessels and nerves that travel through those openings. For effective study of the bones of the head and neck, it is helpful to use photographs and illustrations of these bones, as well as the skull model and palpation of a patient.

Bones and their associated surface tissues also serve as landmarks when taking dental radiographs (see Chapter 2 for more information) and prior to administering a local anesthetic injection (see Chapter 9 for more information).

SKULL

There are 22 bones in the **skull** (skul) of a patient, not including the small bones of the middle ear (Table 3–1). The bones of the skull or braincase can be divided into the **cranium** (**kray-nee-um**) (the part housing the brain) with its **cranial bones** (**kray**-nee-al) and the **face** with its **facial bones.** The bones of the skull, whether facial or cranial, can be single or paired. These bones create the facial features, are involved in the temporomandibular joints, and participate with growth in the formation of dentition. Many texts use the alternative terms "neurocranium" for the cranial bones since they enclose the brain and "viscerocranium" for the facial bones.

Growth takes place in all the bones of the skull. Growth of the upper face takes place at the sutures between the maxillary bones and other bones, as well as at the bony surfaces. Growth in the lower face takes place at the bony surfaces of the mandible and at the head of its condyle. Inadequate or disproportionate growth of the upper face and mandible may leave inadequate room for the developing dentition and cause other occlusal problems. This failure of growth can be addressed by orthodontics and possibly endocrine therapy and surgery.

All the bones of the skull are immovable, except the mandible with its temporomandibular

Table 3–1   CRANIAL AND FACIAL BONES*

Cranial Bones		Facial Bones	
Occipital bone	Single ✓	Vomer	Single
Frontal bone	Single ✓	Lacrimal bones	Paired
Parietal bones	Paired	Nasal bones	Paired
Temporal bones	Paired	Inferior nasal conchae	Paired
Sphenoid bone	Single	Zygomatic bones	Paired
Ethmoid bone	Single	Maxillary bones	Paired
		Mandible	Single

*Note that there are single and paired bones.

Table 3–2 SUTURES OF THE SKULL AND THEIR BONY ARTICULATIONS

Suture	Bony Articulations
Coronal suture	Frontal and parietal bones
Sagittal suture	Parietal bones
Lambdoidal suture	Occipital and parietal bones
Squamosal suture	Temporal and parietal bones
Temporozygomatic suture	Zygomatic and temporal bones
Median palatine suture	Palatine bones
Transverse palatine suture	Maxillae and palatine bones

joint. The articulation of many of the bones in the skull is by sutures (Table 3–2). The skull also has a movable articulation with the bony vertebral column in the neck area.

Many of the skull bones have openings for important nerves and blood vessels of the head and neck (Table 3–3). Skull bones also have many associated processes that are involved in important structures of the face and head (Table 3–4). This chapter may be reviewed after reading the chapters on the blood vessels and nerves, as well as those chapters on the muscles of the head and neck.

It is easier to study the skull by first looking at its various views: the superior, anterior, lateral, and inferior views. Then the skull should be studied by looking at its individual bones and their various landmarks: the cranial bones, facial bones, and bones of the neck. The features of the skull bones such as the fossae and paranasal sinuses should then be studied. This chapter follows this format of study.

Superior View of the Skull

When the skull is viewed from above, four bones are visible (Figure 3–1). At the front of the skull is the single **frontal bone** (**frunt**-il). At the sides are the

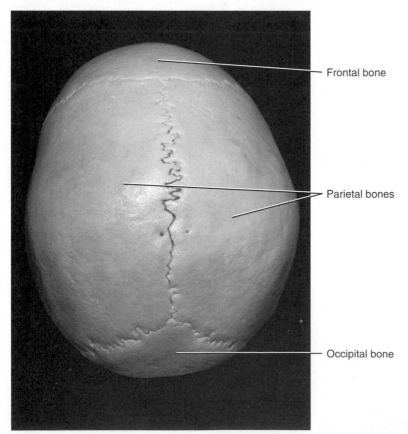

Frontal bone

Parietal bones

Occipital bone

FIGURE 3–1 ■ Superior view of the bones of the skull.

Table 3–3　BONY OPENINGS IN THE SKULL AND THEIR ASSOCIATED NERVES AND BLOOD VESSELS

Bony Opening	Location	Nerves and Vessels
Carotid canal	Temporal bone	Internal carotid artery
Cribriform plate with foramina	Ethmoid bone	Olfactory nerves
External acoustic meatus	Temporal bone	(Opening to tympanic cavity)
Foramen lacerum	Sphenoid, occipital, and temporal bones	(Cartilage)
Foramen magnum	Occipital bone	Spinal cord, vertebral arteries, and eleventh cranial nerve
Foramen ovale	Sphenoid bone	Mandibular division of the fifth cranial nerve
Foramen rotundum	Sphenoid bone	Fifth cranial nerve
Foramen spinosum	Sphenoid bone	Middle meningeal artery
Greater palatine foramen	Palatine bone	Greater palatine nerve and vessels
Hypoglossal canal	Occipital bone	Twelfth cranial nerve
Incisive foramen	Maxilla	Nasopalatine nerve and branches of the sphenopalatine artery
Inferior orbital fissure	Sphenoid bone and maxilla	Infraorbital and zygomatic nerves, infraorbital artery, and ophthalmic vein
Infraorbital foramen and canal	Maxilla	Infraorbital nerve and vessels
Internal acoustic meatus	Temporal bone	Seventh and eighth cranial nerves
Jugular foramen	Occipital and temporal bones	Internal jugular vein and ninth, tenth, and eleventh cranial nerves
Lesser palatine foramen	Palatine bone	Lesser palatine nerve and vessels
Mandibular foramen	Mandible	Inferior alveolar nerve and vessels
Mental foramen	Mandible	Mental nerve and vessels
Optic canal and foramen	Sphenoid bone	Optic nerve and ophthalmic artery
Petrotympanic fissure	Temporal bone	Chorda tympani nerve
Pterygoid canal	Sphenoid bone	Area nerves and vessels
Stylomastoid foramen	Temporal bone	Seventh cranial nerve
Superior orbital fissure	Sphenoid bone	Third, fourth, and sixth cranial nerves and ophthalmic nerve and vein

paired **parietal bones** (pah-**ri**-it-al). At the back of the skull is the single **occipital bone** (ok-**sip**-it-al).

SUTURES ON SUPERIOR VIEW

Three sutures among these four skull bones are also visible on the superior view (Figure 3–2; see Table 3–2). The suture extending across the skull, between the frontal and parietal bones, is the **coronal suture** (kor-**oh**-nahl). A second suture, the **sagittal suture** (**saj**-i-tel), extends from the front to the back of the skull, between the paired parietal bones. The third suture, located between the single

occipital bone and the paired parietal bones, is the **lambdoidal suture** (lam-**doid**-al).

Anterior View of the Skull

When the skull is viewed from the front, certain bones of the skull (or portions of these bones) are visible (Figure 3–3). These bones include the single frontal, ethmoid, vomer, and sphenoid bones and the mandible, and also the paired lacrimal, nasal, inferior nasal conchal, zygomatic, and maxillary bones.

Table 3–4 PROCESSES AND ASSOCIATED STRUCTURES OF THE SKULL BONES

Processes of the Skull	Skull Bones	Associated Structures
Alveolar process	Mandible	Contain roots of mandibular teeth
Alveolar process	Maxilla	Contains roots of maxillary teeth
Coronoid process	Mandible	Portion of ramus
Frontal process	Maxilla	Forms medial infraorbital rim
Frontal process	Zygomatic bone	Forms anterior lateral orbital wall
Greater wing	Sphenoid bone	Anterior process to sphenoid bone body
Lesser wing	Sphenoid bone	Posterolateral process to sphenoid bone body
Mastoid process	Temporal bone	Composed of mastoid air cells
Maxillary process	Zygomatic bone	Forms infraorbital rim and portion of anterior lateral orbital wall
Palatine process	Maxilla	Forms anterior hard palate
Postglenoid process	Temporal bone	Posterior to temporomandibular joint
Pterygoid process	Sphenoid bone	Consists of medial and lateral pterygoid plates
Styloid process	Temporal bone	Serves as attachment for muscles and ligaments
Temporal process	Zygomatic bone	Portion of zygomatic arch
Zygomatic process	Frontal bone	Lateral to orbit
Zygomatic process	Maxilla	Forms lateral portion of infraorbital rim
Zygomatic process	Temporal bone	Portion of zygomatic arch

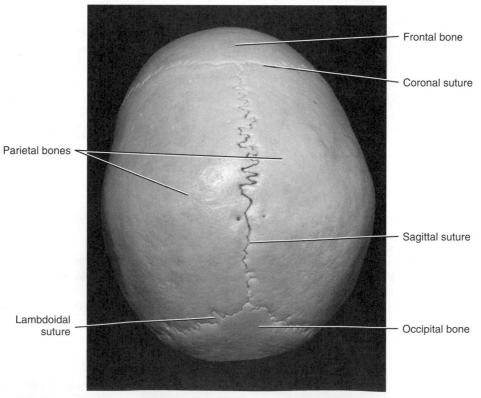

FIGURE 3–2 ■ Superior view of the skull and its suture lines.

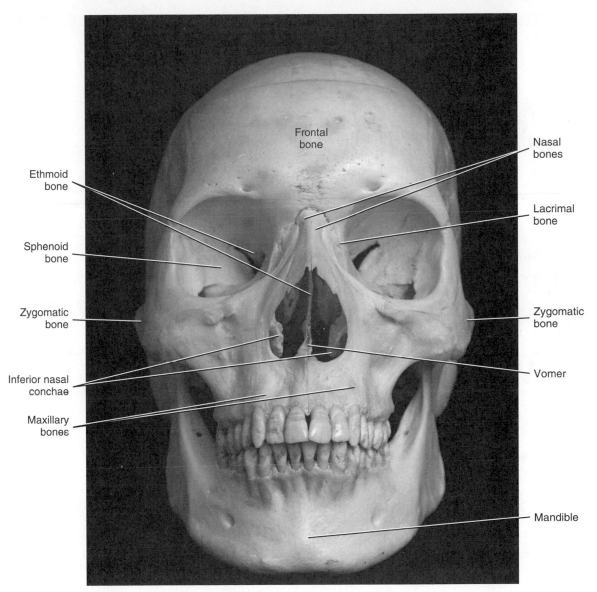

Frontal bone

Nasal bones

Ethmoid bone

Lacrimal bone

Sphenoid bone

Zygomatic bone

Zygomatic bone

Vomer

Inferior nasal conchae

Maxillary bones

Mandible

FIGURE 3–3 ■ Anterior view of the bones of the skull.

FACIAL BONES ON ANTERIOR VIEW

The **facial bones** visible on the anterior view of the skull include the **lacrimal bone** (**lak**-ri-mal), **nasal bone** (**nay**-zil), **vomer** (**vo**-mer), **inferior nasal concha** (**nay**-zil **kong**-kah), **zygomatic bone** (zy-go-**mat**-ik), **maxilla** (mak-**sil**-ah), and **mandible** (**man**-di-bl) (Figure 3–4). The **palatine bones** (**pal**-ah-tine) are not visible on this view and are not strictly considered facial bones, but for ease of learning are included under the heading of facial bones. This main division of the bones of the skull is discussed further in this chapter.

ORBIT AND ASSOCIATED STRUCTURES

The **orbit** (**or**-bit) or eye cavity, which contains and protects the eyeballs, is a prominent feature of the anterior view (Figure 3–5). Many bones of the skull form the walls and apex of the orbits (Table 3–5). The larger **orbital walls** (**or**-bit-al) are composed of the orbital plates of the frontal bone (making the roof or superior wall), ethmoid bone (forming the greatest portion of the medial wall), and lacrimal bone (at the anterior medial corner of the orbit) and the orbital surfaces of the maxilla (floor or inferior wall) and

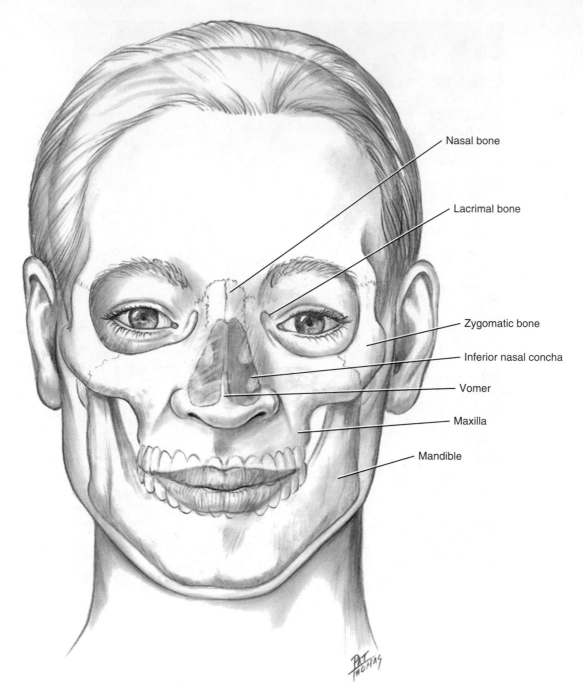

Nasal bone

Lacrimal bone

Zygomatic bone

Inferior nasal concha

Vomer

Maxilla

Mandible

FIGURE 3–4 ■ Anterior view of the facial bones and overlying facial tissues.

zygomatic bone (anterior part of the lateral wall). The orbital surface of the greater wing of the sphenoid bone is also included (the posterior part of the lateral wall).

The **orbital apex** (**or**-bit-al) or the deepest portion of the orbit is composed of the lesser wing of the sphenoid bone (forming the base) and the palatine bone (a small inferior portion) (Figure 3–6; see Table 3–5). The round opening in the orbital apex is the **optic canal** (**op**-tik), which lies between the two roots of the lesser wing of the sphenoid bone (Table 3–3). The optic

FIGURE 3–5 ■ Anterior view of the left orbit of the skull and its walls.

| Table 3–5 | BONES OF THE SKULL THAT FORM THE ORBIT |

Portion of Orbit	Skull Bones
Roof or superior wall	Frontal bone
Medial wall	Ethmoid and lacrimal bones
Lateral wall	Zygomatic and sphenoid bones
Apex or base	Sphenoid and palatine bones

nerve passes through the optic canal to reach the eyeball. The ophthalmic artery also extends through the canal to reach the eye.

There are two orbital fissures noted on the anterior aspect: the superior orbital fissure and inferior orbital fissure (Figure 3 7; see Table 3–3). Lateral to the optic canal is the curved and slitlike **superior orbital fissure** (**or**-bit-al), between the greater and lesser wings of the sphenoid bone. Like the optic canal, the superior

FIGURE 3–6 ■ Anterior view of the left orbit and the orbital apex.

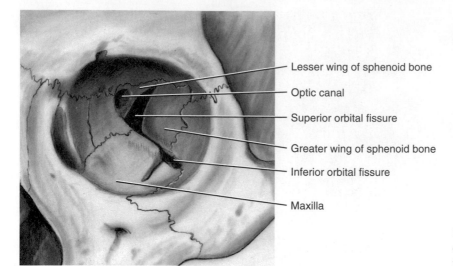

Lesser wing of sphenoid bone

Optic canal

Superior orbital fissure

Greater wing of sphenoid bone

Inferior orbital fissure

Maxilla

FIGURE 3–7 ■ Anterior view of the left orbit and the orbital fissures.

orbital fissure connects the orbit with the cranial cavity. The oculomotor or third cranial nerve, the trochlear or fourth cranial nerve, the abducens or sixth cranial nerve, and the ophthalmic nerve (from the trigeminal or fifth cranial nerve) and vein travel through this fissure.

The **inferior orbital fissure** (**or**-bit-al) can also be seen between the greater wing of the sphenoid bone and the maxilla. The inferior orbital fissure connects the orbit with the infratemporal and pterygopalatine fossae (discussed later in this chapter). The infraorbital and zygomatic nerves, branches of the maxillary nerve, and infraorbital artery enter the orbit through this fissure. The inferior ophthalmic vein travels through this fissure to join the pterygoid plexus of veins.

NASAL CAVITY AND ASSOCIATED STRUCTURES

The **nasal cavity** (**nay**-zil **kav**-it-ee) can also be viewed from the anterior aspect (Figure 3–8). The **nasion** (**nay**-ze-on), a midpoint landmark, is located at the junction of the frontal and nasal bones. The anterior opening of the nasal cavity, the **piriform aperture** (**pir**-i-form), is large and triangular. The **bridge of the nose** is formed from the paired nasal bones. The lateral boundaries of the nasal cavity are formed by the maxillae.

Each lateral wall of the nasal cavity has three projecting structures that extend inward from the maxilla, which are called the **nasal conchae** (**nay**-zil **kong**-kay) (Figure 3–8). These are the superior, middle, and inferior nasal conchae. Each extends scroll-like into the nasal cavity.

The superior nasal concha and middle nasal concha are formed from the ethmoid bone. The inferior nasal concha is a separate facial bone. Beneath each concha is a groove known as a **nasal meatus** (**nay**-zil me-**ate**-us). Each of these meatus has openings through which the paranasal sinuses or nasolacrimal duct communicates with the nasal cavity.

The vertical partition of the nasal cavity, the **nasal septum** (**nay**-zil **sep**-tum), divides the nasal cavity into two portions (Figure 3–9). Anteriorly, the nasal septum is formed by both the nasal septal cartilage inferiorly and the perpendicular plate of the ethmoid bone superiorly. The posterior portions of the nasal septum are formed by the vomer.

Lateral View of the Skull

When viewed from the side, the skull shows both cranial bones and facial bones. A division between the **cranial bones** and **facial bones** can be reinforced by making an imaginary diagonal line that passes downward and backward from the supraorbital ridge of the frontal bone to the tip of the mastoid process of the temporal bone (Figure 3–10). These two main divisions of the bones of the skull are discussed further in this chapter.

On the lateral surface of the skull are two separate parallel ridges or **temporal lines** (**tem**-poh-ral), crossing both the frontal and parietal

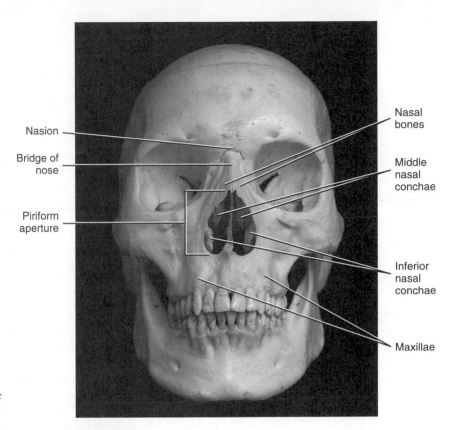

Nasion

Bridge of
nose

Piriform
aperture

Nasal
bones

Middle
nasal
conchae

Inferior
nasal
conchae

Maxillae

FIGURE 3–8 ■ Anterior view of
the skull and the nasal cavity.

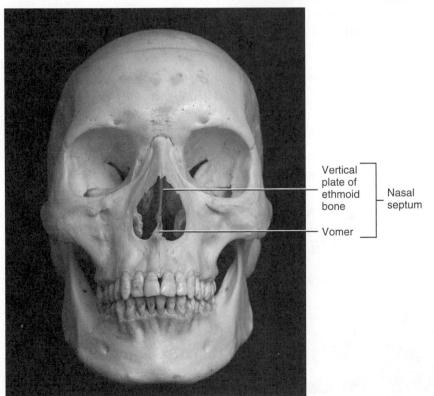

Vertical
plate of
ethmoid
bone

Vomer

Nasal
septum

FIGURE 3–9 ■ Anterior view of
the skull and the nasal septum.

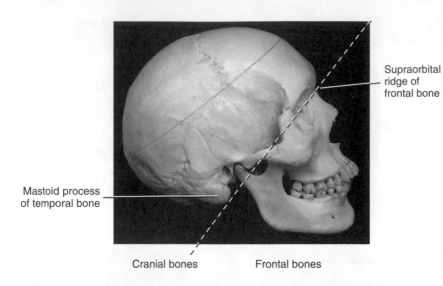

Mastoid process
of temporal bone

Supraorbital
ridge of
frontal bone

Cranial bones   Frontal bones

FIGURE 3–10 ■ Lateral view of the skull and an imaginary diagonal line separating the cranial bones and facial bones.

bones (Figure 3–11). The superior ridge is the superior temporal line. The inferior ridge or inferior temporal line is the superior boundary of the temporal fossa and where the fan-shaped temporalis muscle attaches.

CRANIAL BONES ON LATERAL VIEW

From the lateral view, the **cranium** (**kray**-nee-um) is easily seen, which includes the **cranial bones**: the **occipital** (ok-**sip**-it-al), **frontal** (**frunt**-il), **parietal** (pah-**ri**-it-al), **temporal** (**tem**-poh-ral), **sphenoid** (**sfe**-noid), and **ethmoid** bones (**eth**-moid). This main division of the bones of the skull is discussed further in this chapter.

Also present on the lateral view of the cranium are the associated sutures (Figure 3–12; see Table

3–2). These sutures include the **coronal suture** (kor-**oh**-nahl), an articulation between the frontal and parietal bones, and the **lambdoidal suture** (lam-**doid**-al), an articulation between the parietal and occipital bones. Also present is the arched **squamosal suture** (**skway**-mus-al), between the temporal and parietal bones.

FOSSAE ON LATERAL VIEW

The **temporal fossa** (**tem**-poh-ral) is easily seen on the lateral aspect of the skull (Figure 3–13). The temporal fossa is formed by several bones of the skull and contains the body of the temporalis muscle. Inferior to the temporal fossa is the **infratemporal fossa** (in-frah-**tem**-poh-ral). Deep to the infratemporal fossa and harder to see is the

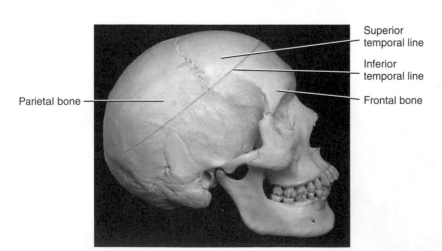

Parietal bone

Superior
temporal line

Inferior
temporal line

Frontal bone

FIGURE 3–11 ■ Lateral view of the skull and superior and inferior temporal lines.

FIGURE 3–12 ■ Lateral view of the cranial bones and their suture lines.

pterygopalatine fossa (**teh**-ri-go- **pal**-ah-tine). The temporal, infratemporal, and pterygopalatine fossae are discussed later in this chapter and contain many important head and neck structures.

ZYGOMATIC ARCH AND TEMPORO-MANDIBULAR JOINT ON LATERAL VIEW

Farther inferior on the lateral aspect are many important bony landmarks (Figure 3–14).

The **zygomatic arch** (zi-go-**mat**-ik) or cheek bone is visible, formed by the union of the broad temporal process of the zygomatic bone and the slender zygomatic process of the temporal bone (see Table 3–4). The suture between these two bones is the **temporozygomatic suture** (tem-por-oh-zi-go-**mat**-ik). The zygomatic arch serves as the origin for the masseter muscle.

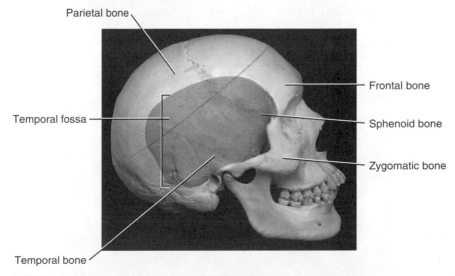

FIGURE 3–13 ■ Lateral view of the skull and temporal fossa.

Zygomatic
arch

Temporal process
of zygomatic bone

Temporal bone

Temporozygomatic
suture

Temporomandibular
joint

Zygomatic process
of temporal bone

Mandible

FIGURE 3–14 ■ Lateral view of the skull showing the zygomatic arch and the temporomandibular joint.

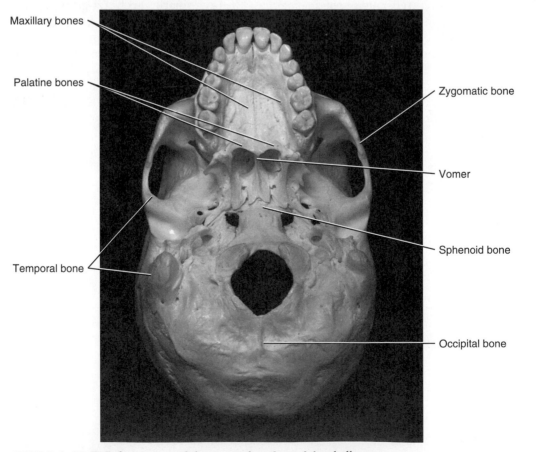

Maxillary bones

Palatine bones

Zygomatic bone

Vomer

Sphenoid bone

Temporal bone

Occipital bone

FIGURE 3–15 ■ Inferior view of the external surface of the skull.

The **temporomandibular joint** (tem-poh-ro-man-**dib**-you-lar) is also noted and is a movable articulation between the temporal bone and the mandible. The specifics of this joint are discussed in Chapter 5. Further landmarks of these bones are covered later in this chapter.

Inferior View of the External Surface of the Skull

Most of the structures of the inferior aspect of the skull surface are more easily viewed on the skull model if the mandible is temporarily removed. The **maxillary, zygomatic, vomer, temporal, sphenoid, occipital,** and **palatine bones** are visible on this inferior view of the skull's external surface (Figure 3–15).

HARD PALATE AND ASSOCIATED STRUCTURES

At the anterior portion of the skull's inferior aspect is the **hard palate** (**pal**-it), bordered by the **alveolar process of the maxilla** (al-**ve**-o-lar, mak-**sil**-ah) with its **maxillary teeth** (**mak**-sil-lare-ee) (Figure 3–16; see Table 3–4). The hard palate is formed by the two palatine processes of the maxillae and the two horizontal plates of the palatine bones.

Two prominent sutures are present on the hard palate (see Table 3–2). One suture is the **median palatine suture** (**pal**-ah-tine), a midline articulation between the two palatine processes of the maxillae anteriorly and the two horizontal plates of the palatine bones posteriorly. The other suture is the **transverse palatine suture** (**pal**-ah-tine), an articulation between the two palatine processes of the maxillae and the two horizontal plates of the palatine bones.

The hard palate forms the floor of the nasal cavity, as well as the roof of the mouth (Figure 3–16). The posterior edge of the hard palate forms the inferior border of two funnel-shaped cavities, the **posterior nasal apertures** (**nay**-zil) or choanae (ko-**a**-nay). The superior border of

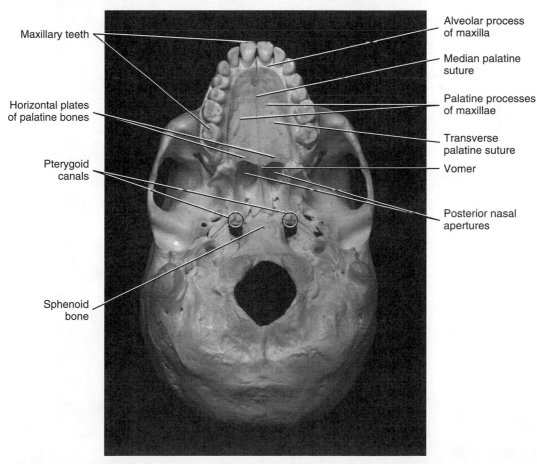

FIGURE 3–16 ■ External surface of the skull with the hard palate highlighted.

each aperture is formed by the vomer and the sphenoid bone. The posterior edge of the vomer forms the medial border of the posterior nasal apertures. The posterior nasal apertures are the posterior openings of the nasal cavity.

Near the superior border of each posterior nasal aperture is a small canal, the **pterygoid canal** (**teh**-ri-goid) (Figure 3–16; see Table 3–3). The pterygoid canal extends to open into the **pterygopalatine fossa** (**teh**-ri-go-**pal**-ah-tine) and carries the pterygoid nerve and blood vessels (the fossa is discussed later in this chapter).

MIDDLE PORTION OF THE EXTERNAL SKULL SURFACE

The middle portion of the inferior aspect of the external skull surface has many important surface prominences and depressions on the **sphenoid bone** (Figure 3–17). The lateral borders of the posterior nasal apertures are formed

on each side by the **pterygoid process** (**teh**-ri-goid) of the sphenoid bone (see Table 3–4).

Each pterygoid process consists of a thin **medial pterygoid plate** (**teh**-ri-goid) and a flattened **lateral pterygoid plate.** The depression between the medial and lateral plates is called the **pterygoid fossa.** At the inferior portion of the medial plate of the pterygoid process is a thin curved process, the **hamulus** (**ha**-mu-lis). The sphenoid bone and its landmarks are covered later in this chapter.

FORAMINA OF THE EXTERNAL SKULL SURFACE

The underside of the skull has a large number of foramina (Figure 3–18; see Table 3–3). These openings provide entrances and exits for the arteries and veins that supply the brain and facial tissues (see Chapter 6 for more information on the blood vessels and associated foramina and canals). They are also the way the cranial nerves

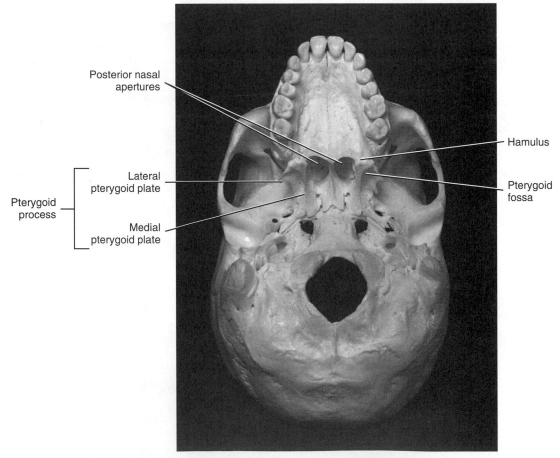

Posterior nasal apertures

Hamulus

Lateral pterygoid plate

Pterygoid fossa

Pterygoid process

Medial pterygoid plate

FIGURE 3–17 ■ Structures on the middle portion of the external skull surface.

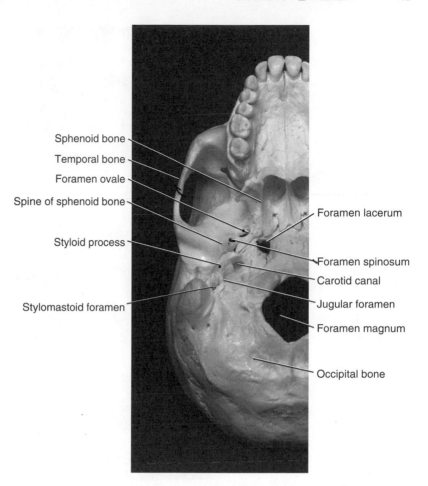

Sphenoid bone
Temporal bone
Foramen ovale
Spine of sphenoid bone
Styloid process
Stylomastoid foramen

Foramen lacerum
Foramen spinosum
Carotid canal
Jugular foramen
Foramen magnum
Occipital bone

FIGURE 3–18 ■ Foramina and associated structures of the external skull
surface.

pass to and from the brain (see Chapter 8 for
more information on the cranial nerves and their
associated foramina and canals).

The larger anterior oval opening on the sphenoid bone is the **foramen ovale (ova**-lee), for the
mandibular division of the trigeminal or fifth
cranial nerve. The smaller and more posterior
opening is the **foramen spinosum (spine**-o-
sum), which carries the middle meningeal artery
into the cranial cavity. The foramen spinosum
receives its name from the nearby **spine of the
sphenoid bone,** which is at the posterior extremity of the sphenoid bone.

Also on the external surface of the skull is the
large irregularly shaped **foramen lacerum (lah-
ser**-um), which in life is filled with cartilage
(Figure 3–18). Posterolateral to the foramen
lacerum is a round opening in the petrous portion of the temporal bone, the **carotid canal
(kah-rot**-id). The carotid canal carries the inter-

nal carotid artery and sympathetic carotid plexus.
A pointed bony projection, the **styloid process
(sty**-loid), is visible lateral and posterior to the
carotid canal (see Table 3–4). Immediately posterior to the styloid process is the **stylomastoid
foramen (sty-lo-mas**-toid), an opening through
which the facial or seventh cranial nerve exits
from the skull to the face.

The **jugular foramen (jug**-you-lar), just medial to the styloid process, is more easily seen if the
skull model is tilted to one side. The jugular foramen is the opening through which pass the internal
jugular vein and three cranial nerves: the glossopharyngeal or ninth cranial nerve, vagus or tenth
cranial nerve, and spinal accessory or eleventh
cranial nerve.

The largest opening on the inferior view is the
foramen magnum (mag-num) of the occipital
bone, through which pass the spinal cord, vertebral
arteries, and accessory or eleventh cranial nerve.

Frontal bone

Cribriform plate of ethmoid bone

Superior orbital fissure

Optic canal

Sphenoid bone

Foramen rotundum

Temporal bone

Foramen ovale

Parietal bone

Carotid canal

Foramen spinosum

Hypoglossal canal

Internal acoustic meatus

Foramen magnum

Jugular foramen

Occipital bone

FIGURE 3–19 ■ Superior view of the internal surface of the skull showing foramina.

Superior View of the Internal Surface of the Skull

The internal surface of the skull is viewed by carefully removing the top half of the skull model. The **frontal, ethmoid, sphenoid, temporal, occipital,** and **parietal bones** are visible from this view of the internal surface of the skull (Figure 3–19).

FORAMINA OF THE INTERNAL SKULL SURFACE

Also present are the inside openings of the **optic canal, superior orbital fissure, foramen ovale, foramen spinosum, carotid canal, jugular foramen,** and **foramen magnum,** as discussed before when viewing the external skull surface (see Figure 3–19; see Table 3–3). Additionally, many other foramina are present on the internal surface of the skull. The perforated **cribriform**

plate (**krib**-ri-form), with foramina for the olfactory nerves, and the **foramen rotundum** (row-**tun**-dum), for the maxillary division of the fifth cranial or trigeminal nerve, are also seen from this view. Finally, also present are the **hypoglossal canal** (hi-poh-**gloss**-al), for the twelfth cranial or hypoglossal nerve, and the **internal acoustic meatus** (ah-**koos**-tik), for the seventh cranial or facial nerve and the eighth cranial or vestibulo-cochlear nerve.

CRANIAL BONES

The **cranium** (**kray**-nee-um) is formed from the **cranial bones** (**kray**-nee-al). The cranial bones include the single occipital, frontal, sphenoid, and ethmoid bones and the paired parietal and temporal bones (Figure 3–20).

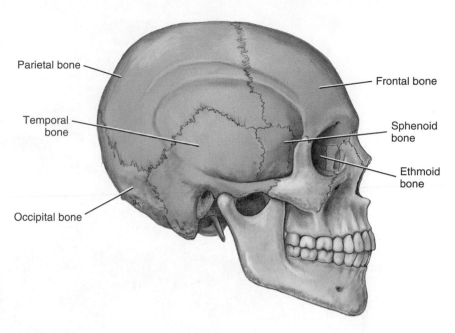

Parietal bone

Frontal bone

Temporal
bone

Sphenoid
bone

Ethmoid
bone

Occipital bone

FIGURE 3–20 ■ Lateral view
of the skull and the cranial
bones.

Occipital Bone

The **occipital bone** (ok-**sip**-it-al) is a single cranial bone located in the most posterior portion
of the skull (Figure 3–21). The occipital bone
articulates with the parietal, temporal, and sphenoid bones of the skull. The occipital bone can
easily be studied from an inferior view of its
external surface.

INFERIOR VIEW OF EXTERNAL SURFACE OF THE OCCIPITAL BONE

On the external surface of the occipital bone
from an inferior view, it can be seen that the
foramen magnum (**mag**-num) is completely
formed by this bone (Figure 3–22; see Table 3–3).
Lateral and anterior to the foramen magnum are
the paired **occipital condyles** (ok-**sip**-it-al),
curved and smooth projections. The occipital

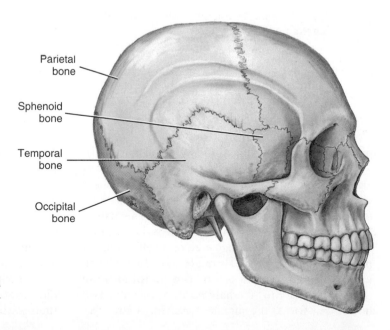

Parietal
bone

Sphenoid
bone

Temporal
bone

Occipital
bone

FIGURE 3–21 ■ Lateral view of the skull
with the occipital bone and its bony articulations.

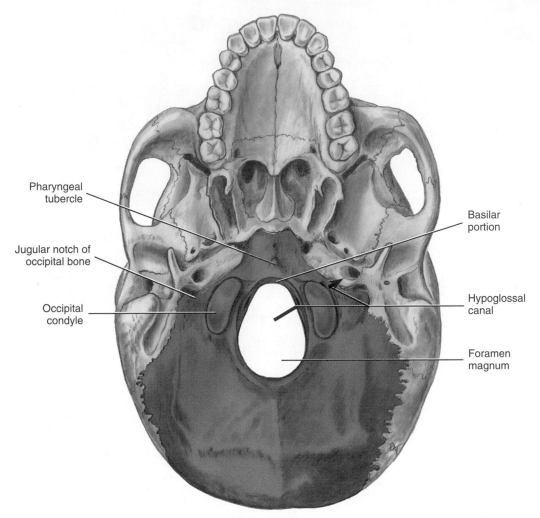

Pharyngeal
tubercle

Basilar
portion

Jugular notch of
occipital bone

Occipital
condyle

Hypoglossal
canal

Foramen
magnum

FIGURE 3–22 ■ Inferior view of the external surface of the skull with the occipital bone highlighted.

condyles have a movable articulation with the atlas, the first cervical vertebra of the vertebral column (discussed later in this chapter). On the stout basilar portion (**bas**-i-lar), a four-sided plate anterior to the foramen magnum, is a midline projection, the pharyngeal tubercle (fah-**rin**-je-al).

When tilting the skull model, the openings anterior and lateral to the foramen magnum are visible on the inferior view of the occipital bone (see Table 3–3). These openings are the paired **hypoglossal canals** (hi-poh-**gloss**-al) (Figure 3–22, *arrow*). The hypoglossal or twelfth cranial nerve is transmitted through the hypoglossal canals. The **jugular notch of the occipital bone** (**jug**-you-lar), the medial portion of the two bones that forms the jugular foramen, is also pre-

sent (a portion of the temporal bone is the other).

Frontal Bone

The **frontal bone** (**frunt**-il) is a single cranial bone that forms both the forehead and the superior portion of the orbits (Figure 3–23). The frontal bone articulates with the parietal bones, sphenoid bone, lacrimal bones, nasal bones, ethmoid bone, zygomatic bones, and maxillae. The frontal bone's portion of the superior temporal line and inferior temporal line is visible when the bone is viewed from the lateral aspect. Internally, the frontal bone contains the paired paranasal sinuses, the **frontal sinuses** (**sy**-nus-es) (discussed

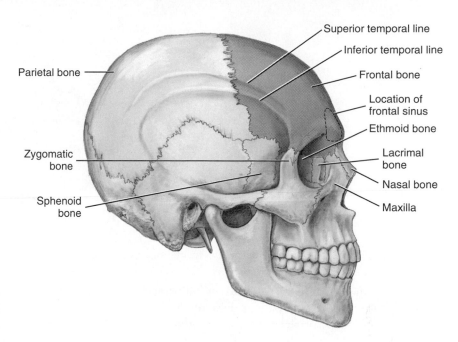

FIGURE 3–23 ■ Lateral view of the skull with the frontal bone and its bony articulations.

later in this chapter). The frontal bone can also be studied from anterior and inferior views.

ANTERIOR VIEW OF FRONTAL BONE

On the anterior aspect (Figure 3–24), certain landmarks are visible on the frontal bone. The orbital plates of the frontal bone create the superior wall or orbital roof. The curved elevations

over the superior portion of the orbit are the **supraorbital ridges** (soo-prah-**or**-bit-al), subjacent to the eyebrows. The supraorbital ridges are more prominent in adult males. The **supraorbital notch** is located on the medial portion of the supraorbital ridge and is where the supraorbital artery and nerve travel from the orbit to the forehead. The supraorbital notch is located about

FIGURE 3–24 ■ Anterior view of the frontal bone.

FIGURE 3–25 ■ Inferior view of the frontal bone with the lacrimal fossa highlighted.

an inch from the midline and when palpated with pressure can produce patient discomfort.

Between the supraorbital ridges is the **glabella** (glah-**bell**-ah), the smooth elevated area between the eyebrows, which tends to be flat in children and adult females and forms a rounded prominence in adult males. Lateral to the orbit there is a projection, the orbital surface of the **zygomatic process of the frontal bone** (zi-go-**mat**-ik) (see Table 3–4).

INFERIOR VIEW OF FRONTAL BONE

From the inferior view of the frontal bone, each **lacrimal fossa** (**lak**-ri-mal) is visible (Figure 3–25).

The lacrimal fossa is located just inside the lateral portion of the supraorbital ridge. This fossa contains the **lacrimal gland,** which produces lacrimal fluid or tears. After lubricating the eye, the lacrimal fluid empties into the nasal cavity through the nasolacrimal duct.

Parietal Bones

The **parietal bones** (pah-**ri**-it-al) are paired cranial bones and articulate with each other at the **sagittal suture** (**saj**-i-tel) (Figure 3–26; see Table

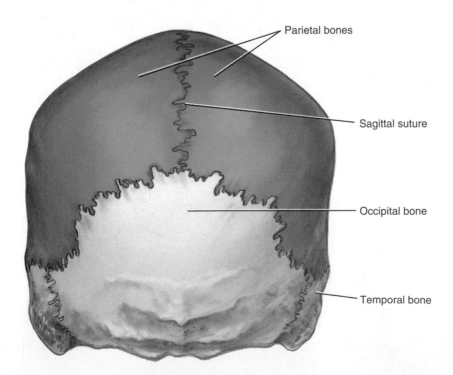

FIGURE 3–26 ■ Posterior view of the skull with the parietal bone and some of its bony articulations.

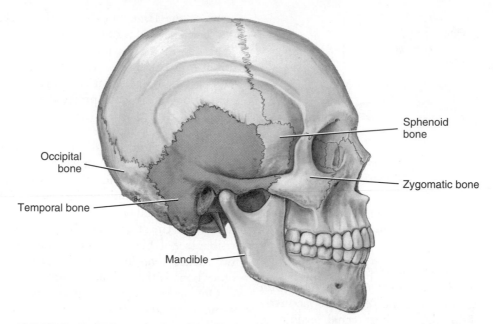

FIGURE 3–27 ■ Lateral view of the skull with the temporal bone and its bony articulations.

3–2). The parietal bones also articulate with the occipital, frontal, temporal, and sphenoid bones.

Temporal Bones

The **temporal bones** (**tem**-poh-ral) are paired cranial bones that form the lateral walls of the skull (Figure 3–27). Each temporal bone articulates with one zygomatic and one parietal bone, the occipital and sphenoid bones, and the mandible. Each temporal bone is composed of three portions: the squamous, tympanic, and petrous portions.

PORTIONS OF TEMPORAL BONE

The portions of the temporal bone can be viewed from the lateral aspect of the skull (Figure 3–28). The large, fan-shaped, flat portion on each of the temporal bones is the **squamous portion of the temporal bone** (**skwa**-mus). The second portion is the small, irregularly shaped **tympanic portion of the temporal bone** (tim-**pan**-ik), which is associated with the ear canal. The third portion is the **petrous portion of the temporal bone** (**pet**-rus), which is inferiorly located and helps form the cranial floor.

SQUAMOUS PORTION OF TEMPORAL BONE

In addition to helping form the braincase, the **squamous portion of the temporal bone** forms the zygomatic process of the temporal bone (zi-go-

mat-ik), which forms part of the zygomatic arch (Figure 3–29; see Table 3–4). This portion of the temporal bone also forms the cranial portion of the temporomandibular joint. This joint is discussed in detail in Chapter 5. On the inferior surface of the zygomatic process of the temporal bone is the **articular fossa** (ar-**tik**-you-ler) or mandibular fossa.

Anterior to the articular fossa is the **articular eminence** (ar-**tik**-you-ler), and posterior is the **postglenoid process** (post-**gle**-noid) (see Table 3–4). The articular fossa and eminence are portions of the temporal bone that articulate with the mandible at the temporomandibular joint.

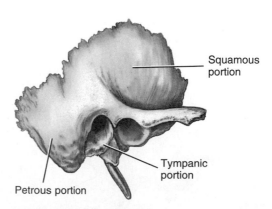

FIGURE 3–28 ■ Lateral view of the portions of the temporal bone: squamous portion, tympanic portion, and petrous portion.

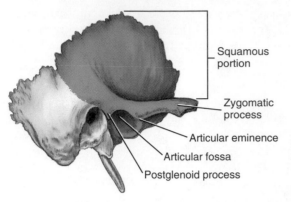

FIGURE 3–29 ■ Lateral view of the temporal bone with the squamous portion highlighted.

TYMPANIC PORTION OF TEMPORAL BONE

The **tympanic portion of the temporal bone** forms most of the **external acoustic meatus** (ah-**koos**-tik), a short canal leading to the tympanic cavity, located posterior to the articular fossa (Figure 3–30; see Table 3–3). Also posterior to the articular fossa, the tympanic portion is separated from the petrosal portion by a fissure, the **petrotympanic fissure** (pe-troh-tim-**pan**-ik), through which the chorda tympani nerve emerges.

PETROUS PORTION OF TEMPORAL BONE

On the inferior aspect of the **petrous portion of the temporal bone** (**pet**-rus), posterior to the external acoustic meatus, is a large roughened projection, the **mastoid process** (**mass**-toid) (Figure 3–31; see Table 3–4). The mastoid process is composed of air spaces or **mastoid air cells** that communicate with the middle ear cavity. The mastoid process also serves as the site for attach-

ment of the large muscles of the neck, such as the sternocleidomastoid muscle.

Medial to the mastoid process is the **mastoid notch** (**mass**-toid) (Figure 3–31A and B). Inferior and medial to the external acoustic meatus is a long pointed bony projection, the **styloid process** (**sty**-loid), a structure that serves for the attachment of muscles and ligaments (see Table 3–4). The **stylomastoid foramen** (sty-lo-**mass**-toid) carries the facial or seventh cranial nerve and is named for its location between the styloid process and mastoid process (see Table 3–3). When the skull model is tilted, the **jugular notch of the temporal bone** (**jug**-you-lar) is visible (see Table 3–3), the lateral portion of the two bones that form the jugular foramen (the other bone is the occipital bone).

On the intracranial surface is the **internal acoustic meatus** (ah-**koos**-tik), which carries the vestibulocochlear or eighth cranial nerve and the facial or seventh cranial nerve (see Figure 3–21; see Table 3–3). Both of these cranial nerves enter the skull from the brain. The vestibulocochlear nerve remains inside the petrous portion of the temporal bone, which houses the inner ear. In contrast, the facial nerve takes a convoluted path through the bone, eventually emerging at the stylomastoid foramen.

Sphenoid Bone

The next cranial bone of the skull to be considered is the single **sphenoid bone** (**sfe**-noid) (Figures 3–32 and 3–33). The sphenoid bone is a midline bone that articulates with the frontal, parietal, ethmoid, temporal, zygomatic, maxillary, palatine, vomer, and occipital bones. This bone is

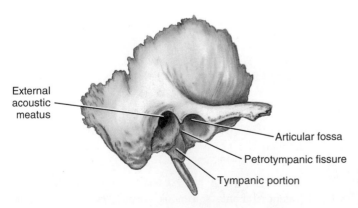

FIGURE 3–30 ■ Lateral view of the temporal bone with the tympanic portion highlighted.

A

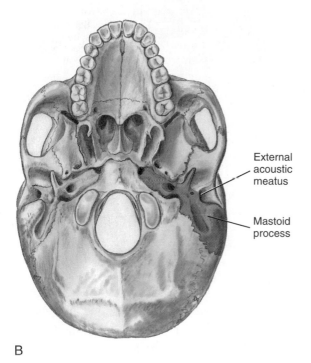

B

FIGURE 3–31 ■ A: Inferior view of the temporal bone with the petrous portion highlighted. B: Location of the petrous portion of the temporal bone demonstrated on an inferior view of the skull.

very complex, with some portions of it encountered in almost every significant area of the skull. The sphenoid bone has important foramina and different portions: the body and its processes.

FORAMINA OF THE SPHENOID BONE

Many foramina or fissures are located in the sphenoid bone, such as the **superior orbital**

fissure, foramen ovale, foramen rotundum, and **foramen spinosum,** which carry important nerves and blood vessels of the head and neck (Figures 3–32 and 3–33; see Table 3–3).

BODY OF THE SPHENOID BONE

The middle portion of the sphenoid bone is the **body of the sphenoid bone** (sfe-noid), which articulates on its anterior surface with the ethmoid bone (Figures 3–32 and 3–33). The body of sphenoid bone articulates posteriorly with the basilar portion of the occipital bone. The body contains the paired paranasal sinuses, the **sphenoid sinuses** (sfe-noid **sy**-nus-es) (discussed later in this chapter).

PROCESSES OF THE SPHENOID BONE

The body of the sphenoid bone has three paired processes that arise from it: the lesser wing, greater wing, and pterygoid process (Figures 3–32 to 3–34; see Table 3–4). The anterior process is the **lesser wing of the sphenoid bone,** which makes up the base of the orbital apex. The posterolateral process is the **greater wing of the sphenoid bone.**

Inferior to the greater wing of the sphenoid bone is the **pterygoid process** (teh-ri-goid), an area for the attachment of some of the muscles of mastication. The pterygoid process consists of two plates, the flattened **lateral pterygoid plate** and thinner **medial pterygoid plate,** with the **pterygoid fossa** between them. The **hamulus** (**ha**-mu-lis), a thin curved process, is the inferior termination of the medial pterygoid plate.

A sharp pointed area, the **spine of the sphenoid bone,** is located at the posterior corner of each greater wing of the sphenoid bone. Each greater wing is divided into two smaller surfaces by the **infratemporal crest** (in-frah-**tem**-poh-ral), the temporal and infratemporal surfaces.

Ethmoid Bone

The **ethmoid bone** (**eth**-moid) is a single midline cranial bone of the skull (Figure 3–35). The ethmoid articulates with the frontal, sphenoid, lacrimal, and maxillary bones and adjoins the vomer at its inferior and posterior border.

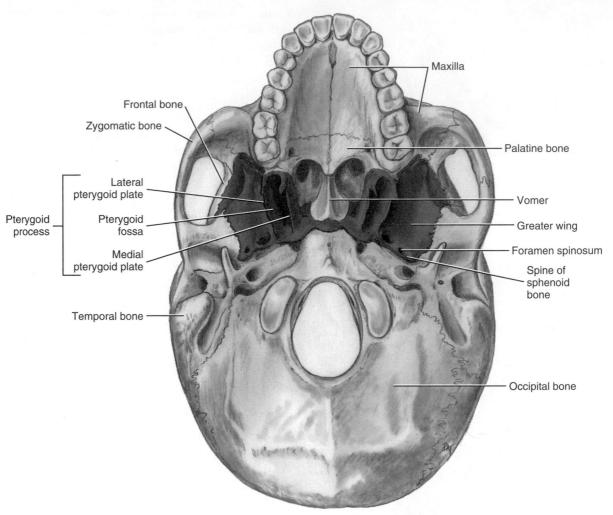

FIGURE 3–32 ■ Inferior view of the external surface of the skull with the sphenoid bone highlighted.

PLATES OF THE ETHMOID BONE AND ASSOCIATED STRUCTURES

The ethmoid bone has two unpaired plates, the midline vertical **perpendicular plate** (per-pen-**dik**-you-lar) and the horizontal **cribriform plate** (**krib**-ri-form), which it crosses. The perpendicular plate is easily seen in the nasal cavity and aids the vomer and nasal septal cartilage in forming the nasal septum (Figure 3–35). The cribriform plate, visible from the inside of the cranial cavity and present on the superior aspect of the bone, is perforated by foramina to allow the passage of olfactory nerves for the sense of smell (Figures 3–36 and 3–37).

The **ethmoid sinuses** (**eth**-moid **sy**-nus-es) or ethmoid air cells are a variable number of small

cavities in the lateral mass of the ethmoid bone and are discussed later in this chapter. A vertical midline continuation of the perpendicular plate into the cranial cavity is the **crista galli** (**kris**-tah **gal**-lee). The crista galli serves as an attachment for layers covering the brain.

NASAL CONCHAE AND ASSOCIATED STRUCTURES

The lateral portions of the ethmoid bone form the **superior nasal conchae** (**nay**-zil **kong**-kee) and **middle nasal conchae** in the nasal cavity and the paired orbital plates (Figures 3–37 and 3–38). The **orbital plate of the ethmoid bone** (**or**-bit-al) forms the medial orbital wall. Between the orbital plate and the conchae are the **ethmoid**

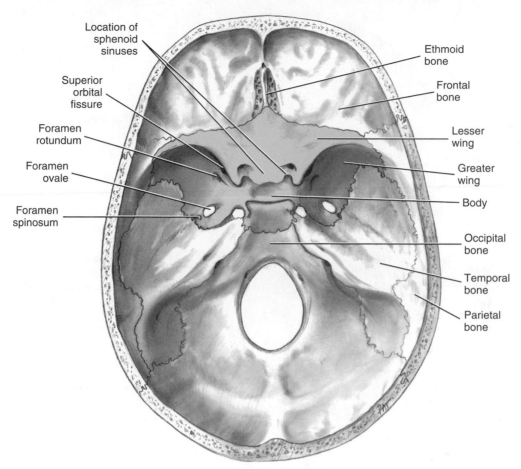

Location of
sphenoid
sinuses

Superior
orbital
fissure

Foramen
rotundum

Foramen
ovale

Foramen
spinosum

Ethmoid
bone

Frontal
bone

Lesser
wing

Greater
wing

Body

Occipital
bone

Temporal
bone

Parietal
bone

FIGURE 3–33 ■ Superior view of the internal surface of the skull with the sphenoid bone highlighted.

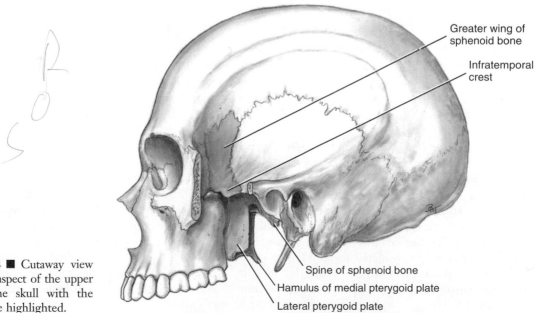

Greater wing of
sphenoid bone

Infratemporal
crest

Spine of sphenoid bone

Hamulus of medial pterygoid plate

Lateral pterygoid plate

FIGURE 3–34 ■ Cutaway view of the lateral aspect of the upper portion of the skull with the sphenoid bone highlighted.

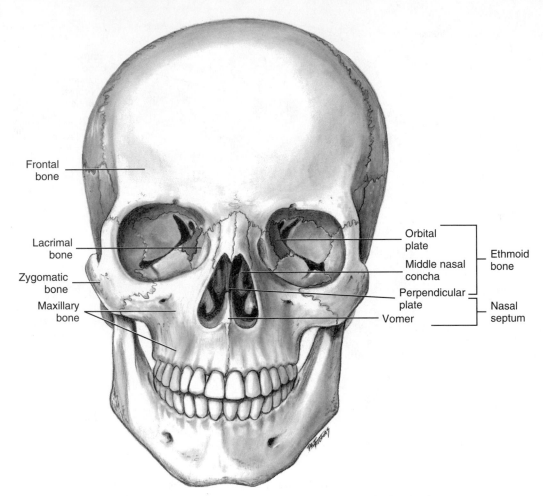

Frontal
bone

Lacrimal
bone

Zygomatic
bone

Maxillary
bone

Orbital
plate

Middle nasal
concha

Perpendicular
plate

Vomer

Ethmoid
bone

Nasal
septum

FIGURE 3–35 ■ Anterior view of the skull with the ethmoid bone highlighted.

sinuses, which consist of air-filled spaces (discussed later in this chapter).

FACIAL BONES

The **facial bones** create the facial features and serve as a base for dentition. The facial bones include the single vomer and mandible and the paired lacrimal, nasal, inferior nasal conchal, zygomatic, and maxillary bones (see Figure 3–4). For ease of learning, the palatine bones will be considered under the heading of facial bones, but they are not strictly considered facial bones.

Many bones of the face are shared by two or more soft tissue components of the face. For exam-

ple, the frontal bone forms both the forehead and the areas around the eyes. This is important to remember since an abnormality in one facial bone often involves many soft tissue components (discussed later in this chapter).

Vomer

The **vomer** (vo-mer) is a single facial bone of the skull that forms the posterior portion of the nasal septum. It is located in the midsagittal plane inside the nasal cavity. The articulations of the vomer are easily seen on a lateral view of the bone (Figure 3–39). The vomer articulates with the ethmoid bone on its anterosuperior border, the nasal cartilage anteriorly, the palatine bones and maxillae

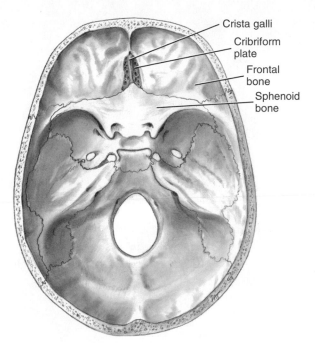

FIGURE 3–36 ■ Superior view of the internal surface of the skull with the ethmoid bone highlighted.

inferiorly, and the sphenoid bone on its posterosuperior border. The posteroinferior border is free of any bony articulation. The vomer has no muscle attachments.

Lacrimal Bones, Nasal Bones, and Inferior Nasal Conchae

The paired **lacrimal bones** (**lak**-ri-mal) are irregular thin plates of bone that form a small portion of the anterior medial wall of the orbit (Figure 3–40). Each lacrimal bone articulates with the ethmoid, frontal, and maxillary bones. The **nasolacrimal duct** (nay-so-**lak**-rim-al dukt) is formed at the junction of the lacrimal and maxillary bones. Lacrimal fluid or tears from the lacrimal gland are drained through this duct into the inferior nasal meatus.

The **nasal bones** (**nay**-zil) are paired facial bones that form the bridge of the nose, articulating with each other in the midline above the piriform aperture. The nasal bones fit between the

FIGURE 3–37 ■ Oblique anterior view of the ethmoid bone with its perpendicular, cribriform, and orbital plates.

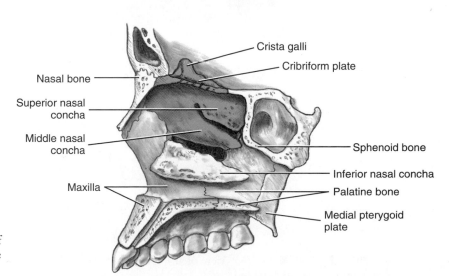

FIGURE 3–38 ■ Lateral wall of the right nasal cavity with the ethmoid bone highlighted.

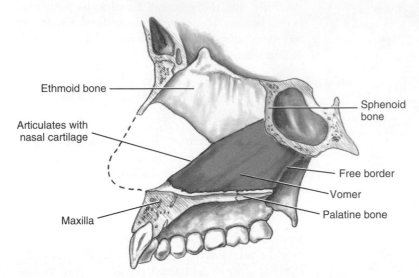

Ethmoid bone

Articulates with
nasal cartilage

Maxilla

Sphenoid
bone

Free border

Vomer

Palatine bone

FIGURE 3–39 ■ Medial wall of the
left nasal cavity with the vomer highlighted (outline of nasal cartilage).

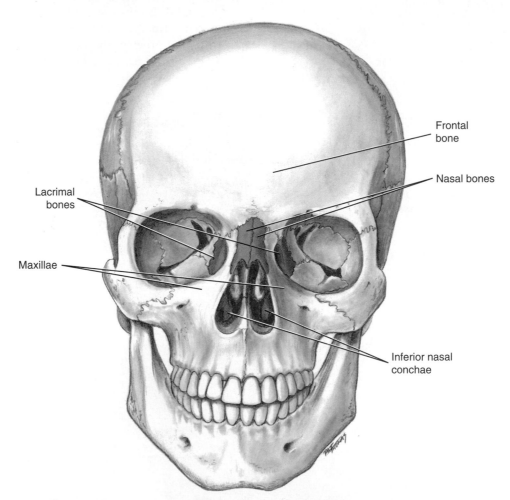

Frontal
bone

Nasal bones

Lacrimal
bones

Maxillae

Inferior nasal
conchae

FIGURE 3–40 ■ Anterior view of the skull with the nasal bones, lacrimal bones, and inferior
nasal conchae highlighted.

frontal processes of the maxillae and thus articulate with the frontal bone superiorly and the maxillae laterally (Figure 3–40).

The **inferior nasal conchae** (**nay**-zil **kong**-kee) are paired facial bones that project off the maxilla to form part of the lateral walls of the nasal cavity (Figure 3–40). Unlike the superior and middle nasal conchae that also project off the maxillae, the inferior nasal conchae are separate facial bones. Each inferior nasal concha is composed of thin spongy bone curved upon itself like a scroll. These bones articulate with the ethmoid, lacrimal, palatine, and maxillary bones. The inferior nasal conchae do not have any muscle attachments.

Zygomatic Bones

The **zygomatic bones** (zi-go-**mat**-ik) are paired facial bones of the skull that form the cheek bones or malar surfaces (Figures 3–41 and 3–42). The zygomatic bones articulate with the frontal, temporal, sphenoid, and maxillary bones. Each zygomatic bone has a diamond shape composed of three processes with similarly named associated bony articulations: the frontal, temporal, and maxillary processes.

PROCESSES OF THE ZYGOMATIC BONE

Each process of the zygomatic bone forms important structures of the skull (Figures 3–41 and 3–42, Table 3–4). The orbital surface of the **frontal process of the zygomatic bone** (**frunt**-il) forms the anterior lateral orbital wall. The **temporal process of the zygomatic bone** (**tem**-poh-ral) forms the zygomatic arch together with the zygomatic process of the temporal bone. The orbital surface of the **maxillary process of the zygomatic bone** (**mak**-sil-lare-ee) forms a por-

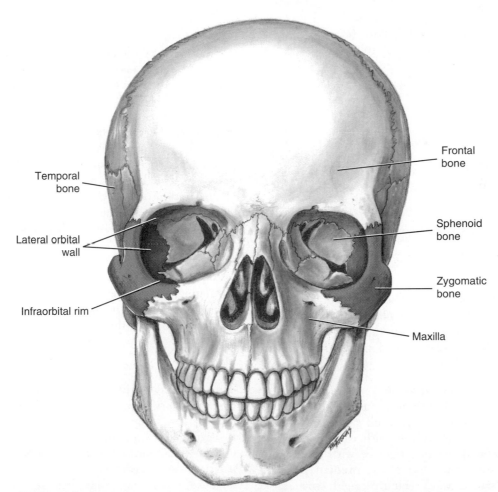

FIGURE 3–41 ■ Anterior view of the skull with the zygomatic bones highlighted.

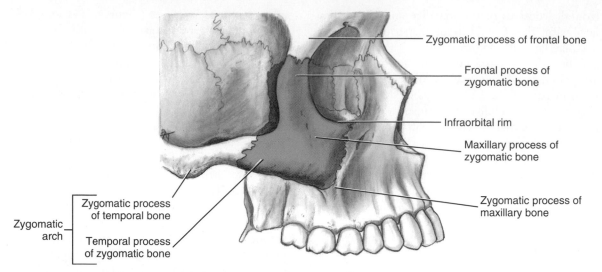

Zygomatic process of frontal bone

Frontal process of zygomatic bone

Infraorbital rim

Maxillary process of zygomatic bone

Zygomatic process of maxillary bone

Zygomatic process of temporal bone

Zygomatic arch

Temporal process of zygomatic bone

FIGURE 3–42 ■ Lateral view of the upper portion of the skull with the zygomatic bone highlighted.

tion of the **infraorbital rim** (in-frah-**or**-bit-al rim) and a small portion of the anterior part of the lateral orbital wall.

Palatine Bones

The **palatine bones** (**pal**-ah-tine) are paired bones of the skull that are not strictly considered facial bones, but they will be considered under this heading for ease of learning. Each palatine bone consist of two plates, the horizontal and vertical plates.

PLATES OF THE PALATINE BONE

Both the horizontal and vertical plates can be seen from a posterior view of a palatine bone (Figure 3–43). The **horizontal plates of the palatine bones** form the posterior portion of the hard palate. The **vertical plates of the palatine bones** form part of the lateral walls of the nasal cavity, and each plate contributes a small lip of bone to the orbital apex.

SUTURE OF THE PALATINE BONES

The palatine bones serve as a link between the maxillae and the sphenoid bone with which they articulate, as well as with each other. The two horizontal plates articulate with each other at the posterior portion of the **median palatine suture** (**pal**-ah-tine) (Figure 3–44; see Table 3–2).

FORAMINA OF THE PALATINE BONES

There are two important foramina in the palatine bones that transmit nerves and blood vessels to this region, the greater and lesser palatine foramina (see Figure 3–44, Table 3–3). The **greater palatine foramen** (**pal**-ah-tine) is located in the posterolateral region of each of the palatine bones, usually at the apex of the maxillary third molar. The greater palatine foramen transmits the greater palatine nerve and blood vessels and is a landmark for the administration of a local anesthetic for the greater palatine nerve block (see Chapter 9).

A smaller opening nearby, the **lesser palatine foramen** (**pal**-ah-tine), transmits the lesser palatine nerve and blood vessels to the soft palate and tonsils. Both foramina are openings of the pterygopalatine canal that carries the descending palatine nerves and blood vessels from the pterygopalatine fossa to the palate.

Maxilla

The upper jaw or **maxilla** (mak-**sil**-ah) consists of two maxillary bones or **maxillae** (mak-**sil**-lay) that are fused together (Figure 3–45). The maxillae articulate with the frontal, lacrimal, nasal, inferior nasal conchal, vomer, sphenoid, ethmoid, palatine, and zygomatic bones. Each maxilla includes a body and four processes: the frontal, zygomatic, palatine, and alveolar processes.

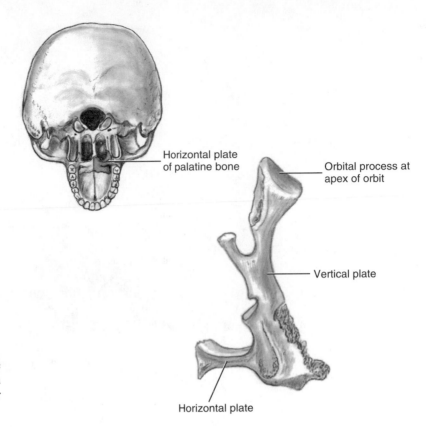

Horizontal plate
of palatine bone

Orbital process at
apex of orbit

Vertical plate

Horizontal plate

FIGURE 3–43 ■ Posterior view of the right palatine bone with its location demonstrated on a posterior-inferior view of the skull.

The **body of the maxilla** has orbital, nasal, infratemporal, and facial surfaces. The bodies contain air-filled spaces or paranasal sinuses, the **maxillary sinuses** (**mak**-sil-lare-ee **sy**-nuses) (discussed later in this chapter). The maxilla can be studied from its three views: the anterior, lateral, and inferior views.

ANTERIOR VIEW OF THE MAXILLA

The **frontal process of the maxilla** (**frunt**-il) articulates with the frontal bone and forms the medial orbital rim with the lacrimal bone on its anterior surface (Figures 3–45, 3–46, and 3–47; see Table 3–4). Each maxilla's orbital surface is separated from the sphenoid bone by the **inferior**

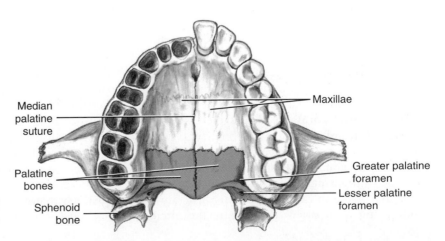

Median
palatine
suture

Maxillae

Palatine
bones

Greater palatine
foramen

Lesser palatine
foramen

Sphenoid
bone

FIGURE 3–44 ■ Inferior view of the hard palate with the palatine bones highlighted.

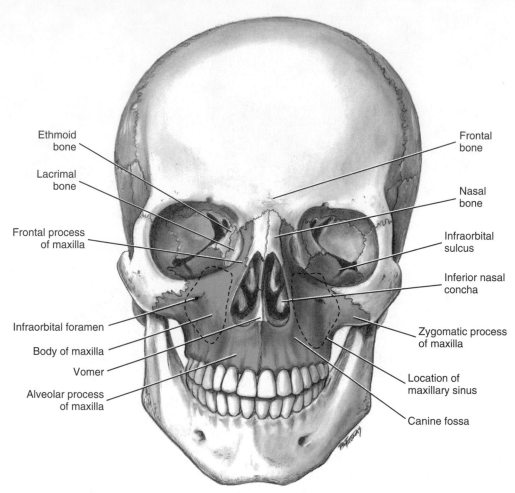

FIGURE 3–45 ■ Anterior view of the skull with the maxilla and its bony articulations (articulation of the maxilla with the pterygoid process of the sphenoid bone and palatine bones cannot be seen in this view).

orbital fissure (**or**-bit-al) (see Figure 3–7, Table 3–3). The inferior orbital fissure carries the infraorbital and zygomatic nerves, infraorbital artery, and inferior ophthalmic vein. The groove in the floor of the orbital surface is the **infraorbital sulcus** (in-frah-**or**-bit-al).

The infraorbital sulcus becomes the **infraorbital canal** (in-frah-**or**-bit-al) and then terminates on the facial surface of the maxilla as the **infraorbital foramen** (see Table 3–3). This foramen transmits the infraorbital nerve and blood vessels. The infraorbital foramen is a landmark for the administration of a local anesthetic for the infraorbital block (see Chapter 9). Palpation of the infraorbital foramen will cause a mild aching in a patient. Inferior to the infraorbital foramen is an elongated depression, the **canine fossa** (**kay**-nine). The canine fossa is just posterosuperior to the roots of the maxillary canine teeth.

Each tooth of the maxillary arch is covered by a prominent facial ridge of bone, a portion of the **alveolar process of the maxilla** (al-**ve**-o-lar) (see Table 3–4). The facial ridge over the maxillary canine, the **canine eminence** (**kay**-nine), is especially prominent. The maxillary bone over the facial surface of the maxillary teeth is less dense than the mandible over similar teeth. This allows a greater incidence of clinically adequate local anesthesia for the maxillary teeth when the drug is administered as a local infiltration (see Chapter 9).

① Middle cranial fossa		⑧ External oblique line
② Orbit		⑨ Angle of mandible
③ Zygomatic arch		⑩ Glenoid fossa
④ Palate		⑪ Articular eminence
⑤ Styloid process		⑫ Vertebra
⑥ Septa in maxillary sinus		⑬ Maxillary sinus
⑦ Maxillary tuberosity		⑭ Ear lobe

B

FIGURE 3–46 ■ A: Panoramic radiograph. (Modified from Bath-Balogh M, Fehrenbach MJ. *Illustrated Dental Embryology, Histology, and Anatomy.* WB Saunders, Philadelphia, 1997.) B: Panoramic anatomy of the midface. (Modified from Olson SS. *Dental Radiography Laboratory Manual.* WB Saunders, Philadelphia, 1995.)

LATERAL VIEW OF THE MAXILLA

The **zygomatic process of the maxilla** (zy-go-**mat**-ik) articulates with the zygomatic bone laterally, completing the **infraorbital rim** (in-frah-**or**-bit-al) (Figures 3–46 and 3–47; see Table 3–4). Some of the landmarks noted in the anterior view of the maxilla are also present.

INFERIOR VIEW OF THE MAXILLAE

On the inferior surface, each **palatine process of the maxilla** (**pal**-ah-tine) articulates with the other to form the anterior, major portion of the hard palate (Figures 3–46 and 3–48; see Table 3–4). The suture between these two palatine processes of the maxillae is the anterior portion

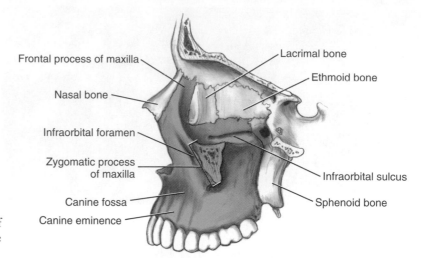

FIGURE 3–47 ■ Cutaway view of the lateral aspect of the skull with the maxilla highlighted.

of the **median palatine suture** (see Table 3–2). In the patient, this is covered by the median palatine raphe, a midline fibrous band of tissue.

In the anterior midline portion of the palatine process, just posterior to the maxillary central incisors, is the **incisive foramen** (in-**sy**-ziv) (see

Table 3–3). This foramen carries the branches of the right and left nasopalatine nerves and blood vessels from the nasal cavity to the palate. The incisive foramen is a landmark for the administration of a local anesthetic for the nasopalatine nerve block (see Chapter 9). The soft tissue bulge

FIGURE 3–48 ■ Posterior-inferior view of the maxillae and hard palate.

over the incisive foramen in the patient is called the **incisive papilla.**

The **alveolar process of the maxilla** (al-**ve**-o-lar) usually contains the roots of the maxillary teeth (Figures 3–46 and 3–48; see Table 3–4). The alveolar process of the maxilla can become resorbed in a patient who is completely edentulous in the maxillary arch (resorption occurs to a lesser extent in partially edentulous cases), possibly leading to problems with the maxillary sinuses (discussed later in this chapter). The body of the maxilla is not resorbed with tooth loss, but its walls may become thinner in this case.

The density of the maxillary bone in an area determines the route that a dental infection takes with abscess and fistula formation (see Chapter 12). Finally, the differences in alveolar process density determine the easiest and most convenient areas of bony fracture used during tooth extraction. Thus the maxillary teeth are mechanically easier to remove by fracturing the thinner facial surface rather than the thicker lingual surface.

On the posterior portion of the body of the maxilla is a rounded, roughened elevation, the **maxillary tuberosity** (**mak**-sil-lare-ee), just posterior to the most distal molar of the maxillary dentition (Figures 3–46 to 3–48). The superiolateral portion of the maxillary tuberosity is perforated by one or more **posterior superior alveolar foramina** (al-**ve**-o-lar), where the poste-

rior superior alveolar nerve and blood vessel branches enter the bone from the back. The maxillary tuberosity is a landmark for the administration of a local anesthetic for the posterior superior alveolar block (see Chapter 9).

Mandible

The lower jaw or **mandible** (**man**-di-bl) is a single facial bone that is the only freely movable bone of the skull (Figures 3–49 and 3–50). This bone is also the largest and strongest facial bone. The mandible has a movable articulation with the temporal bones at each temporomandibular joint (see Chapter 5 for more information). The mandible is more effectively studied when it is temporarily removed from the skull model. The mandible can be studied from three views: the anterior, lateral, and medial views.

ANTERIOR VIEW OF THE MANDIBLE

On the anterior surface of the mandible are many important landmarks (Figures 3–51 to 3–53). The **mental protuberance** (**ment**-il pro-**too**-ber-ins), the bony prominence of the chin, is located beneath the roots of the mandibular incisors. The mental protuberance is more pronounced in males but can be visualized and palpated in females. In the midline on the surface of the mandible is a faint ridge, an indication of the mandibular

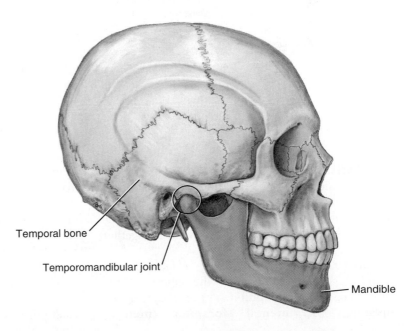

FIGURE 3–49 ■ Lateral view of the skull showing the mandible and the temporomandibular joint.

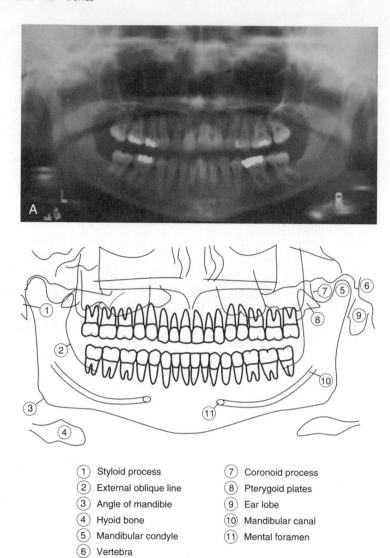

1. Styloid process
2. External oblique line
3. Angle of mandible
4. Hyoid bone
5. Mandibular condyle
6. Vertebra
7. Coronoid process
8. Pterygoid plates
9. Ear lobe
10. Mandibular canal
11. Mental foramen

B

FIGURE 3–50 ■ A: Panoramic radiograph. (Modified from Bath-Balogh M, Fehrenbach MJ. *Illustrated Dental Embryology, Histology, and Anatomy*. WB Saunders, Philadelphia, 1997.) B: Panoramic anatomy of the lower face. (Modified from Olson SS. *Dental Radiography Laboratory Manual*. WB Saunders, Philadelphia, 1995.)

symphysis (**sim**-fi-sis), where the bone is formed by the fusion of right and left processes. Like other symphyses in the body, this is a midline articulation where the bones are joined by fibrocartilage, but this articulation fuses together in early childhood.

Farther posteriorly on the surface of the mandible, typically between the apices of the first and second mandibular premolars, is an opening, the **mental foramen** (**ment**-il)

(Figures 3–50 to 3–52; see Table 3–3). As the mandibular growth proceeds in young children, the mental foramen alters direction from anterior to posterosuperior. The mental foramen allows the entrance of the mental nerve and blood vessels into the mandibular canal (discussed later in this chapter).

The mental foramen's posterosuperior opening in adults signifies the changed direction of the emerging mental nerve. This is an important

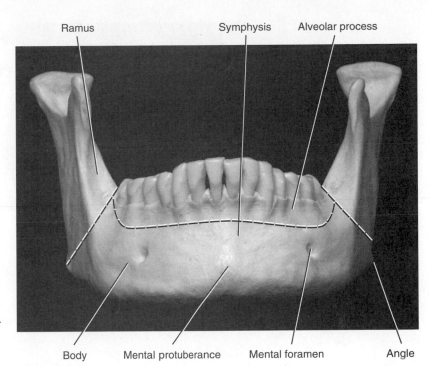

Ramus Symphysis Alveolar process

Body Mental protuberance Mental foramen Angle

FIGURE 3–51 ■ Anterior view of the mandible and its associated landmarks.

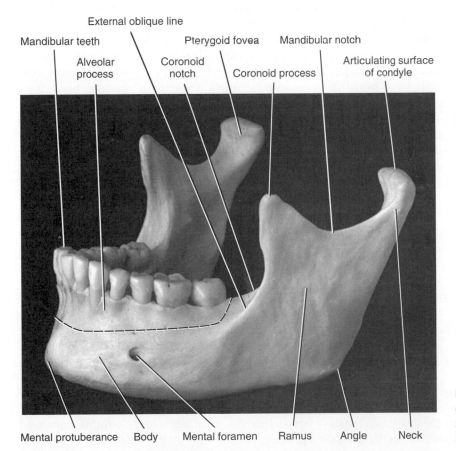

External oblique line

Mandibular teeth Pterygoid fovea Mandibular notch

Alveolar process Coronoid notch Coronoid process Articulating surface of condyle

Mental protuberance Body Mental foramen Ramus Angle Neck

FIGURE 3–52 ■ Slightly oblique lateral view of the mandible and its associated landmarks.

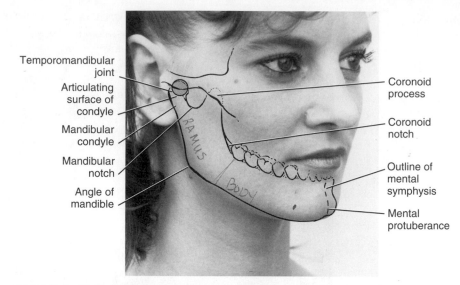

Temporomandibular joint

Articulating surface of condyle

Mandibular condyle

Mandibular notch

Angle of mandible

RAMUS

BODY

Coronoid process

Coronoid notch

Outline of mental symphysis

Mental protuberance

FIGURE 3–53 ■ Lateral view of the face showing the landmarks of the mandible. (From Bath-Balogh M, Fehrenbach MJ. *Illustrated Dental Embryology, Histology, and Anatomy.* WB Saunders, Philadelphia, 1997.)

landmark to note on an oral radiograph prior to the administration of a local anesthetic for a mental or incisive block (see Chapter 9). It is also important not to confuse the mental foramen on a radiograph with a periapical lesion related to the teeth or other oral lesions.

The heavy horizontal portion of the lower jaw below the mental foramen is called the **body of the mandible** (Figure 3–51). Superior to this, the portion of the lower jaw usually containing the roots of the mandibular teeth is the **alveolar process of the mandible** (al-ve-o-lar) (Figure 3–52; see Table 3–4). In children, the body of the mandible, along with the alveolar process, elongates to provide space for the additional teeth as one nears adulthood.

If a patient becomes completely edentulous in the mandibular arch (or to some extent in partial edentulous cases), the lower alveolar process can become resorbed. This resorption can occur to such an extent that the mental foramen is virtually on the superior border of the mandible, instead of opening on the anterior surface, changing its relative position. The body of the mandible is not affected and remains thick and rounded.

The alveolar process of the mandibular incisors is less dense than the body of the mandible in that area and even less dense than the alveolar process of the posterior teeth, allow-

ing local infiltration of the mandibular incisors by a local anesthetic with varying degrees of success (see Chapter 9). The density of the mandibular bone in an area also determines the route that a dental infection takes with abscess and fistula formation (see Chapter 12). Finally, the differences in alveolar process density determine the easiest and most convenient areas of bony fracture used during tooth extraction. Thus the mandibular third molar is mechanically easier to remove by fracturing the thinner lingual surface (being careful of the nearby lingual nerve) rather than the thicker buccal surface.

LATERAL VIEW OF THE MANDIBLE

On the lateral aspect of the mandible, the stout, flat plate of the **ramus** (**ray**-mus) extends superiorly and posteriorly from the **body of the mandible** on each side (Figure 3–52). During growth of the body, the body of the mandible and alveolar process elongates posterior to the mental foramen, providing space for three additional permanent teeth. The ramus, which serves as the primary area for the attachment of the muscles of mastication, grows superior and posterior, displacing the mental protuberance of the chin inferiorly and anteriorly as one nears adulthood.

The anterior border of the ramus is a thin, sharp margin that terminates in the **coronoid process** (**kor**-ah-noid) (see Table 3–4). The main portion of the anterior border of the ramus forms a concave forward curve called the **coronoid notch.** The coronoid notch is a landmark for the administration of a local anesthetic for the inferior alveolar block (see Chapter 9). Inferior to the coronoid notch, the anterior border of the ramus becomes the **external oblique line** (ob-**leek**). The external oblique line is a crest where the ramus joins the body of the mandible.

The posterior border of the ramus is thickened and extends from the **angle of the mandible** to a projection, the **condyle of the mandible** with its neck (Figures 3–50 to 3–53). The **articulating surface of the condyle** (ar-**tik**-you-late-ing) is an oval head involved in the temporomandibular joint. Between the coronoid process and the condyle is a depression, the **mandibular notch** (man-**dib**-you-lar).

MEDIAL VIEW OF THE MANDIBLE

Visible on the internal or medial view of the mandible are the **body of the mandible, alveolar process of the mandible** (al-**ve**-o-lar) (see Table 3–4), and **ramus** (**ray**-mus) (Figure 3–54). In addition, near the midline of the mandible is a cluster of small projections called the **genial tubercles** (ji-**ni**-il) or mental spines, which is another muscle attachment area.

At the lateral edge of each mandibular alveolar process is a rounded roughened area, the **retromolar triangle** (re-tro-**moh**-lar), just posterior to the most distal molar of the mandibular dentition. The retromolar triangle is a bony landmark that when covered with soft tissue is the retromolar pad in a patient.

Along each medial surface of the body of the mandible is the **mylohyoid line** (my-lo-**hi**-oid) or mylohyoid ridge that extends posteriorly and superiorly, becoming more prominent as it ascends each body. The mylohyoid line is the point of attachment of the mylohyoid muscle that forms the floor of the mouth. The roots of the posterior mandibular teeth often extend internally below the mylohyoid line.

A shallow depression, the **sublingual fossa** (sub-**ling**-gwal), which contains the sublingual salivary gland, is located superior to the anterior portion of the mylohyoid line. Below the posterior portion of the mylohyoid line and below the posterior mandibular teeth is a deeper depression, the **submandibular fossa** (sub-man-**dib**-you-lar), which contains the submandibular salivary gland.

On the internal surface of the ramus is a central opening, the **mandibular foramen** (man-**dib**-you-lar), which is the opening of the **mandibular canal** (Figure 3–54; see Table 3–3). The inferior

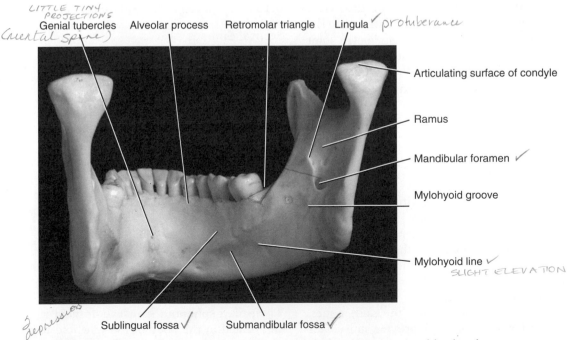

FIGURE 3–54 ■ Internal or medial view of the mandible and its associated landmarks.

alveolar nerve and blood vessels exit the mandible through the mandibular foramen after traveling in the mandibular canal. With age and tooth loss, the alveolar process is absorbed so that the mandibular canal is nearer the superior border. Sometimes with excessive alveolar process absorption, the mandibular canal disappears entirely and leaves the inferior alveolar nerve without its bony protection, although it is still covered by soft tissues.

Rarely, a patient may have a bifid inferior alveolar nerve, in which case a second mandibular foramen, more inferiorly placed, exists and can be detected by noting a doubled mandibular canal on a radiograph (see Chapter 8 for more information). It is important to keep this anatomical variant concerning the mandibular foramen in mind when administering a local anesthetic for the inferior alveolar block (see Chapter 9).

Overhanging the mandibular foramen is a bony spine, the **lingula** (ling-gul-ah), which serves as an attachment for the sphenomandibular ligament associated with the temporomandibular joint (see Chapter 5 for more information). A small groove, the **mylohyoid groove** (my-lo-**hi**-oid), passes forward and downward from the mandibular foramen. The mylohyoid nerve and blood vessels travel in the mylohyoid groove.

The **articulating surface of the condyle** (ar-**tik**-you-late-ing) can be seen in this view. This is where the mandible articulates with the temporal bone at the temporomandibular joint (see Chapter 5 for more information). Below the articular surface of the condyle on the anterior surface is a triangular depression, the **pterygoid fovea** (**teh**-ri-goid **fo**-vee-ah) (see Figure 3–52).

PARANASAL SINUSES

The **paranasal sinuses** (pare-ah-**na**-zil **sy**-nuses) are paired, air-filled cavities in bone (Figures 3–55 and 3–56). These sinuses are lined with mucous membranes. The paranasal sinuses include the frontal, sphenoid, ethmoid, and maxillary sinuses. The sinuses communicate with the nasal cavity through small ostia or openings in the lateral nasal wall.

The sinuses serve to lighten the skull bones, act as sound resonators, and provide mucus for the nasal cavity. Yet the mucous membranes of the sinuses can become inflamed and congested with mucus as in a *primary sinusitis* (sy-nu-**si**-tis). A primary sinusitis can involve allergies or an infection occurring in the sinus. The symptoms of sinusitis are headache, usually near the involved sinus, and foul-smelling nasal or pharyngeal discharge, possibly with some systemic signs of infection such as fever and weakness. The skin over the involved sinus can be tender, hot, and red due to the inflammatory process in the area.

This congestion of the sinus space with mucus can lead to blockage of the ostia, preventing normal air exchange and drainage into the nasal cavity. In extreme cases of sinusitis, surgery is performed to enlarge the ostia in the lateral walls of the nasal cavity, creating adequate drainage.

An infection in one sinus can travel through the nasal cavity to other sinuses, leading to serious complications for the patient. Since the maxillary posterior teeth are in close proximity to the maxillary sinus, this can also create clinical problems if there are any disease processes, such as an infection, in any of these teeth (discussed later and in Chapter 12). These clinical problems can include a *secondary sinusitis* (sy-nu-**si**-tis), inflammation of the sinuses from another source, such as an infection of the adjacent teeth. A *perforation* (per-fo-**ray**-shun), an abnormal hole in the wall of the sinus, also can occur with infection.

Frontal Sinuses

The paired **frontal sinuses** (**frunt**-il **sy**-nuses) are located in the frontal bone just superior to the nasal cavity (see Figures 3–23 and 3–25). These two paranasal sinuses are asymmetrical (around 2–3 centimeters in diameter), but the left and right sinuses are always separated by a septum. Each frontal sinus communicates with and drains into the nasal cavity by a constricted canal to the middle nasal meatus, the **frontonasal duct** (frunt-o-**na**-zil dukt). Standing near the patient during an extraoral examination, visually inspect and use bilateral palpation of the frontal sinuses (Figure 3–57).

Sphenoid Sinuses

The paired **sphenoid sinuses** (**sfe**-noid **sy**-nuses) are located in the body of the sphenoid bone and cannot be palpated during an extraoral examina-

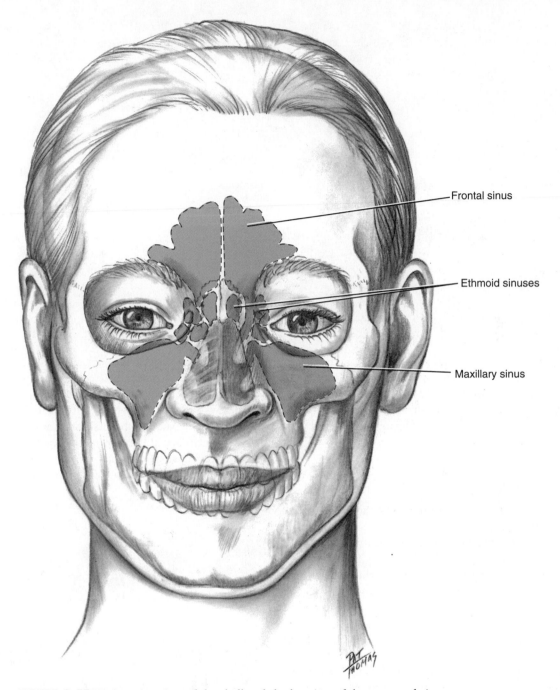

Frontal sinus

Ethmoid sinuses

Maxillary sinus

FIGURE 3–55 ■ Anterior view of the skull and the location of the paranasal sinuses.

tion (see Figure 3–33). These two paranasal sinuses are frequently asymmetrical (around 1.5–2.5 centimeters in diameter). The sphenoid sinuses communicate with and drain into the nasal cavity through an opening superior to each superior nasal concha.

Ethmoid Sinuses

The **ethmoid sinuses** (**eth**-moid **sy**-nuses) or ethmoid air cells are a variable number of small cavities in the lateral mass of the ethmoid bone and cannot be palpated during an extraoral exam-

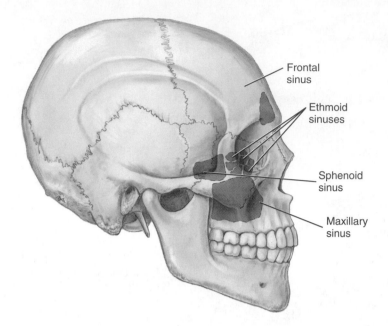

FIGURE 3–56 ■ Lateral view of the skull and the location of the paranasal sinuses.

ination (see Figure 3–37). These paranasal sinuses are roughly divided into the anterior, middle, and posterior ethmoid air cells. The posterior ethmoid air cells open into the superior meatus of the nasal cavity, and the middle and anterior ethmoid air cells open into the middle meatus.

Maxillary Sinuses

The **maxillary sinuses** (**mak**-sil-lare-ee **sy**-nuses) are paired paranasal sinuses, each located in the body of the maxilla, just posterior to the maxillary canine and premolars (see Figures 3–45 and 3–46). The size varies according to individuals and their ages. These pyramid-shaped sinuses are the largest of the paranasal sinuses, and each one has an apex, three walls, a roof, and a floor. A portion of the sinuses can be seen on radiographs of the maxillary posterior teeth. During an extraoral examination, visually inspect and use bilateral palpation of the maxillary sinuses (Figure 3–58).

The apex of the pyramid of the maxillary sinus points into the zygomatic arch, and the medial wall is formed by the lateral wall of the nasal cavity. The anterior wall corresponds to the anterior or facial wall of the maxilla, and the posterior wall is the infratemporal surface of the maxilla, the maxillary tuberosity. The roof of the maxillary sinus is the orbital floor, and the floor

is the alveolar process of each maxilla. Each maxillary sinus is divided into communicating compartments by bony walls or septa.

Because of the close proximity of the maxillary sinus to the alveolar process containing the roots of the maxillary posterior teeth, the periodontal tissues of these teeth may be in direct contact with the mucosa of the maxillary sinus. This

FIGURE 3–57 ■ Palpation of the frontal sinuses.

FIGURE 3–58 ■ Palpation of the maxillary sinuses.

close proximity can cause serious clinical problems such as secondary sinusitis and perforation during infection (see Chapter 12 for more information), extraction, or trauma related to the maxillary posterior teeth. The discomfort associated with a primary maxillary sinus infection can mimic the same discomfort with an endodontic or periodontal infection of the maxillary posterior teeth.

With age, the enlarging maxillary sinus may surround the roots of the maxillary posterior teeth and extend its margins into the body of the zygoma. If the maxillary posterior teeth are lost, the maxillary sinus may expand even more, thin-

ning the bony floor of the alveolar process, so that only a thin shell of bone is present.

The maxillary sinus drains into the middle meatus on each side. Drainage of the maxillary sinus is complicated and may promote a prolonged or chronic sinusitis because the ostium of each sinus is higher than the floor of the sinus cavity. Surgery may need to be performed in the case of chronic maxillary sinusitis.

FOSSAE OF THE SKULL

Three deeper depressions or *fossae* are present on the external surface of the skull. The bony boundaries for these paired fossae, the temporal, infratemporal, and pterygopalatine fossae, should be located on the skull model and skull diagrams (Table 3–6). These fossae are important landmarks of the skull for locating muscles, blood vessels, and nerves (Table 3–7).

Temporal Fossa

The **temporal fossa** (**tem**-poh-ral) is a flat, fan-shaped depression on the lateral surface of the skull (Figure 3–59; see also Figure 3–13). The temporal fossa is formed by parts of five bones: the zygomatic, frontal, greater wing of the sphenoid, temporal, and parietal bones.

The boundaries of the temporal fossa are: superiorly and posteriorly, the inferior temporal

Table 3–6	BOUNDARIES OF FOSSAE OF THE SKULL		
Boundaries of Fossae	**Temporal Fossa**	**Infratemporal Fossa**	**Pterygopalatine Fossa**
Superior	Inferior temporal line	Greater wing of sphenoid bone	Inferior surface of sphenoid bone body
Anterior	Frontal process of zygomatic bone	Maxillary tuberosity	Maxillary tuberosity
Medial	Surface of temporal bone	Lateral pterygoid plate	Vertical plate of palatine bone
Lateral	Zygomatic arch	Mandibular ramus and zygomatic arch	Pterygomaxillary fissure
Inferior	Infratemporal crest of sphenoid bone	No bony border	Pterygopalatine canal
Posterior	Inferior temporal line	No bony border	Pterygoid process of sphenoid bone

Table 3–7 MUSCLES, BLOOD VESSELS, AND NERVES OF FOSSAE OF THE SKULL

	Temporal Fossa	Infratemporal Fossa	Pterygopalatine Fossa
Muscles	Temporalis muscle	Pterygoid muscles	
Blood vessels	Area blood vessels	Pterygoid plexus and maxillary artery (second part) and branches, including middle meningeal artery, inferior alveolar artery, and posterior superior alveolar artery	Maxillary artery (third part) and branches, including infraorbital and sphenopalatine arteries
Nerves	Area nerves	Mandibular nerve, including inferior alveolar and lingual nerves	Pterygopalatine ganglion and maxillary nerve

line; anteriorly, the frontal process of the zygomatic bone; medially, the surface of the temporal bone; and laterally, the zygomatic arch. Inferiorly, the boundary between the temporal fossa and the infratemporal fossa is the infratemporal crest on the greater wing of the sphenoid bone.

The temporal fossa includes a narrow strip of the parietal bone, the squamous portion of the temporal bone, the temporal surface of the frontal bone, and the temporal surface of the greater wing of the sphenoid bone. The temporal fossa contains the body of the temporalis muscle and area blood vessels and nerves.

Infratemporal Fossa

The **infratemporal fossa** (in-frah-**tem**-poh-ral) is a paired depression that is inferior to the anterior part of the temporal fossa (see Figure 3–59). The temporal fossa and infratemporal fossa are divided by the infratemporal crest on the greater wing of the sphenoid bone. The infratemporal fossa can also be viewed from the inferior aspect of the skull model after temporarily removing the mandible (Figure 3–60).

The boundaries of the infratemporal fossa include: superiorly, the greater wing of the sphe-

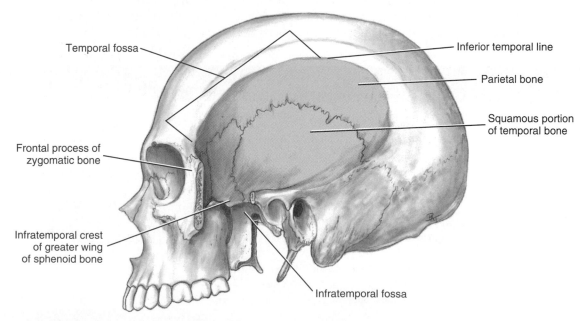

FIGURE 3–59 ■ Lateral view of the skull and the temporal fossa and its boundaries (with portions of the zygomatic and temporal bones removed).

Maxillary tuberosity

Infratemporal crest
of greater wing
of sphenoid bone

Infratemporal fossa

Inferior orbital fissure

Zygomatic arch

Lateral pterygoid
plate of
sphenoid bone

Foramen ovale

Foramen spinosum

FIGURE 3–60 ■ Inferior view of the skull (with the mandible removed) and the infratemporal fossae and boundaries.

noid bone; anteriorly, the maxillary tuberosity; medially, the lateral pterygoid plate; and laterally, the ramus of the mandible and zygomatic arch. There is no bony inferior or posterior boundary.

Many structures pass from the infratemporal fossa into the orbit through the inferior orbital fissure, which is located at the anterior, superior end of the fossa. Other structures pass into the infratemporal fossa from the cranial cavity.

The infratemporal fossa contains the mandibular division of the fifth cranial or trigeminal nerve (including the inferior alveolar and lingual nerves), which enters by way of the foramen ovale (see Table 3–3). The fossa also contains the pterygoid plexus and the pterygoid muscles.

The maxillary artery and its branches are also located here, including the middle meningeal artery, which goes into the cranial cavity through the foramen spinosum, the inferior alveolar artery which enters the mandible through the mandibular foramen, and the posterior alveolar artery which enters the maxilla through the posterior superior alveolar foramina (see Table 3–3).

Pterygopalatine Fossa

The **pterygopalatine fossa** (**teh**-ri-go-**pal**-ah-tine) is a cone-shaped depression, deep to the infratemporal fossa (Figure 3–61). This small but

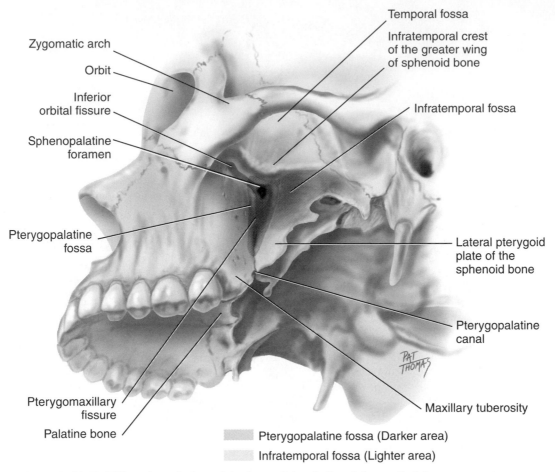

Zygomatic arch

Orbit

Inferior
orbital fissure

Sphenopalatine
foramen

Pterygopalatine
fossa

Pterygomaxillary
fissure

Palatine bone

Temporal fossa

Infratemporal crest
of the greater wing
of sphenoid bone

Infratemporal fossa

Lateral pterygoid
plate of the
sphenoid bone

Pterygopalatine
canal

Maxillary tuberosity

Pterygopalatine fossa (Darker area)

Infratemporal fossa (Lighter area)

FIGURE 3–61 ■ Oblique lateral view of the base of the skull and the roof of the pterygopalatine fossa and its boundaries.

important fossa is located between the pterygoid process and the maxillary tuberosity, close to the apex of the orbit.

The boundaries of the pterygopalatine fossa are: superiorly, the inferior surface of the body of the sphenoid bone; anteriorly, the maxillary tuberosity; medially, the vertical plate of the palatine bone; laterally, the pterygomaxillary fissure; inferiorly, the pterygopalatine canal; and posteriorly, the pterygoid process of the sphenoid bone.

The pterygopalatine fossa contains the maxillary artery and nerve and their branches arising here, including the infraorbital and sphenopalatine arteries, the maxillary division of the trigeminal or fifth cranial nerve and branches, and the pterygopalatine ganglion (see Table 3–3). The

foramen rotundum is the entrance route for the maxillary nerve. A second foramen, the pterygoid canal, in the pterygoid process, transmits autonomic fibers to the ganglion. The pterygopalatine canal connects with the greater and lesser palatine foramina of the palatine bones of the hard palate.

BONES OF THE NECK

Cervical Vertebrae

The **cervical vertebrae** (ser-vi-kal ver-teh-bray) are located in the vertebral column between the skull and the thoracic vertebrae. There are seven cervical vertebrae. All vertebrae have a central

FIGURE 3–62 ■ Posterior view of the skull and the first and second cervical vertebrae.

Occipital bone
Occipital condyles
Atlas (first cervical vertebra)
Axis (second cervical vertebra)

vertebral foramen (**ver**-teh-brahl) for the spinal cord and associated tissues. In contrast to other vertebrae, the cervical vertebrae are characterized by the presence of a **transverse foramen** in the **transverse process** on each side of the vertebral foramen. The vertebral artery runs through these transverse foramina.

Damage to any of the vertebrae can affect dental treatment as the patient may experience a range of problems, from difficulty in movement to paralysis. Only the first two cervical vertebrae will be described because their anatomy is unusual and they are located near the skull.

FIRST CERVICAL VERTEBRA

The first cervical vertebra or **atlas** (**at**-lis) articulates with the skull at the occipital condyles of the occipital bone (Figure 3–62). The atlas has the form of an irregular ring consisting of two **lateral masses** (masez) connected by a short **anterior arch** and a longer **posterior arch** (Figure 3–63). This cervical bone lacks a body and a spine.

The lateral masses can be effectively palpated by placing fingers between the two mastoid processes and the angles of the mandible. More medially, the lateral masses present large concave

superior articular processes (ar-**tik**-you-lar) for the corresponding occipital condyles of the skull. The lateral masses also have circular **inferior articular processes** for articulation with the second cervical vertebra.

SECOND CERVICAL VERTEBRA

The second cervical vertebra or **axis** (**ak**-sis) is characterized by the **dens** (denz) or odontoid process (Figure 3–64). The dens articulates anteriorly with the anterior arch of the first cervical vertebra (Figure 3–65). The body of the axis is inferior to the dens. The spine of the axis is located posterior to the body. The body and the adjoining transverse process present **superior articular processes** (ar-**tik**-you-lar) for an additional articulation with the inferior articulating surfaces of the atlas. The inferior aspect of the axis presents **inferior articular processes** for articulating with the articular processes of the third cervical vertebra.

Hyoid Bone

The **hyoid bone** (**hi**-oid) is suspended in the neck. It forms the base of the tongue and larynx. Many muscles attach to the hyoid bone (see Chapter 4 for more information). The hyoid bone is superior

Superior articular process
Transverse foramen
Transverse process
Vertebral foramen
Anterior arch
Lateral mass
Posterior arch

FIGURE 3–63 ■ Superior view of the first cervical vertebra, the atlas.

Dens

Body

Superior articular process

Transverse foramen

Transverse process

Vertebral foramen

Inferior articular process

Spine

FIGURE 3–64 ■ Posterosuperior view of the second cervical vertebra, the axis.

and anterior to the thyroid cartilage of the larynx. This bone is typically at the level of the third cervical vertebra but is raised during swallowing and other activities. The hyoid bone can be effectively palpated by feeling below and medial to the angles of the mandible. Do not confuse the hyoid bone with the thyroid cartilage (the 'Adam's apple').

The hyoid bone does not articulate with any other bones, giving it its characteristic mobility, which is needed for mastication, swallowing, and speech. This bone is horizontally suspended from the end of the styloid process by the stylohyoid ligament and is connected by the broad thyrohyoid membrane with the thyroid cartilage (see Chapter 4 for more information).

The U-shaped hyoid bone consists of five parts as seen from an anterior view (Figure 3–65). The anterior portion is the midline **body of the hyoid bone.** There is also a pair of projections on each side of the hyoid bone, the **greater cornu** and **lesser cornu.** These horns serve as attachments for muscles and ligaments.

ABNORMALITIES OF BONE

Abnormalities of bone can include bony enlargements and fractures that may heal with abnormal contours. The dental professional needs to record any abnormal areas of bone and make any appropriate referrals. It is important to remember that since many bones of the face are shared by two or more soft tissue components of the face, an abnormality of one facial bone often involves many soft tissue components. A fracture of the frontal bone may clinically involve both the forehead and the eyes.

Bony enlargements can lead to facial asymmetry (Figure 3–66) or nodular intraoral areas (Figure 3–67). Some, such as palatal or mandibular tori, are normal variations, but others can be due to endocrine diseases, causing abnormal bone growth. Bone can also enlarge with tumorous growth of bone or other tissues, such as dental tissues, as in the case of an ameloblastoma.

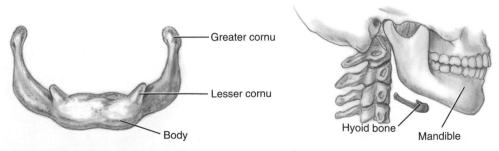

Greater cornu

Lesser cornu

Body

Hyoid bone

Mandible

FIGURE 3–65 ■ Anterior view of the hyoid bone with its location demonstrated on a lateral view of the lower skull and the upper vertebral bones.

FIGURE 3–67 ■ Nodular bony enlargements may occur in the oral cavity, such as in this case of a palatal torus, a benign growth of bone.

FIGURE 3–66 ■ Bony enlargements may lead to facial asymmetry, such as in this patient with an ameloblastoma, a tumor of dental tissues in the mandible.

Bone may also fracture with severe blows to the face. Fractures of the facial skeleton tend to occur at its points of buttress with the cranium. These buttress points include the medial aspect of the orbit, articulation of the zygoma with the frontal and temporal bones, articulation of the pterygoid plates, and the palatine bones and maxillae. If the fracture is bilateral, the entire facial skeleton can be pushed posteriorly, resulting in upper respiratory tract obstruction. These fractures may heal poorly and result in abnormal bony contours.

IDENTIFICATION EXERCISES

Identify the structures on the following diagrams by filling in the blanks with the correct anatomical term. You can check your answers by looking back at the figure indicated in parentheses for each identification diagram.

1. (Figure 3–4)

NASAL BONE

LACRIMAL BONE

ZYGOMATIC BONE

INFERIOR NASAL CONCHA

VOMER

MAXILLA

MANDIBLE

2. (Figure 3–7)

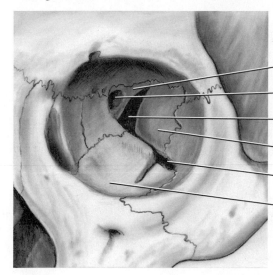

lesser wing of sphenoid bone

optic canal

superior orbital fissure

greater wing of sphenoid bone

inferior orbital fissure

maxilla

3. (Figure 3–20)

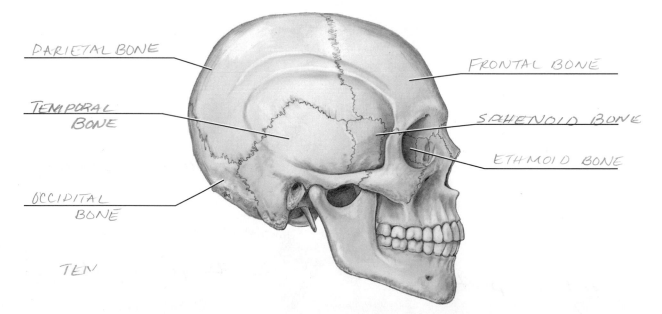

PARIETAL BONE

TEMPORAL BONE

OCCIPITAL BONE

TEN

FRONTAL BONE

SPHENOID BONE

ETHMOID BONE

4. (Figure 3–22)

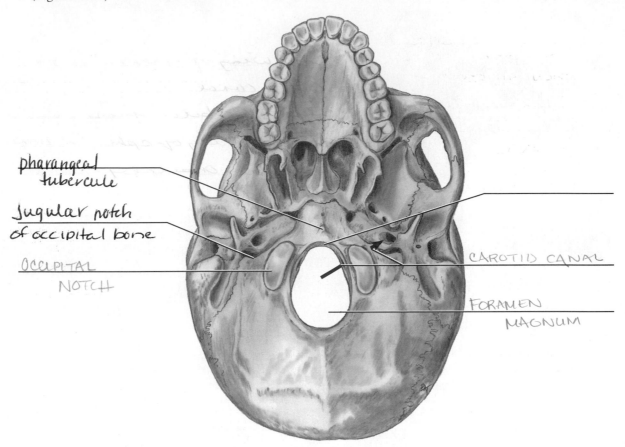

pharangeal
tubercule

Jugular notch
of occipital bone

OCCIPITAL
NOTCH

CAROTID CANAL

FORAMEN
MAGNUM

5. (Figure 3–28)

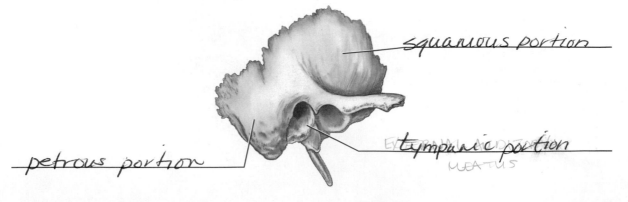

squamous portion

petrous portion

tympanic portion

EXTERNAL
MEATUS

6. (Figure 3–32)

PTERYGOID PROCESS

MEDIAL PTERYGOID PLATES

PTERYGOID FOSSA

LATERAL PTERYGOID PLATE

FRONTAL BONE

ZYGOMATIC BONE

MAXILLA

Palatine bone

VOMER

GREATER OR GREAT WINGS WINGS

FORAMEN SPINOSUM

Spine of Sphenoid

MASTOID PROCESS

OCCIPITAL BONE

7. (Figure 3–33)

Sphenoid Sinuses

SUPERIOR ORBITAL FISSURE

FORAMEN ROTUNDUM

FORAMEN OVALAE

FORAMEN SPINOSUM

ETHMOID BONE OR CRISTA GALLI

FRONTAL BONE

LESSER WINGS

GREATER WINGS

BODY

OCCIPITAL

TEMPORAL

PARIETAL

8. (Figure 3–35)

FRONTAL BONE

LACRIMAL BONE

ZYGOMATIC BONE

MAXILLARY BONE

Orb. plate

mid nasal concha

ETHMOID BONE

perp. plate

Vomer

NASAL SEPTUM

9. (Figure 3–38)

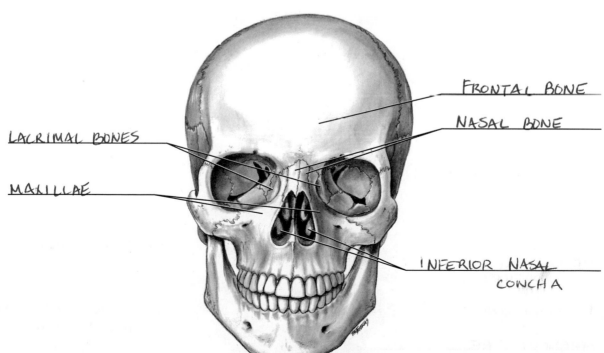

CRISTA GALLI

CRIBIFORM PLATE

NASAL BONE

SUP. NASAL CONCHA

MIDDLE NASAL CONCHA

SPHENOID BONE

INF. NASAL CONCHA

PALATINE BONE

MAXILLA

MEDIAL PTERYGOID
PLATE

10. (Figure 3–40)

FRONTAL BONE

NASAL BONE

LACRIMAL BONES

MAXILLAE

INFERIOR NASAL
CONCHA

11. (Figure 3–42)

ZYGO PROCESS OF FRONTAL BONE

FRONTAL OF ZYGOMATIC

INFRAORBITAL RIM

MAX. PROCESS OF ZYGOMATIC BONE

ZYGOMATIC PROCESS OF MAX. BONE

Zygo process of Temporal

TEMPORAL PROCESS OF ZYGO

ZYGOMATIC ARCH

12. (Figure 3–44)

MAXILLARY BONE

MEDIAL PALATINE SUTURE

PALATINE BONE'S

SPHENOID BONE

GREATER PALATINE FORAMEN

LESSER PALATINE FORAMEN

13. (Figure 3–45)

ETHMOID BONE

LACRIMAL BONE

Frontal process of Max

infraorbital foramen
body of maxilla
vomer
alveolar process
of maxilla

Frontal Bone

Nasal Bone

Infraorbital Sulcus

Inferior Nalsal Concha

Zygo. process of Max.

Loc. of Max sinus

Canine fossa

14. (Figure 3–47)

Frontal process of max.

Nasal bone

Infraorbital foramen

Zygo. process of max

Canine fossa
Canine eminence

lacrimal bone
ethmoid bone

infraorbital sulcus

sphenoid bone

15. (Figures 3–52, 3–55)

16. (Figure 3–60)

17. (Figure 3–62)

18. (Figure 3–65)

hyoid bone

REVIEW QUESTIONS

1. Which of the following features is located on the temporal bone?
   A. Superior temporal line
   B. Foramen rotundum
   C. External acoustic meatus
   D. Cribriform plate
   E. Orbital plate

2. The area immediately posterior to the most distal tooth in the upper arch is called the
   A. Retromolar triangle
   B. Postglenoid process
   C. Cribriform plate
   D. Maxillary tuberosity
   E. Hamular process

3. In addition to the zygomatic bone, which of the following bones has a process that forms the zygomatic arch?
   A. Temporal bone
   B. Maxilla
   C. Sphenoid bone
   D. Palatine bone

4. Which of the following is the name of the articulation of the parietal bones and the occipital bone?
   A. Coronal suture
   B. Squamosal suture
   C. Sagittal suture
   D. Lambdoidal suture

5. Which of the following bony landmarks form an articulation?
   A. Occipital condyles with the atlas
   B. Occipital condyles with the axis
   C. Mandibular fossa with the coronoid notch
   D. Mandibular fossa with the coronoid process

6. Which of the following features is located on the lateral surface of the mandible?
   A. Lingula
   B. Submandibular fossa
   C. Genial tubercles
   D. External oblique line
   E. Mandibular foramen

7. The orbital apex is composed of the lesser wing of the sphenoid bone and the
   A. Ethmoid bone
   B. Frontal bone
   C. Maxilla
   D. Palatine bone
   E. Lacrimal bone

8. Which of the following landmarks is formed by the maxillae?
   A. Mental spine
   B. Median palatine suture
   C. Retromolar triangle
   D. Hamulus
   E. Inferior orbital fissure

9. Which of the following is located in the infratemporal fossa?
   A. Masseter muscle
   B. Pterygopalatine ganglion
   C. Posterior superior alveolar artery
   D. Maxillary division of the fifth cranial nerve

10. The concavity on the anterior border of the coronoid process of the ramus is called the
    A. Mandibular notch
    B. Coronoid notch
    C. Temporal fossa
    D. Infratemporal fossa

11. Which of the following landmarks serves to help locate the hyoid bone?
    A. Level of the first cervical vertebra
    B. Superior and anterior to the thyroid cartilage
    C. Articulation with the cartilage of the larynx
    D. Inferior and posterior to the Adam's apple

12. Which of the following forms the floor of each maxillary sinus?
    A. Alveolar process of the maxilla
    B. Facial wall of the maxilla
    C. Infratemporal surface of the maxilla
    D. Lateral wall of the nasal cavity

13. Which of the following processes is located just inferior and medial to the external acoustic meatus?
    A. Pterygoid process
    B. Styloid process
    C. Mastoid process
    D. Hamulus

14. The spaces under the three conchae of the lateral walls of the nasal cavity are called
    A. Ostia
    B. Ducts
    C. Meatus
    D. Inferior nasal conchae
    E. Vestibules

15. Which of the following bones and their processes form the hard palate?
    A. Maxillary processes of the maxillae and the horizontal plates of the palatine bones
    B. Palatal processes of the maxillae and the maxillary plates of the palatine bones
    C. Horizontal plates of the palatine bones and the palatine processes of the maxillae
    D. Maxillary plates of the palatine bones and the horizontal processes of the maxillae

16. Which of the following nerves is associated with the stylomastoid foramen?
    A. Fifth cranial nerve
    B. Seventh cranial nerve
    C. Ninth cranial nerve
    D. Tenth cranial nerve
    E. Eleventh cranial nerve

17. Which of the following bones of the skull is paired?
    A. Sphenoid bone
    B. Ethmoid bone
    C. Occipital bone
    D. Vomer
    E. Parietal bone

18. Which of the following plates is perforated to allow the passage of the olfactory nerves for the sense of smell?
    A. Medial plate of the sphenoid bone
    B. Lateral plate of the sphenoid bone
    C. Perpendicular plate of the ethmoid bone
    D. Cribriform plate of the ethmoid bone

19. Which of the following bones of the skull is considered a cranial bone?
    A. Vomer
    B. Maxilla
    C. Sphenoid bone
    D. Zygomatic bone
    E. Mandible

20. In which portion of the temporal bone is the temporomandibular joint located?
    A. Squamous portion
    B. Tympanic portion
    C. Petrous portion
    D. Mastoid portion

21. Which is a single bone located at the midline of the skull?
    A. Temporal
    B. Zygomatic
    C. Sphenoid
    D. Inferior nasal conchae

22. Which of the following is a normal, short, windowlike opening in bone?
    A. Fossa
    B. Foramen
    C. Fissure
    D. Perforation

23. Which of the following bones helps form the jugular foramen along with the jugular notch of the temporal bone?
    A. Occipital
    B. Mandible
    C. Parietal
    D. Sphenoid

24. Which of the following is a faint ridge noted where the right and left mandibular processes fused together in early childhood?
    A. Mylohyoid line
    B. Mental protuberance
    C. Mandibular symphysis
    D. External oblique line

25. In which bone are the infraorbital foramen and canal located?
    A. Frontal
    B. Maxilla
    C. Sphenoid
    D. Zygomatic

REVIEW ACTIVITIES

1. Standing in front of a mirror, point out the bones of the skull that you can locate, such as the frontal and temporal bones.

2. Holding a skull, locate the bones of the head, such as the sphenoid and vomer.

3. Point out the bones of the skull that you can locate in a patient (or peer) who is lying in a dental chair or on a couch so that the person can see them in a hand mirror.

4. Point out on a skull the bones that form the orbit, such as the ethmoid and lacrimal bones.

5. Point out on a skull the bones that form the zygomatic arch and palate.

6. Point out on a skull the foramina and associated structures on the inferior view of the external and internal skull surfaces.

7. Point out on a skull the landmarks of the external and internal surfaces of the maxilla and mandible.

8. Standing in front of a mirror looking at your face, point out the surface landmarks of the maxilla and mandible, as well as the location of the paranasal sinuses.

9. Point out on a skull the location of the three fossae, using a dental probe or tongue depressor.

10. Standing in front of a mirror that shows your neck, point out the hyoid bone.

Muscles

CHAPTER OUTLINE

This chapter discusses the following topics:

I. Muscular System
II. Muscles of the Head and Neck
   A. Cervical Muscles
   B. Muscles of Facial Expression
   C. Muscles of Mastication
   D. Hyoid Muscles
   E. Muscles of the Tongue
   F. Muscles of the Pharynx

LEARNING OBJECTIVES

After studying this chapter, the reader should be able to:

1. Define and pronounce all the key words and anatomical terms in this chapter.
2. Locate and identify the muscles of the head and neck on a diagram, a skull, and a patient.
3. Describe the origin, insertion, and action of the muscles of the head and neck.
4. State the nerve(s) innervating each of the muscles of the head and neck.
5. Discuss the processes of mastication, speech, and swallowing in regard to anatomical considerations.
6. Correctly complete the identification exercises and review questions and activities for this chapter.
7. Integrate the knowledge about the muscles of the head and neck into the clinical practice of patient examination and related muscular diseases.

KEY WORDS

Action (**ak**-shun) Movement accomplished by a muscle when the muscle fibers contract.

Facial paralysis (pah-**ral**-i-sis) Loss of action of the facial muscles.

Insertion (in-**sir**-shun) End of the muscle that is attached to the more movable structure.

Muscle (**mus**-il) Type of body tissue that shortens under neural control, causing soft tissue and bony structures to move.

Origin (**or**-i-jin) End of the muscle that is attached to the least movable structure.

MUSCULAR SYSTEM

A *muscle* (**mus**-il) in the muscular system shortens under neural control, causing soft tissue and bony structures of the body to move. Each muscle has two ends attached to these structures, and they are categorized according to their role in movement. The *origin* (**or**-i-jin) is the end of the muscle that is attached to the least movable structure. The *insertion* (in-**sir**-shun) is the other end of the muscle and is attached to the more movable structure.

Generally, the insertion of the muscle moves toward the origin when the muscle is contracted. The movement that is accomplished when the muscle fibers contract is the *action* (**ak**-shun) of the muscle. The muscles have specific innervation that is discussed in this chapter, but a more thorough explanation of the nervous system can be found in Chapter 8. The blood supply to the muscular area is discussed in Chapter 6. It is important to remember that unlike innervation to the muscles, which is a one-to-one relationship, arterial supply is regional. Arteries supply all structures in their vicinity, and muscles receive blood from all close-by arteries.

MUSCLES OF THE HEAD AND NECK

The dental professional needs to determine the location and action of many muscles of the head and neck in order to perform a thorough patient examination. This information is important since the placement of many other structures, such as bones, blood vessels, nerves, and lymph nodes, is related to the location of the muscles. The muscles may also malfunction and be involved in temporomandibular joint disorders, occlusal dysfunction, and certain nervous system diseases. Muscles of the head and neck and their attachments also are a consideration in the spread of dental infections (see Chapter 12 for more information).

The muscles of the head and neck are divided into seven main groups: the cervical muscles, muscles of facial expression, muscles of mastication, hyoid muscles, muscles of the tongue, muscles of the soft palate, and muscles of the pharynx. There are also muscle groups to the ears, eyes, and nose that are not included in this chapter.

CERVICAL MUSCLES

The two **cervical muscles** (ser-vi-kal) considered in this text are both superficial and easily palpated on the neck. These cervical muscles are the sternocleidomastoid and trapezius muscles.

Sternocleidomastoid Muscle

One of the largest and most superficial cervical muscles is the paired **sternocleidomastoid muscle (SCM)** (stir-no-klii-do-**mass**-toid), or sternomastoid muscle. The SCM is thick and serves as a primary muscular landmark of the neck during an extraoral examination of a patient. The SCM is effectively palpated when the patient moves the head to the side (Figure 4–1). The SCM divides the neck region into anterior and posterior cervical triangles (see Chapter 2).

Sternocleidomastoid muscle

FIGURE 4–1 ■ Palpating the sternocleidomastoid muscle of a patient by having the patient turn the head to the opposite side (muscle highlighted).

FIGURE 4–2 ■ Origin and insertion of the sternocleidomastoid muscle.

External acoustic meatus

Mastoid process of temporal bone

Sternocleidomastoid muscle

Clavicle

Sternum

ORIGIN AND INSERTION. The SCM originates from the medial portion of the clavicle and the sternum's superior and lateral surfaces and passes posteriorly and superiorly to insert on the mastoid process of the temporal bone (Figure 4–2). This insertion is just posterior and inferior to the external acoustic meatus of each ear.

ACTION. If one SCM contracts, the head and neck bend to the same side, and the face and front of the neck rotate to the opposite side. If both muscles contract, the head will flex at the neck and extend at the junction between the neck and skull.

INNERVATION. The SCM is innervated by the eleventh cranial or accessory nerve.

Trapezius Muscle

The other important superficial cervical muscle is the paired **trapezius muscle** (trah-**pee**-zee-us), which covers the lateral and posterior surfaces of the neck. The trapezius muscle is a broad, flat, triangular muscle.

ORIGIN AND INSERTION. The trapezius muscle originates from the external surface of the occipi-

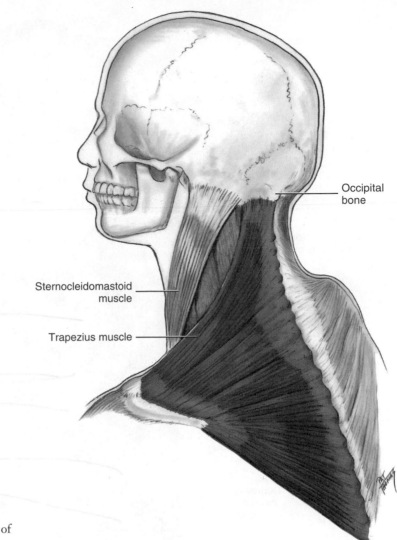

Occipital
bone

Sternocleidomastoid
muscle

Trapezius muscle

FIGURE 4–3 ■ Origin and insertion of
the trapezius muscle.

tal bone and the posterior midline of the cervical
and thoracic regions. This muscle inserts on
the lateral third of the clavicle and parts of the
scapula (Figure 4–3).

ACTION. The cervical fibers of the trapezius
muscle act to lift the clavicle and scapula, as when
the shoulders are shrugged.

INNERVATION. The trapezius muscle is innervated by the eleventh cranial or accessory nerve
and the third and fourth cervical nerves.

MUSCLES OF FACIAL EXPRESSION

The **muscles of facial expression** are paired
muscles in the superficial fascia of the facial tis-

sues (Figures 4 4 and 4–5). All the muscles of
facial expression originate from bone (rarely the
fascia) and insert on skin tissue. These muscles
also cause wrinkles at right angles to the muscle's
action line. Again, the use of your mirror image
as various facial expressions are made is very
helpful in learning about these muscles. It is true
that smiling is easier than frowning, as our
grandmothers would say. It does take only 17
muscles to smile, but it takes a lot of extra effort
by your facial muscles (43, to be exact) to frown.

ORIGIN AND INSERTION. The locations of the
muscles of facial expression are varied. These
muscles may be further grouped according to
whether they are situated in the scalp, eye, or
mouth region. The specific origin and insertion

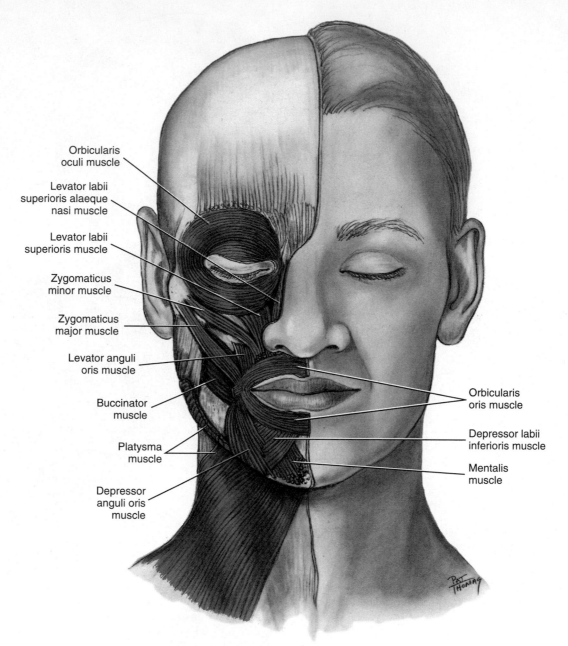

Orbicularis
oculi muscle

Levator labii
superioris alaeque
nasi muscle

Levator labii
superioris muscle

Zygomaticus
minor muscle

Zygomaticus
major muscle

Levator anguli
oris muscle

Buccinator
muscle

Platysma
muscle

Depressor
anguli oris
muscle

Orbicularis
oris muscle

Depressor labii
inferioris muscle

Mentalis
muscle

FIGURE 4–4 ■ Frontal view of most of the muscles of facial expression.

of each muscle of facial expression are listed in Table 4–1.

ACTION. During facial expression, the muscles of facial expression all act in various combinations, similar to the muscles of mastication, to vary the appearance of the face (Table 4–2). An inability to form facial expressions on one side of the face may be the first sign of damage to the nerve of these muscles.

INNERVATION. All the muscles of facial expression are innervated by the seventh cranial or facial nerve, each nerve serving one side of the face. Damage to the facial nerve results in *facial paralysis* (pah-**ral**-i-sis) of facial expression on the involved side (Figure 4–6). Paralysis is the loss of voluntary muscle action. The facial nerve can become damaged permanently or temporarily (see Chapter 8 for more information). This

Corrugator
supercilii muscle

Orbicularis
oculi muscle

Levator labii
superioris alaeque
nasi muscle

Levator labii
superioris muscle

Zygomaticus
minor muscle

Levator anguli
oris muscle

Zygomaticus
major muscle

Orbicularis
oris muscle

Risorius muscle

Depressor labii
inferioris muscle

Mentalis muscle

Depressor anguli
oris muscle

Platysma muscle

FIGURE 4–5 ■ Lateral view of most of the muscles of facial expression.

damage can occur with a stroke (cerebrovascular accident), Bell's palsy, and parotid salivary gland cancer (malignant neoplasm) since the facial nerve travels through the gland. The gland can also be damaged permanently by surgery or temporarily by trauma, as with an incorrectly given inferior alveolar local anesthetic block (see Chapter 9). These situations of paralysis not only inhibit facial expression but also seriously impair the patient's ability to speak, either permanently or temporarily.

Muscles of Facial Expression in the Scalp Region

EPICRANIAL MUSCLE

The **epicranial muscle** (ep-ee-**kray**-nee-al) or epicranius is a muscle of facial expression located in the scalp region. This muscle has two bellies, the frontal and occipital bellies. The bellies are separated by a large, spread-out scalpal tendon. This muscle and its tendon are one of the layers that form the scalp.

Table 4–1   ORIGIN AND INSERTION OF THE MUSCLES OF FACIAL EXPRESSION

Muscles	Origin	Insertion
Epicranial	Frontal belly: epicranial aponeurosis	Frontal belly: eyebrow and root of nose
	Occipital belly: occipital and temporal bone	Occipital belly: epicranial aponeurosis
Orbicularis oculi	Orbital rim, frontal and maxillary bones	Lateral region of eye, some encircle eye
Corrugator supercilii	Frontal bone	Eyebrow
Orbicularis oris	Encircle mouth	Angle of mouth
Buccinator	Maxilla, mandible, and pterygomandibular raphe	Angle of mouth
Risorius	Fascia superficial to masseter muscle	Angle of mouth
Levator labii superioris	Maxilla	Upper lip
Levator labii superioris alaeque nasi	Maxilla	Ala of nose and upper lip
Zygomaticus major	Zygomatic bone	Angle of mouth
Zygomaticus minor	Zygomatic bone	Upper lip
Levator anguli oris	Maxilla	Angle of mouth
Depressor anguli oris	Mandible	Angle of mouth
Depressor labii inferioris	Mandible	Lower lip
Mentalis	Mandible	Chin
Platysma	Clavicle and shoulder	Mandible and muscles of mouth

Table 4–2   MUSCLES OF FACIAL EXPRESSION AND THEIR ASSOCIATED FACIAL EXPRESSIONS

Muscles	Facial Expression
Epicranial	Surprise
Orbicularis oculi	Closing eyelid
Corrugator supercilii	Frowning
Orbicularis oris	Closing or pursing lips
Buccinator	Chewing
Risorius	Smiling widely
Levator labii superioris	Raising upper lip
Levator labii superioris alaeque nasi	Raising upper lip and dilating nostrils in a sneer
Zygomaticus major	Smiling
Zygomaticus minor	Raising upper lip
Levator anguli oris	Smiling
Depressor anguli oris	Frowning
Depressor labii inferioris	Lowering lower lip
Mentalis	Raising chin and protruding lower lip
Platysma	Grimacing

ORIGIN AND INSERTION. The frontal belly arises from the **epicranial aponeurosis** (ap-o-new-**row**-sis) or galea aponeurotica, a scalpal tendon (Figure 4–7). The epicranial aponeurosis is located over the area where the parietal and occipital bones meet, the most superior portion of the skull. The frontal belly then inserts into the skin tissue of the eyebrow and root of the nose. The occipital belly originates from the occipital bone and mastoid process of the temporal bone and then inserts in the epicranial aponeurosis.

ACTION. The epicranial muscle raises the eyebrows and scalp, as when a person shows surprise (Figure 4–8).

Muscles of Facial Expression in the Eye Region

The muscles of facial expression in the eye region include the orbicularis oculi and corrugator supercilii muscles (Figure 4–9).

ORBICULARIS OCULI MUSCLE
The **orbicularis oculi muscle** (or-bik-you-**laa**-

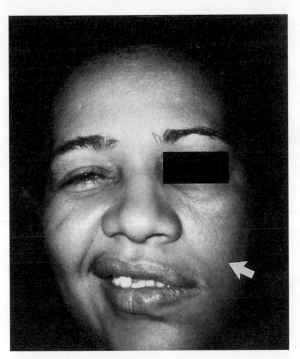

FIGURE 4–6 ■ Patient trying to smile with unilateral paralysis of the facial muscles due to muscle damage. Patient is unable to show facial expression on that side *(arrow)*.

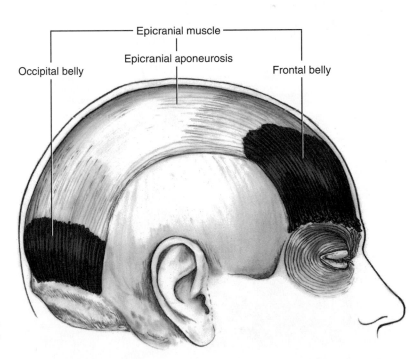

Epicranial muscle

Epicranial aponeurosis

Occipital belly

Frontal belly

FIGURE 4–7 ■ Origin and insertion of the frontal belly and occipital belly of the epicranial muscle.

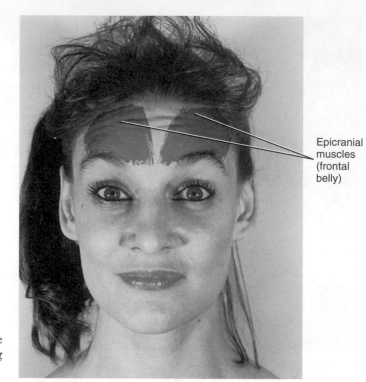

Epicranial muscles (frontal belly)

FIGURE 4–8 ■ Facial expression of surprise on a patient using the epicranial muscle, raising the eyebrows and scalp (muscle highlighted).

Corrugator supercilii muscle

Orbicularis oculi muscle (superior portion cut)

FIGURE 4–9 ■ Orbicularis oculi muscle and corrugator supercilii muscle.

ris **oc**-yule-eye) is a muscle of facial expression that encircles the eye.

ORIGIN AND INSERTION. The orbicularis oculi muscle originates on the orbital rim, nasal process of the frontal bone, and frontal process of the maxilla. Most of the fibers insert in the skin tissue at the lateral region of the eye, although some of the inner fibers completely encircle the eye.

ACTION. The orbicularis oculi muscle closes the eyelid. If all the fibers are active, the eye can be squinted, and wrinkles form in the lateral portions of the eye ('crow's feet').

CORRUGATOR SUPERCILII MUSCLE

The **corrugator supercilii muscle** (cor-rew-**gay**-tor soo-per-**sili**-eye) is a muscle of facial expression in the eye region, deep to the superior portion of the orbicularis oculi muscle.

ORIGIN AND INSERTION. The corrugator supercilii muscle originates on the frontal bone in the supraorbital region. The muscle then passes superiorly and laterally to insert in the skin tissue of the eyebrow.

ACTION. The corrugator supercilii muscle draws the skin tissue of the eyebrow medially and inferiorly toward the nose. This movement causes vertical wrinkles in the forehead, as when a person frowns (see Figure 4–14B).

Muscles of Facial Expression in the Mouth Region

The muscles of facial expression in the mouth region include the orbicularis oris, buccinator, risorius, levator labii superioris, levator labii superioris alaeque nasi, zygomaticus major, zygomaticus minor, levator anguli oris, depressor anguli oris, depressor labii inferioris, mentalis, and platysma muscles.

ORBICULARIS ORIS MUSCLE

The **orbicularis oris muscle** (or-bik-you-**laa**-ris **or**-is) is an important muscle of facial expression in the mouth region.

ORIGIN AND INSERTION. The orbicularis oris muscle encircles the mouth and inserts in the skin tissue at the angle of the mouth (Figure 4-10). In the upper lip, fibers also insert on the ridges of the philtrum.

ACTION. The orbicularis oris muscle closes the lips. When the fibers are very active, the lips are pursed.

Orbicularis oris muscle

FIGURE 4–10 ■ Orbicularis oris muscle.

BUCCINATOR MUSCLE

The **buccinator muscle** (buck-**sin**-nay-tor) is a muscle of facial expression that forms the anterior portion of the cheek.

ORIGIN AND INSERTION. The buccinator muscle originates from three areas: the alveolar processes of the maxilla and mandible and a fibrous structure, the **pterygomandibular raphe** (**teh**-ri-go-man-**dib**-yule-lar **ra**-fe) (Figure 4–11). The pterygomandibular raphe extends from the hamulus and passes inferiorly to attach to the posterior end of the mandible's mylohyoid line. The buccinator and superior pharyngeal constrictor muscles of the pharynx are attached to each other at the raphe. The pterygomandibular raphe is noted in the oral cavity as the **pterygomandibular fold.** The buccinator runs horizontally to insert into the skin tissue at the angle of the mouth. Thus the buccinator muscle has different fiber groups, the deep vertical fibers between the alveolar processes and the superficial horizontal fibers from the raphe to the corner of the mouth.

ACTION. The buccinator muscle pulls the angle of the mouth laterally and shortens the cheek both vertically and horizontally. This action causes the muscle to keep food pushed back on the occlusal surface of teeth, as when a person chews. By keeping the food in the correct position when chewing, the buccinator muscle assists the muscles of mastication.

RISORIUS MUSCLE

The **risorius muscle** (ri-**soh**-ree-us) is a thin muscle of facial expression in the mouth region.

ORIGIN AND INSERTION. The risorius muscle originates from fascia superficial to the masseter muscle and passes anteriorly to insert in the skin tissue at the angle of the mouth (Figure 4–12).

ACTION. The risorius muscle widens the mouth, as when a person smiles widely.

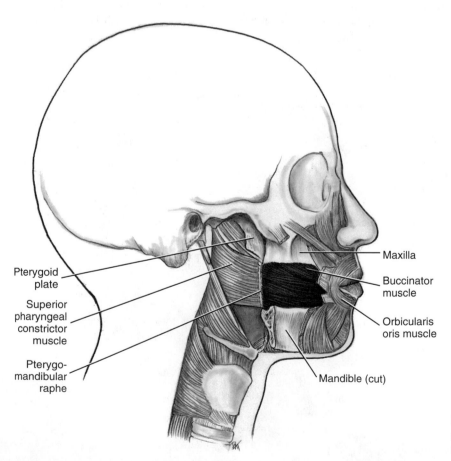

Pterygoid plate

Superior pharyngeal constrictor muscle

Pterygo-mandibular raphe

Maxilla

Buccinator muscle

Orbicularis oris muscle

Mandible (cut)

FIGURE 4–11 ■ Origin and insertion of the buccinator muscle.

Masseter
muscle

Platysma
muscle

Orbicularis
oris muscle

Risorius muscle

FIGURE 4–12 ■ Origin and insertion of the
risorius muscle.

LEVATOR LABII SUPERIORIS MUSCLE

A broad, flat muscle of facial expression in the
mouth region is the **levator labii superioris
muscle** (le-**vate**-er **lay**-be-eye soo-per-ee-**or**-is).

ORIGIN AND INSERTION. The levator labii superioris muscle originates from the infraorbital rim
of the maxilla. The muscle then passes inferiorly
to insert in the skin tissue of the upper lip
(Figure 4–13).

ACTION. The levator labii superioris muscle
elevates the upper lip (Figure 4–14A).

LEVATOR LABII SUPERIORIS ALAEQUE NASI MUSCLE

The **levator labii superioris alaeque nasi
muscle** (le-**vate**-er **lay**-be-eye soo-per-ee-**or**-is
a-lah-cue **naz**-eye) is also a muscle of facial
expression in the mouth region.

ORIGIN AND INSERTION. The levator labii superioris alaeque nasi muscle originates from the
frontal process of the maxilla. The muscle then
passes inferiorly to insert into two areas: the skin
tissue of the ala (or wing) of the nose and the
upper lip (see Figure 4–13).

ACTION. The levator labii superioris alaeque
nasi muscle elevates the upper lip and ala of the
nose, thus also dilating the nostrils, as in a sneer-
ing expression (Figure 4–14B).

ZYGOMATICUS MAJOR MUSCLE

Another muscle of facial expression in the
mouth region is the **zygomaticus major muscle**
(zy-go-**mat**-i-kus **may**-jer).

ORIGIN AND INSERTION. The zygomaticus major
muscle originates from the zygomatic bone, lateral to the zygomaticus minor muscle. The muscle
then passes anteriorly and inferiorly to insert in
the skin tissue at the angle of the mouth (see
Figure 4–13).

ACTION. The zygomaticus major muscle elevates the angle of the upper lip and pulls it laterally, as when a person smiles (see Figure 4–14A).

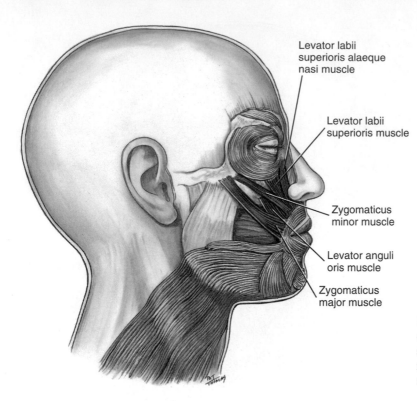

Levator labii superioris alaeque nasi muscle

Levator labii superioris muscle

Zygomaticus minor muscle

Levator anguli oris muscle

Zygomaticus major muscle

FIGURE 4–13 ■ Levator labii superioris alaeque nasi muscle, levator labii superioris muscle, zygomaticus minor muscle, levator anguli oris muscle, and zygomaticus major muscle.

ZYGOMATICUS MINOR MUSCLE

The **zygomaticus minor muscle** (zy-go-**mat**-i-kus **my**-ner) is a small muscle of facial expression in the mouth region, medial to the zygomaticus major muscle.

ORIGIN AND INSERTION. The zygomaticus minor muscle originates on the body of the zygomatic bone. The muscle then inserts in the skin tissue of the upper lip adjacent to the insertion of the levator labii superioris muscle (see Figure 4–13).

ACTION. The zygomaticus minor elevates the upper lip (see Figure 4–14A).

LEVATOR ANGULI ORIS MUSCLE

Deep to both the zygomaticus major and zygomaticus minor muscles is the **levator anguli oris muscle** (le-**vate**-er **an**-gu-lie **or**-is), another muscle of facial expression in the mouth region.

ORIGIN AND INSERTION. The levator anguli oris muscle originates on the canine fossa of the maxilla, usually superior to the root of the maxillary canine. The muscle then passes inferiorly to insert in skin tissues at the angle of the mouth (see Figure 4–13).

ACTION. The levator anguli oris muscle elevates the angle of the mouth, as when a person smiles (see Figure 4–14A).

DEPRESSOR ANGULI ORIS MUSCLE

The **depressor anguli oris muscle** (de-**pres**-er **an**-gu-lie **or**-is) is a triangular muscle of facial expression in the lower mouth region.

ORIGIN AND INSERTION. The depressor anguli oris muscle originates on the lower border of the mandible and passes superiorly to insert in the skin tissue at the angle of the mouth (Figure 4–15).

Levator labii
superioris
muscle

Levator anguli
oris muscle

Risorius
muscle

Zygomaticus
minor muscle

Zygomaticus
major muscle

A

Corrugator
supercilii
muscle

Levator labii
superioris
alaeque
nasi muscle

Depressor
anguli oris
muscle

B

FIGURE 4–14 ■ A: Patient using the risorius muscle, levator labii superioris muscle, levator anguli oris muscle, zygomaticus minor muscle, and zygomaticus major muscle when smiling (muscles highlighted and labeled). B: Patient using the corrugator supercilii muscle, levator labii superioris alaeque nasi muscle, and depressor anguli oris muscle while looking disgusted (muscles highlighted and labeled).

FIGURE 4–15 ■ Depressor labii inferioris muscle and depressor anguli oris muscle.

ACTION. The depressor anguli oris muscle depresses the angle of the mouth, as when a person frowns (see Figure 4–14B).

DEPRESSOR LABII INFERIORIS MUSCLE

Deep to the depressor anguli oris muscle is the **depressor labii inferioris muscle** (de-**pres**-er **lay**-be-eye in-**fere**-ee-o-ris), another muscle of facial expression in the mouth region.

ORIGIN AND INSERTION. The depressor labii inferioris muscle also originates from the lower border of the mandible and passes superiorly to insert in the skin tissue of the lower lip (see Figure 4-15).

ACTION. The depressor labii inferioris muscle depresses the lower lip, exposing the mandibular incisor teeth.

MENTALIS MUSCLE

The **mentalis muscle** (men-**ta**-lis) is a short, thick muscle of facial expression superior and medial to the mental nerve in the mouth region.

ORIGIN AND INSERTION. The mentalis muscle originates on the mandible near the midline and inserts in the skin tissue of the chin (Figure 4–16).

ACTION. The mentalis muscle raises the chin, causing the displaced lower lip to protrude and narrowing the oral vestibule. These fibers when active may dislodge a complete denture in an edentulous patient who has lost alveolar ridge height.

PLATYSMA MUSCLE

The **platysma muscle** (plah-**tiz**-mah) is a muscle of facial expression that runs from the neck all the way to the mouth, covering the anterior cervical triangle.

ORIGIN AND INSERTION. The platysma muscle originates in the skin tissue superficial to the clavicle and shoulder. The muscle then passes anteriorly to insert on the lower border of the mandible and the muscles surrounding the mouth (Figure 4–17).

ACTION. The platysma muscle raises the skin of the neck and also pulls the corner of the mouth down, as when a person grimaces (Figure 4–18).

FIGURE 4–16 ■ Mentalis muscle.

Orbicularis
oris muscle

Mentalis
muscle

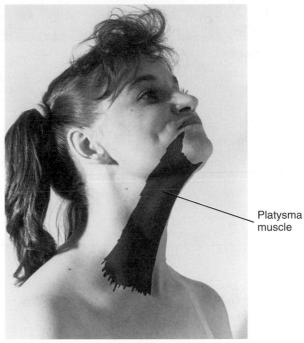

FIGURE 4–18 ■ Patient using the platysma muscle to raise the skin of the neck and pull the corner of the mouth down, as when a person grimaces (muscle highlighted).

Platysma
muscle

MUSCLES OF MASTICATION

The **muscles of mastication** (mass-ti-**kay**-shun) are four pairs of muscles attached to the mandible: the masseter, temporalis, medial pterygoid, and lateral pterygoid muscles.

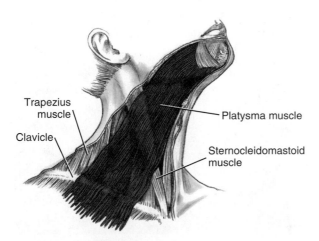

Trapezius
muscle

Clavicle

Platysma muscle

Sternocleidomastoid
muscle

FIGURE 4–17 ■ Origin and insertion of the platysma muscle.

ORIGIN AND INSERTION. The origin and insertion of each muscle are discussed (Table 4–3).

ACTION. The muscles of mastication are responsible for closing the jaws, moving the lower jaw forward or backward, and shifting the lower jaw to one side. These jaw movements involve the movement of the mandible, while the rest of the skull remains relatively stable. These muscles of mastication work with the temporomandibular joint to accomplish these movements of the mandible (see Chapter 5 for more information). The dental professional needs to understand the association of the muscles of mastication with the movements of the mandible: depression, elevation, protrusion, retraction, and lateral deviation (Table 4–4).

INNERVATION. All the muscles of mastication are innervated by the mandibular division of the fifth cranial or trigeminal nerve.

Masseter Muscle

The most obvious muscle of mastication is the **masseter muscle (mass**-et-er) (see Figure 2–6)

Table 4–3 ORIGIN AND INSERTION OF THE MUSCLES OF MASTICATION

Muscles	Origin	Insertion
Masseter	Superficial head: anterior two thirds of lower border of zygomatic arch	Superficial head: angle of mandible
	Deep head: posterior one third and medial surface of zygomatic arch	Deep head: ramus of mandible
Temporalis	Temporal fossa	Coronoid process of mandible
Medial pterygoid	Pterygoid fossa of sphenoid bone	Angle of mandible
Lateral pterygoid	Superior head: greater wing of sphenoid bone	Both heads: pterygoid fovea of mandible
	Inferior head: lateral pterygoid plate from sphenoid bone	

since it is the most superficially located and one of the strongest. The masseter muscle is a broad, thick, rectangular muscle on each side of the face, anterior to the parotid salivary gland. This muscle can become enlarged in patients who habitually clench or grind their teeth and even in those who constantly chew gum. This masseteric hypertrophy is asymptomatic and soft and is usually bilateral but can be unilateral. If the hypertrophy is bilateral, there still may be asymmetry of the face due to unequal enlargement of the muscles (Figure 4–19). This enlargement

may be confused with parotid gland disease, dental infections, and maxillofacial neoplasms. However, no other signs are present except those involved in changes in occlusion intraorally, and the swelling corresponds to the outline of the masseter muscle. Most patients seek medical attention because of comments about facial appearance.

During an extraoral examination, stand near the patient and visually inspect and use bilateral palpation of the masseter muscle. Place the fingers of each hand over the masseter muscle and ask the patient to clench the teeth together several times (Figure 4–20). This mus-

Table 4–4 MUSCLES OF MASTICATION WITH ASSOCIATED MOVEMENTS OF MANDIBLE

Muscles	Mandibular Movements
Masseter	Elevation of mandible (during jaw closing)
Temporalis	Elevation of mandible (during jaw closing)
	Retraction of mandible (lower jaw backward)
Medial pterygoid	Elevation of mandible (during jaw closing)
Lateral pterygoid	Inferior heads: slight depression of mandible (during jaw opening)
	One muscle: lateral deviation of mandible (shift lower jaw to opposite side)
	Both muscles: protrusion of mandible (lower jaw forward)

FIGURE 4–19 ■ Bilateral enlargement of the masseter muscle.

FIGURE 4–20 ■ Palpation of the masseter muscle by asking patient to clench the teeth.

cle has two heads, a superficial head and a deep head.

ORIGIN AND INSERTION. The superficial head of the masseter muscle originates from the anterior two thirds of the lower border of the zygomatic arch. The deep head originates from the posterior third and the entire medial

surface of the zygomatic arch. Both these heads of the masseter muscle pass inferiorly to insert on the mandible. The superficial head inserts on the lateral surface of the angle, and the deep head inserts on the ramus above the angle (Figure 4–21).

ACTION. The action of the masseter muscle when there is bilateral contraction of the entire muscle is to elevate the mandible, raising the lower jaw. Elevation of the mandible occurs during the closing of the jaws.

Temporalis Muscle

The **temporalis muscle** (tem-poh-**ral**-is) is a broad, fan-shaped muscle of mastication on each side of the head that fills the temporal fossa, superior to the zygomatic arch.

ORIGIN AND INSERTION. The temporalis muscle originates from the entire temporal fossa that is bound at the top by the inferior temporal line and at the bottom by the infratemporal crest. The muscle then passes inferiorly to insert on the coronoid process of the mandible (Figure 4–22).

ACTION. If the entire temporalis muscle contracts, the main action of the temporalis muscle is to elevate the mandible, raising the lower jaw.

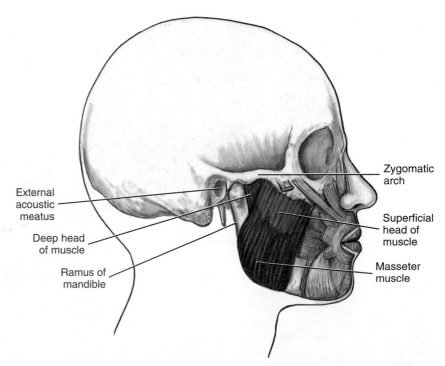

FIGURE 4–21 ■ Masseter muscle with its superficial head and its deep head.

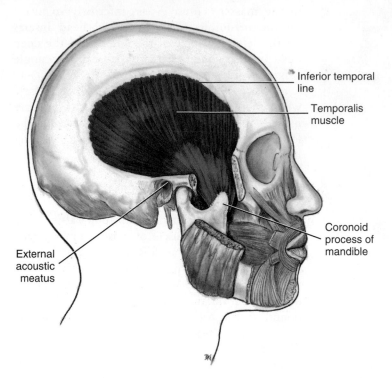

FIGURE 4–22 ■ Origin and insertion of the temporalis muscle (zygomatic arch and superior part of the masseter muscle have been removed).

FIGURE 4–23 ■ Medial pterygoid muscle and lateral pterygoid muscle with its superior head and its inferior head (lower part of the temporalis muscle, zygomatic arch, and most of the mandibular ramus have been removed).

Elevation of the mandible occurs during the closing of the jaws. If only the posterior portion contracts, the muscle moves the lower jaw backward. Moving the lower jaw backward causes retraction of the mandible. Retraction of the jaw often accompanies the closing of the jaws.

Medial Pterygoid Muscle

Deeper, yet similar in form to the superficial masseter muscle, is another muscle of mastication, the **medial pterygoid muscle (teh**-ri-goid) or internal pterygoid muscle.

ORIGIN AND INSERTION. The medial pterygoid muscle originates from the pterygoid fossa on the medial surface of the lateral pterygoid plate of the sphenoid bone. The muscle then passes inferiorly, posteriorly, and laterally to insert on the medial surface of the angle of the mandible (Figure 4–23).

ACTION. The action of the medial pterygoid muscle is to elevate the mandible, raising the lower jaw. Elevation of the mandible occurs during the closing of the jaws. This muscle is weaker than the masseter muscle in this action.

Lateral Pterygoid Muscle

The final muscle of mastication to consider is the **lateral pterygoid muscle (teh**-ri-goid) or external pterygoid muscle. This muscle has two separate heads of origin, the superior head and inferior head. The two heads of the muscle are separated by a slight interval anteriorly but fuse posteriorly. The entire muscle lies within the infratemporal fossa, deep to the temporalis muscle (see Chapter 3).

ORIGIN AND INSERTION. The superior head of the lateral pterygoid muscle originates from the inferior surface of the greater wing of the sphenoid bone (the roof of the infratemporal fossa). The inferior head of the muscle originates from the lateral surface of the lateral pterygoid plate of the sphenoid bone. Both heads of the muscle then unite, passing posteriorly to insert on the anterior surface of the neck of mandibular condyle at the pterygoid fovea (see Figure 4–23). A few of the most superior fibers insert on the capsule of the temporomandibular joint.

ACTION. The inferior head has a slight tendency to depress the mandible, lowering the lower jaw. Depression of the mandible occurs during the opening of the jaws. The main action when both muscles contract is to bring the lower jaw forward, thus causing the protrusion of the mandible. Protrusion of the mandible often occurs during opening of the jaws. If only one lateral pterygoid muscle is contracted, the lower jaw shifts to the opposite side, causing lateral deviation of the mandible.

HYOID MUSCLES

The **hyoid muscles (hi**-oid) assist in the actions of mastication and swallowing. Most of the hyoid muscles are in a superficial position in the neck tissues. The hyoid muscles can be grouped according to whether they are suprahyoid or infrahyoid muscles (Table 4–5).

ORIGIN AND INSERTION. Both groups of the hyoid muscles are attached in some way to the **hyoid bone** (Figure 4–24). The hyoid bone is a horseshoe-shaped bone suspended inferior to the mandible (see Chapter 3 for more information). The hyoid bone does not articulate with any other bone and has only muscular and ligamentary attachments. The designation for each muscle group, suprahyoid or infrahyoid muscles, is based on its vertical position in relationship to the hyoid bone. The specific origin and insertion of each hyoid muscle are discussed (Table 4–6).

Suprahyoid Muscles

The **suprahyoid muscles** (soo-prah-**hi**-oid) are located superior to the hyoid bone (Figures 4–24,

Table 4–5 HYOID MUSCLES AND THEIR GROUP, SUPRAHYOID OR INFRAHYOID, BASED ON THEIR RELATIONSHIP TO THE HYOID BONE

Suprahyoid	Infrahyoid
Digastric	Sternothyroid
Mylohyoid	Sternohyoid
Geniohyoid	Thyrohyoid
Stylohyoid	

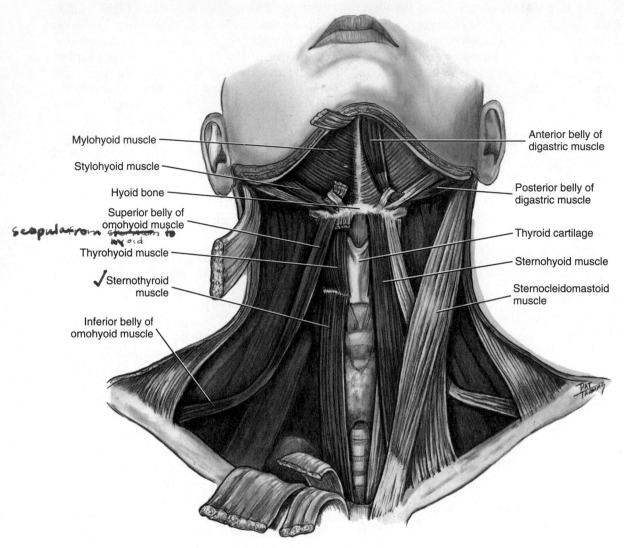

Mylohyoid muscle

Stylohyoid muscle

Hyoid bone

Superior belly of
omohyoid muscle

Thyrohyoid muscle

Sternothyroid
muscle

Inferior belly of
omohyoid muscle

Anterior belly of
digastric muscle

Posterior belly of
digastric muscle

Thyroid cartilage

Sternohyoid muscle

Sternocleidomastoid
muscle

scapula from sternum to
hyoid

FIGURE 4–24 ■ Anterior view of the hyoid bone and the hyoid muscles (except the geniohyoid muscle).

4–25 and 4–26). These muscles may be further-divided according to their anterior or posterior position to the hyoid bone. The **anterior suprahyoid muscle group** includes the anterior belly of the digastric, mylohyoid, and geniohyoid muscles. The **posterior suprahyoid muscle group** includes the posterior belly of the digastric and stylohyoid muscles.

ACTION. There are two actions associated with mastication that result from the contraction of the suprahyoid muscles. One action of both the anterior and posterior suprahyoid muscles is to cause the elevation of the hyoid bone and larynx

if the mandible is stabilized by contraction of the muscles of mastication. This action occurs during swallowing.

The other action associated with mastication results from only the contraction of the anterior suprahyoid muscles, which causes the mandible to depress and the jaws to open when the hyoid bone is stabilized by the contraction of the posterior suprahyoid muscles and infrahyoid muscles, the other hyoid muscle group. Thus normal jaw opening involves the lateral pterygoid muscles, which protrude the mandible, and the anterior suprahyoid muscles, which lower the mandible.

Table 4–6	ORIGIN AND INSERTION OF THE HYOID MUSCLES	
Muscles	**Origin**	**Insertion**
Suprahyoid		
Digastric	Anterior belly: intermediate tendon	Anterior belly: medial surface of mandible
	Posterior belly: mastoid notch of temporal bone	Posterior belly: intermediate tendon
Mylohyoid	Mylohyoid line of mandible	Body of hyoid bone
Geniohyoid	Genial tubercles of mandible	Body of hyoid bone
Stylohyoid	Styloid process of temporal bone	Body of hyoid bone
Infrahyoid		
Sternothyroid	Posterior surface of sternum	Thyroid cartilage
Sternohyoid	Posterior and superior surfaces of sternum	Body of hyoid bone
Omohyoid	Inferior belly: scapula	Inferior belly: superior belly
	Superior belly: inferior belly	Superior belly: body of hyoid bone
Thyrohyoid	Thyroid cartilage	Body and greater cornu of hyoid bone

Some of the suprahyoid muscles have additional specific actions that are also discussed.

DIGASTRIC MUSCLE

The **digastric muscle** (di-**gas**-trik) is a suprahyoid muscle that has two separate bellies, the anterior and posterior bellies. The anterior belly is part of the anterior suprahyoid muscle group, and the posterior belly is part of the posterior suprahyoid muscle group. Each digastric muscle demarcates the superior portion of the anterior cervical triangle, forming (with the mandible) a submandibular triangle on each side of the neck. The right and left anterior bellies of the muscle form a midline submental triangle.

ORIGIN AND INSERTION. The anterior belly of the digastric muscle originates on a tendon loosely attached to the body and greater cornu of the hyoid bone called the **intermediate tendon** (in-ter-**me**-dee-it **ten**-don) and passes superiorly and anteriorly to insert close to the symphysis on the inner surface of the mandible. The posterior belly arises from the mastoid notch, medial to the mastoid process of the temporal bone, and passes anteriorly and inferiorly to insert on the intermediate tendon.

INNERVATION. The digastric muscle's anterior belly is innervated by the mylohyoid nerve, a branch of the mandibular division of the fifth cranial or trigeminal nerve. The posterior belly of the muscle is innervated by the posterior digastric nerve, a branch of the seventh cranial or facial nerve.

MYLOHYOID MUSCLE

The **mylohyoid muscle** (my-lo-**hi**-oid) is an anterior suprahyoid muscle that is deep to the digastric muscle, with fibers running transversely between the two sides of the mandible.

ORIGIN AND INSERTION. The mylohyoid muscle originates from the mylohyoid line on the inner surface of the mandible. The right and left muscles pass inferiorly to unite medially, forming the floor of the mouth. The most posterior fibers of the muscle insert on the body of the hyoid bone.

ACTION. In addition to either elevating the hyoid bone or depressing the mandible, the mylohyoid muscle also forms the floor of the mouth and helps elevate the tongue.

INNERVATION. The mylohyoid muscle is innervated by the mylohyoid nerve, a branch of the mandibular division of the fifth cranial or trigeminal nerve.

STYLOHYOID MUSCLE

The **stylohyoid muscle** (sty-lo-**hi**-oid) is a thin posterior suprahyoid muscle, anterior and

FIGURE 4–25 ■ Lateral view of the hyoid bone and the suprahyoid muscles (except the geniohyoid muscle).

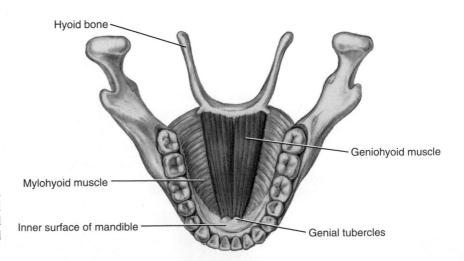

FIGURE 4–26 ■ View from above of the floor of the oral cavity showing the origin and insertion of the geniohyoid muscle.

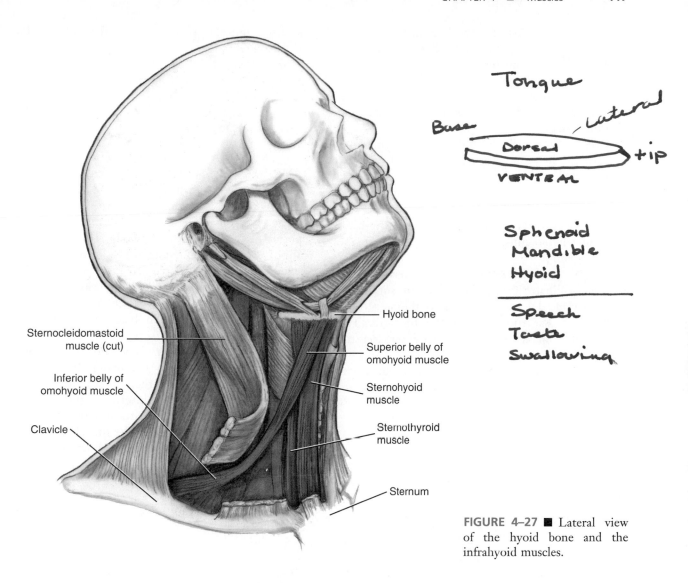

Sternocleidomastoid
muscle (cut)

Inferior belly of
omohyoid muscle

Clavicle

Hyoid bone

Superior belly of
omohyoid muscle

Sternohyoid
muscle

Sternothyroid
muscle

Sternum

FIGURE 4–27 ■ Lateral view of the hyoid bone and the infrahyoid muscles.

superficial to the posterior belly of the digastric muscle.

ORIGIN AND INSERTION. The stylohyoid muscle originates from the styloid process of the temporal bone and passes anteriorly and inferiorly to insert on the body of the hyoid bone.

INNERVATION. The stylohyoid muscle is innervated by the stylohyoid nerve, a branch of the seventh cranial or facial nerve.

GENIOHYOID MUSCLE

The **geniohyoid muscle** (ji-nee-o-**hi**-oid) is an anterior suprahyoid muscle that is deep to the mylohyoid muscle.

ORIGIN AND INSERTION. The geniohyoid muscle originates from the medial surface of the mandible. On this surface of the mandible, the muscle is attached near the symphysis at the genial tubercles (see Figure 4–24). The muscle then passes posteriorly and inferiorly to insert on the body of the hyoid bone.

INNERVATION. The geniohyoid muscle is innervated by the first cervical nerve, conducted by way of the twelfth cranial or hypoglossal nerve.

Infrahyoid Muscles

The **infrahyoid muscles** (in-frah-**hi**-oid) are four pairs of hyoid muscles inferior to the hyoid bone

(Figure 4–27; see also Figure 4–24). The infrahyoid muscles include the sternohyoid, sternothyroid, thyrohyoid, and omohyoid muscles.

ACTION. Most of the infrahyoid muscles depress the hyoid bone. Some of the infrahyoid muscles have additional specific actions that are also discussed.

INNERVATION. All the infrahyoid muscles are innervated by the second and third cervical nerves.

STERNOTHYROID MUSCLE

The **sternothyroid muscle** (ster-no-**thy**-roid) is an infrahyoid muscle located superficial to the thyroid gland.

ORIGIN AND INSERTION. The sternothyroid muscle originates from the posterior surface of the sternum, deep and medial to the sternothyroid muscle, at the level of the first rib. The muscle then passes superiorly to insert on the thyroid cartilage.

ACTION. The sternothyroid muscle depresses the thyroid cartilage and larynx, yet does not directly depress the hyoid bone.

STERNOHYOID MUSCLE

The **sternohyoid muscle** (ster-no-**hi**-oid) is an infrahyoid muscle superficial to the ster-nothyroid muscle, as well as the thyroid gland and cartilage.

ORIGIN AND INSERTION. The sternohyoid muscle originates from the posterior and superior surfaces of the sternum, close to where the sternum joins each clavicle. The muscle then passes superiorly to insert on the body of the hyoid bone.

OMOHYOID MUSCLE

The **omohyoid muscle** (o-mo-**hi**-oid) is an infrahyoid muscle lateral to both the sternothyroid and thyrohyoid muscles. This muscle has a superior belly and an inferior belly. The superior belly of each muscle divides the inferior portion of the anterior cervical triangle into the carotid and muscular triangles. In the posterior cervical triangle, the inferior belly of each muscle serves to demarcate the subclavian triangle (inferiorly) from the occipital triangle (superiorly).

ORIGIN AND INSERTION. The inferior belly of the omohyoid muscle originates from the scapula. The inferior belly then passes anteriorly and superiorly, crossing the internal jugular vein, beneath the SCM, where it attaches by a short tendon to the superior belly. The muscle's superior belly originates from the short tendon attached to the inferior belly and then inserts

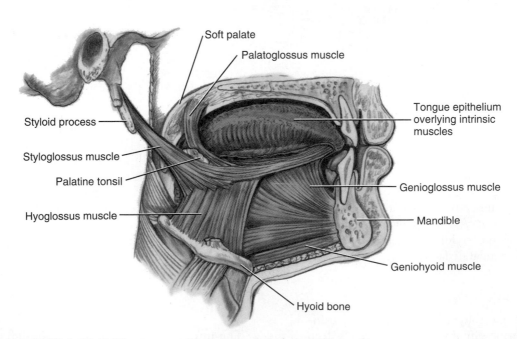

FIGURE 4–28 ■ The tongue with its intrinsic and extrinsic muscles.

on the lateral border of the body of the hyoid bone.

THYROHYOID MUSCLE

The **thyrohyoid muscle** (thy-ro-**hi**-oid), the final infrahyoid muscle to be discussed, is covered by the omohyoid and sternohyoid muscles.

ORIGIN AND INSERTION. The thyrohyoid muscle originates on the thyroid cartilage and inserts on the body and greater cornu of the hyoid bone. This muscle appears as a continuation of the sternothyroid muscle.

ACTION. In addition to depressing the hyoid bone, the thyrohyoid muscle raises the thyroid cartilage and larynx.

MUSCLES OF THE TONGUE

The **muscles of the tongue** can be grouped according to whether they are intrinsic or extrinsic tongue muscles (Figure 4–28). The tongue consists of symmetrical halves divided from each other by the **median septum** (**sep**-tum), a deep fibrous structure in the midline of the tongue. The median septum corresponds to the midline depression on the tongue's dorsal surface called the **median lingual sulcus** (see Chapter 1 for more information). Each half of the tongue has muscular groups arranged in various directions, with the intrinsic and extrinsic tongue muscles intertwining with each other. The tongue is further divided into a base and body with an apex.

ORIGIN AND INSERTION. The intrinsic tongue muscles are all located inside the tongue. The extrinsic tongue muscles all have their origin outside the tongue yet have their insertion inside the tongue.

ACTION. The tongue has complex movements during mastication, speaking, and swallowing. These movements are a result of the combined action of muscles of the tongue. The intrinsic tongue muscles change the shape of the tongue. The extrinsic tongue muscles also move the tongue, while suspending and anchoring the tongue to the mandible, styloid process, and hyoid bone. When studying the muscles of the tongue, try to visualize the movements produced by these muscles. The specific actions of each muscle of the tongue will be given.

Intrinsic Tongue Muscles

There are four sets of **intrinsic tongue muscles** (in-**trin**-sik) that are all located entirely inside the tongue (see Figure 4–28). These muscles of the tongue are named by their orientation. The intrinsic tongue muscles include the superior longitudinal, transverse, vertical, and inferior longitudinal muscles. Anatomists consider the intrinsic tongue muscles to be inseparable, so they are not usually treated as separate muscles.

ORIGIN AND INSERTION. The superior longitudinal muscle is the most superficial of the intrinsic tongue muscles. This muscle runs in an oblique and longitudinal direction in the dorsal surface from the base to the apex. Deep to the superior longitudinal muscle is the **transverse muscle**. The transverse muscle runs in a transverse direction from the median septum to pass outward toward the lateral surface of the tongue. The **vertical muscle** (**ver**-ti-kel) runs in a vertical direction from the dorsal surface inward to the ventral surface in the body of the tongue. The inferior longitudinal muscle is located in the ventral surface of the tongue. This muscle runs in a longitudinal direction from the base to the apex of the tongue.

ACTION. The superior and inferior longitudinal muscles act together to change the shape of the tongue by shortening and thickening it and act singly to help it curl in various directions. The transverse and vertical muscles act together to make the tongue long and narrow.

INNERVATION. All the intrinsic tongue muscles are innervated by the twelfth cranial or hypoglossal nerve.

Extrinsic Tongue Muscles

There are three pairs of **extrinsic tongue muscles** (eks-**trin**-sik) with different origins outside the tongue and all their insertions inside the tongue (see Figure 4–28, Table 4–7). The extrinsic tongue muscles include the genioglossus, styloglossus, and hyoglossus muscles. Some anatomists also include the palatoglossus muscle in this category since it is involved in tongue movement; the palatoglossus muscle is discussed with the muscles of the soft palate in this chapter.

Table 4–7 EXTRINSIC TONGUE MUSCLES WITH THEIR ORIGINS, INSERTIONS, AND ACTIONS

Muscles	Origin	Insertion	Action
Genioglossus	Genial tubercles on mandible	Hyoid bone and tongue	Protrudes tongue and depresses portions
Styloglossus	Styloid process of temporal bone	Tongue	Retracts tongue
Hyoglossus	Greater cornu and body of hyoid bone	Tongue	Depresses tongue

INNERVATION. All the extrinsic tongue muscles are innervated by the twelfth cranial or hypoglossal nerve.

GENIOGLOSSUS MUSCLE

The **genioglossus muscle** (ji-nee-o-**gloss**-us) is a fan-shaped extrinsic tongue muscle superior to the geniohyoid muscle.

ORIGIN AND INSERTION. The genioglossus muscle arises from the genial tubercles (or mental spines) on the internal surface of the mandible. A few of the most inferior fibers insert on the hyoid bone, but most of the fibers insert in the tongue from its base almost to the apex. The right and left muscles are separated by the tongue's median septum.

ACTION. Different parts of the genioglossus muscle can protrude the tongue out of the oral cavity or depress parts of the tongue surface. The protrusive activity of the genioglossus muscle helps to prevent the tongue from sinking back and obstructing respiration; therefore during general anesthesia, the mandible is sometimes pulled forward to achieve the same effect.

STYLOGLOSSUS MUSCLE

The **styloglossus muscle** (sty-lo-**gloss**-us) is another extrinsic tongue muscle.

ORIGIN AND INSERTION. The styloglossus muscle originates from the styloid process of the temporal bone. The muscle then passes inferiorly and anteriorly to insert into two parts of the lateral surface of the tongue, its apex and at the border of the body and base.

ACTION. The styloglossus muscle retracts the tongue, moving it superiorly and posteriorly.

HYOGLOSSUS MUSCLE

The **hyoglossus muscle** (hi-o-**gloss**-us) is the final extrinsic tongue muscle to be considered.

ORIGIN AND INSERTION. The hyoglossus muscle originates on the greater cornu and part of the body of the hyoid bone. The muscle then inserts into the lateral surface of the body of the tongue.

ACTION. The hyoglossus muscle depresses the tongue.

MUSCLES OF THE PHARYNX

The **pharynx** (**far**-inks) is part of both the respiratory and digestive tracts and is connected to both the nasal and oral cavities. The pharynx consists of three portions, the nasopharynx, oropharynx, and laryngopharynx (see Chapter 1 for more information). The **muscles of the pharynx** are involved in speaking, swallowing, and middle ear function. The muscles of the pharynx include the stylopharyngeus, pharyngeal constrictor, and soft palate muscles.

Stylopharyngeus Muscle

The **stylopharyngeus muscle** (sty-lo-fah-**rin**-je-us) is a paired longitudinal muscle of the pharynx.

ORIGIN AND INSERTION. The stylopharyngeus originates from the styloid process of the temporal bone. The muscle then inserts into the lateral and posterior pharyngeal walls (Figure 4–29A and B).

ACTION. The stylopharyngeus muscle elevates the pharynx, simultaneously widening the pharynx.

INNERVATION. The stylopharyngeus muscle is innervated by the ninth cranial or glossopharyngeal nerve.

Pharyngeal Constrictor Muscles

The **pharyngeal constrictor muscles** (fah-**rin**-je-il kon-**strik**-tor) consist of three paired muscles,

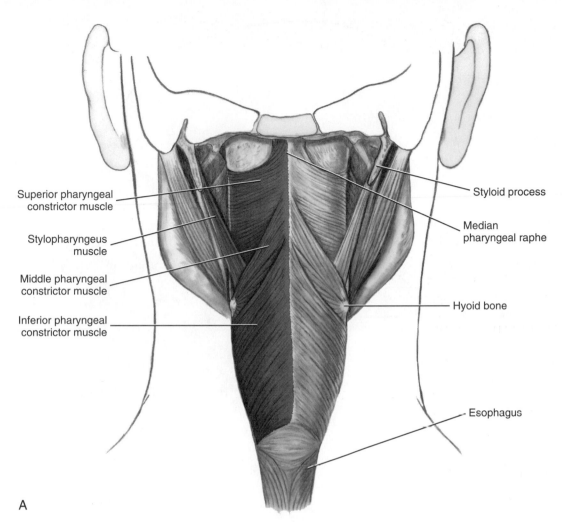

FIGURE 4–29 ■ A: Posterior view of the muscles of the pharynx.

Superior pharyngeal constrictor muscle

Stylopharyngeus muscle

Middle pharyngeal constrictor muscle

Inferior pharyngeal constrictor muscle

Styloid process

Median pharyngeal raphe

Hyoid bone

Esophagus

A

the superior, middle, and inferior pharyngeal constrictor muscles, which form the lateral and posterior walls of the pharynx.

ORIGIN AND INSERTION. The origin of each of the three pharyngeal constrictor muscles is different, although the muscles overlap each other and all have similar insertions (see Figure 4–29A and B). The superior pharyngeal constrictor muscle originates from the pterygoid hamulus, mandible, and pterygomandibular raphe. The middle pharyngeal constrictor muscle originates on the hyoid bone and stylohyoid ligament. The inferior pharyngeal constrictor muscle originates from the thyroid and cricoid cartilages of the larynx. All three pharyngeal constrictor muscles overlap each other, the inferior being most superficial. These muscles then insert into the **median**

pharyngeal raphe (fah-**rin**-je-al **ra**-fe), a midline fibrous band of the posterior wall of the pharynx that is itself attached to the base of the skull.

ACTION. The pharyngeal constrictor muscles raise the pharynx and larynx and help drive food inferiorly into the esophagus during swallowing.

INNERVATION. All three pharyngeal constrictor muscles are innervated by the pharyngeal plexus.

Muscles of the Soft Palate

The **soft palate** (**pal**-it) forms the nonbony posterior portion of the roof of the mouth or the oropharynx and connects laterally with the tongue (see Chapter 1 for more information). The muscles of the soft palate are involved in speaking and swallowing. The **muscles of the**

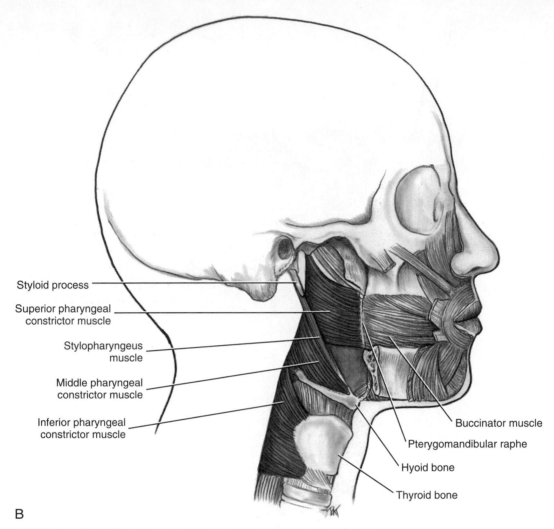

Styloid process

Superior pharyngeal
constrictor muscle

Stylopharyngeus
muscle

Middle pharyngeal
constrictor muscle

Inferior pharyngeal
constrictor muscle

Buccinator muscle

Pterygomandibular raphe

Hyoid bone

Thyroid bone

B

FIGURE 4–29 ■ *Continued.* B: Lateral view of the muscles of the pharynx.

soft palate include the palatoglossus, palatopharyngeus, levator veli palatini, and tensor veli palatini muscles and the muscle of the uvula (Figures 4–30 and 4–31, Table 4–8). Some anatomists consider the palatoglossus muscle to be an extrinsic muscle of the tongue since it is involved in tongue movement, but it will be considered only a muscle of the soft palate in this chapter.

ACTION. When the muscles of the soft palate are relaxed, the soft palate extends posteriorly over the anterior oropharynx. The combined actions of several muscles of the soft palate move the soft palate superiorly and posteriorly to contact the posterior pharyngeal wall that is being moved anteriorly. This movement of both the soft palate and pharyngeal wall brings a separation

between the nasopharynx and oral cavity during swallowing to prevent food from entering the nasal cavity while eating. Specific actions of each muscle of the soft palate will also be discussed.

INNERVATION. All the muscles of the soft palate are innervated by the pharyngeal plexus, except the tensor veli palatini muscle. This muscle is supplied by the mandibular division of the fifth cranial or trigeminal nerve.

PALATOGLOSSUS MUSCLE

The **palatoglossus muscle** (pal-ah-to-**gloss**-us) forms the **anterior faucial pillar** (**faw**-shawl **pil**-er) in the oral cavity, a vertical fold anterior to each palatine tonsil (see Figures 4–28 and 4–31).

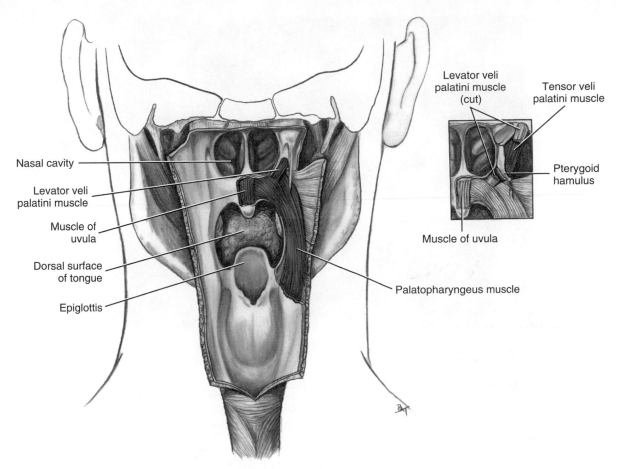

Levator veli palatini muscle (cut)

Tensor veli palatini muscle

Pterygoid hamulus

Muscle of uvula

Nasal cavity

Levator veli palatini muscle

Muscle of uvula

Dorsal surface of tongue

Epiglottis

Palatopharyngeus muscle

FIGURE 4–30 ■ Posterior view of the muscles of the soft palate (pharyngeal constrictor muscles have been cut and mucous membranes partially removed).

ORIGIN AND INSERTION. The palatoglossus muscle originates from the **median palatine raphe** (**pal**-ah-tine **ra**-fe), a midline fibrous band of the palate. The muscle then inserts into the lateral surface of the tongue.

ACTION. The palatoglossus muscle elevates the base of the tongue, arching the tongue against the soft palate, and depresses the soft palate toward the tongue. The muscles on both sides form a sphincter, separating the oral cavity from the pharynx.

PALATOPHARYNGEUS MUSCLE

The **palatopharyngeus muscle** (pal-ah-to-fah-**rin**-je-us) forms the **posterior faucial pillar** (**faw**-shawl **pil**-er) in the oral cavity, a vertical fold posterior to each palatine tonsil (see Figures 4–30 and 4–31).

ORIGIN AND INSERTION. The palatopharyngeus muscle originates in the soft palate and inserts in the walls of the laryngopharynx and on the thyroid cartilage.

ACTION. The palatopharyngeus muscle moves the palate posteroinferiorly and the posterior pharyngeal wall anterosuperiorly to help close off the nasopharynx during swallowing.

LEVATOR VELI PALATINI MUSCLE

The **levator veli palatini muscle** (le-**vate**-er **vee**-lie pal-ah-**teen**-ee) is a muscle mainly situated superior to the soft palate (see Figure 4–30).

ORIGIN AND INSERTION. The levator veli palatini muscle originates from the inferior surface of the temporal bone. The muscle then inserts into the **median palatine raphe** (**pal**-ah-tine **ra**-fe), a midline fibrous band of the palate (see Chapter 1).

Posterior faucial pillar

Anterior faucial pillar

Soft palate

Uvula

Posterior wall of oropharynx

Palatine tonsils

FIGURE 4–31 ■ Intraoral view of the soft palate, uvula, and anterior and posterior faucial pillars with palatine tonsils. These oral landmarks are related to muscular tissue.

ACTION. The levator veli palatini muscle raises the soft palate and helps bring it into contact with the posterior pharyngeal wall to close off the nasopharynx during speech and swallowing.

TENSOR VELI PALATINI MUSCLE

The **tensor veli palatini muscle** (**ten**-ser **vee**-lie pal-ah-**teen**-ee) is a special muscle that stiffens the soft palate (see Figure 4–30). This muscle is

probably active during all palatal movements. Some of its fibers are also responsible for opening the auditory tube to allow air to flow between the pharynx and middle ear cavity.

ORIGIN AND INSERTION. The tensor veli palatini muscle originates from the auditory tube area and the inferior surface of the sphenoid bone. The muscle then passes inferiorly between the medial pterygoid muscle and medial pterygoid plate,

Table 4–8 MUSCLES OF THE SOFT PALATE WITH THEIR ORIGINS, INSERTIONS, AND ACTIONS

Muscles	Origin	Insertion	Action
Palatoglossus (anterior faucial pillar)	Median palatine raphe	Tongue	Elevates and arches tongue, depressing soft palate toward tongue
Palatopharyngeus (posterior faucial pillar)	Soft palate	Laryngopharynx and thyroid cartilage	Moves palate posteroinferiorly and posterior pharyngeal wall anterosuperiorly
Levator veli palatini	Temporal bone	Median palatine raphe	Raises soft palate to contact the posterior pharyngeal wall
Tensor veli palatini	Auditory tube and sphenoid bone	Median palatine raphe	Tenses and slightly lowers soft palate
Muscle of the uvula	Tissue projection that hangs inferiorly from posterior soft palate		Soft palate closely adapts to posterior pharyngeal wall

forming a tendon near the pterygoid hamulus. The tendon winds around the hamulus, using it as a pulley, and then spreads out to insert in the median palatine raphe.

ACTION. The tensor veli palatini muscle tenses and slightly lowers the soft palate.

MUSCLE OF THE UVULA

The **muscle of the uvula** (u-vu-lah) is the final muscle of the soft palate to be considered.

ORIGIN AND INSERTION. The muscle of the uvula lies within the **uvula of the palate** (see Chapter 1 for more information). The uvula is a midline tissue structure that hangs inferiorly from the posterior margin of the soft palate (see Figures 4–30 and 4–31).

ACTION. The muscle of the uvula shortens and broadens the uvula, changing the contour of the posterior portion of the soft palate. This change in contour allows the soft palate to adapt closely to the posterior pharyngeal wall to help close off the nasopharynx during swallowing.

IDENTIFICATION EXERCISES

Identify the structures on the following diagrams by filling in the blanks with the correct anatomical term. You can check your answers by looking back at the figure indicated in parentheses for each identification diagram.

1. (Figure 4–4)

Orbicularis Occuli

levatator labii sup. alaeqear nusi

levatator labii superior

Zygomaticus minor

Zygomaticus major

levatator anguli oris

Buccinator

Platysma

Depressor anguli oris

orbicularis oris

Depresor labii inferiororis

Mentalis

2. (Figure 4–5)

Corrugator supercilii muscle
Orbicularis Oculii
levatutor labii superioris alaeque nasi

Zygomaticus minor
levatutor anguli oris
zygomaticus major
orbicularis oris
risorius
depressor labii inferiororis
mentalis
depressor anguli oris
platysma

3. (Figures 4–22, 4–23)

inferior temporal line
temporalis
superior head lat. pterygoid
inferior head lat pterygoid
medial pterygoid

external acoustic meatus

mandibular condyle.

4. (Figure 4–24)

5. (Figure 4–27)

Hyoid Bone
Sup belly of Omohyoid

6. (Figure 4–28)

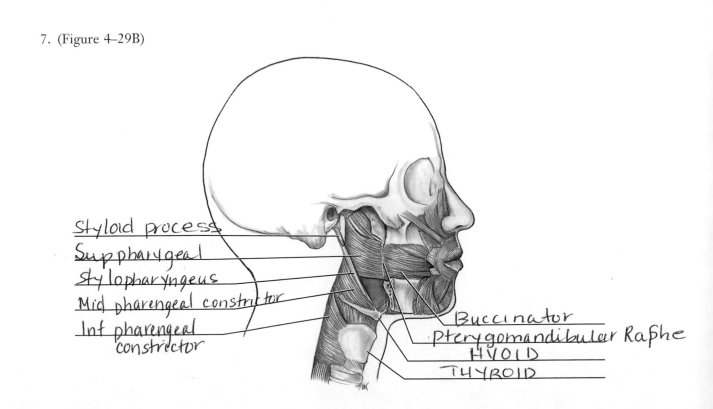

SOFT PALATE

PALATOGLOSSUS MUSCLE

STYLOID PROCESS

STYLOGLOSSAS MUSCLE

PALATINE TONSIL

HYPOGLOSSUS MUSCLE

TONGUE

GENIOGLOSSAS MUSCLE

MANDIBLE

GENIOGLOSSUS MUSCLE

HYOID

7. (Figure 4–29B)

Styloid process

Suppharygeal

Stylopharyngeus

Mid pharengeal constrictor

Inf pharengeal constrictor

Buccinator

Pterygomandibular Raphe

HYOID

THYROID

8. (Figure 4–30)

REVIEW QUESTIONS

1. Both the origin of the frontal belly of the epicranial muscle and the insertion of its occipital belly are at the
   A. Clavicle and sternum
   B. Mastoid process
   C. Epicranial aponeurosis
   D. Pterygomandibular raphe

2. Which of the following muscles is considered a muscle of mastication?
   A. Buccinator muscle
   B. Risorius muscle
   C. Mentalis muscle
   D. Masseter muscle
   E. Corrugator supercilii muscle

3. The origin of a muscle is
   A. The starting point of a muscle
   B. Where the muscle fibers join the bone tendon
   C. The muscle end attached to the least movable structure
   D. The muscle end attached to the most movable structure

4. Which of the following muscle pairs is divided by a median septum?
   A. Geniohyoid muscle
   B. Masseter muscle
   C. Digastric muscle
   D. Transverse muscle of the tongue
   E. Vertical muscle of the tongue

5. Which of the following paired muscles unites medially, forming the floor of the mouth?
   A. Geniohyoid muscle
   B. Omohyoid muscle
   C. Digastric muscle
   D. Mylohyoid muscle
   E. Transverse muscle of the tongue

6. Which of the following muscle groups depress the hyoid bone?
   A. Muscles of mastication
   B. Suprahyoid muscles
   C. Infrahyoid muscles
   D. Intrinsic tongue muscles
   E. Extrinsic tongue muscles

7. Which of the following muscles has two bellies, giving the muscle two different origins?
   A. Lateral pterygoid muscle
   B. Geniohyoid muscle
   C. Thyrohyoid muscle
   D. Stylohyoid muscle

8. Which of the following is the most important muscle used when the patient's lips close around the saliva ejector?
   A. Risorius muscle
   B. Mentalis muscle
   C. Mylohyoid muscle
   D. Buccinator muscle
   E. Orbicularis oris muscle

9. Which of the following muscle groups is involved in elevating the hyoid bone and depressing the mandible?
   A. Muscles of mastication
   B. Suprahyoid muscles
   C. Infrahyoid muscles
   D. Intrinsic tongue muscles
   E. Extrinsic tongue muscles

10. Which of the following muscle groups is innervated by the cervical nerves?
    A. Muscles of mastication
    B. Muscles of facial expression
    C. Suprahyoid muscles
    D. Infrahyoid muscles
    E. Intrinsic tongue muscles

11. Which muscle can make the patient's oral vestibule shallow, thereby making dental work difficult?
    A. Mentalis muscle
    B. Zygomaticus major muscle
    C. Depressor anguli oris muscle
    D. Levator anguli oris muscle

12. Which of the following muscle groups is innervated by the facial nerve?
    A. Intrinsic tongue muscles
    B. Extrinsic tongue muscles
    C. Muscles of facial expression
    D. Muscles of mastication

13. Which of the following muscle groups inserts directly on the hyoid bone?
    A. Geniohyoid, stylohyoid, and omohyoid muscles
    B. Masseter, stylohyoid, and digastric muscles
    C. Masseter, buccinator, and omohyoid muscles
    D. Palatopharyngeus and palatoglossus muscles and muscle of the uvula

14. Which of the following muscles is used when a patient grimaces?
    A. Epicranial muscle
    B. Corrugator supercilii muscle
    C. Risorius muscle
    D. Mentalis muscle

15. Which of the following muscles is an extrinsic muscle of the tongue?
    A. Geniohyoid muscle
    B. Hyoglossus muscle
    C. Mylohyoid muscle
    D. Transverse muscle
    E. Vertical muscle

16. Which of the following muscles compresses the cheeks during chewing, assisting the muscles of mastication?
    A. Risorius muscle
    B. Buccinator muscle
    C. Mentalis muscle
    D. Orbicularis oris muscle

17. The superior pharyngeal constrictor muscle
    A. Originates from the larynx
    B. Inserts on the median pharyngeal raphe
    C. Overlaps the stylopharyngeus muscle
    D. Is a longitudinal muscle of the pharynx

18. Which of the following statements concerning the masseter muscle is correct?
    A. Is the most superficial muscle of facial expression
    B. Originates from the zygomatic arch
    C. Inserts on the medial surface of the mandible's angle
    D. Depresses the mandible during jaw movement

19. Which of the following muscles creates the anterior faucial pillar in the oral cavity?
    A. Palatoglossus muscle
    B. Palatopharyngeus muscle
    C. Stylopharyngeus muscle
    D. Tensor veli palatini muscle

20. Which of the following situations occurs when both sternocleidomastoid muscles are used by the patient?
    A. Neck is drawn laterally
    B. Head flexes at the neck
    C. Chin moves superiorly to the opposite side
    D. Head rotates and is drawn to the shoulders

21. Which muscle does *not* aid in smiling when it contracts?
    A. Zygomatic major muscle
    B. Levator anguli oris muscle
    C. Risorius muscle
    D. Orbicularis oris muscle

22. Which muscle lies just deep to the skin of the neck?
    A. Platysma muscle
    B. Buccinator muscle
    C. Risorius muscle
    D. Mentalis muscle

23. Which muscle is most superior?
    A. Corrugator supercilii muscle
    B. Zygomatic major muscle
    C. Superior pharyngeal constrictor muscle
    D. Superior belly of the omohyoid muscle

24. Which muscle when contracted causes a frown?
    A. Zygomaticus minor muscle
    B. Levator anguli oris muscle
    C. Depressor anguli oris muscle
    D. Risorius muscle

25. Which muscle is most superficial?
    A. Masseter muscle
    B. Medial pterygoid muscle
    C. Lateral pterygoid muscle
    D. Superior pharyngeal constrictor muscle

REVIEW ACTIVITIES

1. Standing in front of a mirror showing the face and neck, locate and palpate the origin and insertion of the SCM and trapezius muscles.

2. Standing in front of a mirror showing the face, locate and palpate the muscles of facial expression and use each one as you locate it.

3. Standing in front of a mirror showing the face, locate and palpate the muscles of mastication.

4. Move through the movements of the jaws (while looking in a mirror that shows the face) and note the muscles of mastication at work for each movement, including the clenching of the teeth.

5. Start two columns on a sheet of paper, one named suprahyoid and the other named infrahyoid, and then list each muscle in relationship to the hyoid bone.

Temporomandibular Joint

5

LEARNING OBJECTIVES

After studying this chapter, the reader should be able to:

1. Define and pronounce all the key words and anatomical terms in this chapter.
2. Locate and identify the specific anatomical landmarks of the temporomandibular joint on a diagram, a skull, and a patient.
3. Describe the movements of the temporomandibular joint and their relationship to the muscles in the head and neck region.
4. Discuss the disorders of the temporomandibular joint.
5. Correctly complete the identification exercises and review questions and activities for this chapter.
6. Integrate the knowledge about the anatomy of the temporomandibular joint into the examination of the joint for disorders.

KEY WORDS

Depression of the mandible (de-**presh**-in) Lowering of the lower jaw.

Joint (joint) Site of a junction or union between two or more bones.

Lateral deviation of the mandible (de-vee-**ay**-shun) Shifting of the lower jaw to one side.

Ligament (**lig**-ah-mint) Band of fibrous tissue connecting bones.

Elevation of the mandible (el-eh-**vay**-shun) Raising of the lower jaw.

Protrusion of the mandible (pro-**troo**-shun) Bringing of the lower jaw forward.

Retraction of the mandible (re-**trak**-shun) Bringing of the lower jaw backward.

Subluxation (sub-luk-**ay**-shun) Acute episode of temporomandibular joint disorder in which both joints become dislocated often due to excessive mandibular protrusion and depression.

Temporomandibular disorder (TMD) (tem-poh-ro-man-**dib**-you-lar) Disorder involving one or both temporomandibular joints.

ANATOMY OF THE TEMPOROMANDIBULAR JOINT

A *joint* (joint) is a site of a junction or union between two or more bones. The **temporomandibular joint (TMJ)** (tem-poh-ro-man-**dib**-you-lar) is a joint on each side of the head that allows for movement of the mandible for speech and mastication. A patient may have a disease process associated with one or both of the temporomandibular joints. Thus the dental professional needs to understand the anatomy of the joint, the normal movements involved with the joint, and any possible disorders associated with the joint.

The temporomandibular joint is innervated by the mandibular division of the fifth cranial or trigeminal nerve. The blood supply to the joint is from branches of the external carotid artery.

BONES OF THE JOINT

The temporomandibular joint has two sets of articulations, one on each side of the head: the two temporal bones and the two condyles of the mandible (Figure 5–1). Both articulating bony surfaces of the joint are covered by fibrocartilage. Chapter 3 has more information on both of these bones of the joint.

Temporal Bone

The **temporal bone (tem**-poh-ral) is a cranial bone that articulates with the mandible at the TMJ (Figure 5–2). The articulating area on the temporal bone of the joint is located on the bone's inferior aspect. This articulating area includes the bone's articular eminence and articular fossa. The **articular eminence** (ar-**tik**-you-ler) is positioned anterior to the articular fossa and consists of a smooth, rounded ridge.

The **articular fossa** (ar-**tik**-you-ler) or mandibular fossa is posterior to the articular eminence and consists of a depression on the temporal bone, posterior and medial to the zygomatic process of the temporal bone (zy-go-**mat**-ik). Posterior to the articular fossa is a sharper ridge, the postglenoid process (post-**gle**-noid).

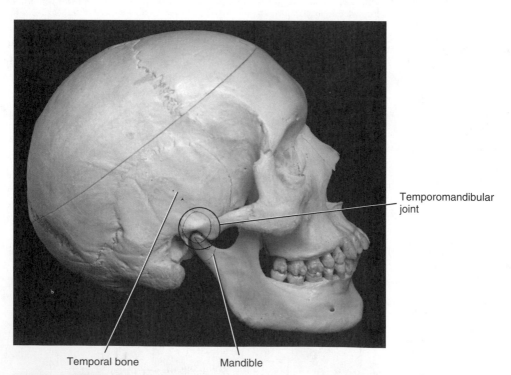

Temporomandibular joint

Temporal bone   Mandible

FIGURE 5–1 ■ Lateral view of the skull showing the temporomandibular joint with the temporal bone and mandible.

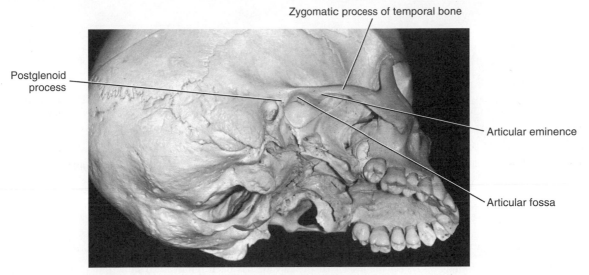

FIGURE 5–2 ■ Inferolateral view of the skull with the temporal bone.

Mandible

The **mandible (man**-di-bl) is a facial bone that articulates with the temporal bone at the head of the **condyle of the mandible** with its **articulating surface of the condyle** (ar-**tik**-you-late-ing) (Figure 5–3). Posterior to the condyle is the **coronoid process (kor**-ah-noid). The depression of the **mandibular notch** (man-**dib**-you-lar) is located between the condyle and coronoid process (Figure 3–53, lateral view of the face, showing landmarks of the mandible).

JOINT CAPSULE

A fibrous **joint capsule** completely encloses the TMJ (Figure 5–4). The capsule wraps around the margin of the temporal bone's articular eminence and articular fossa superiorly. Inferiorly, the capsule

FIGURE 5–3 ■ Anterolateral view of the mandible.

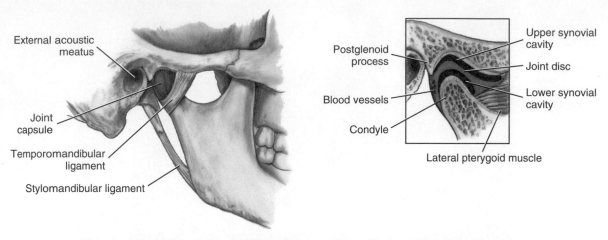

FIGURE 5–4 ■ Lateral view of the joint capsule of the temporomandibular joint and its lateral temporomandibular ligament. Note on the inset that the capsule has been removed to show the upper and lower synovial cavities and their relationship to the joint disc.

wraps around the circumference of the mandibular condyle, including the condyle's neck.

DISC OF THE JOINT

The fibrous **disc of the joint** (disk) or meniscus of the joint is located between the temporal bone and condyle of the mandible on each side (see Figure 5–4). On parasagittal section, the disc appears caplike on the mandibular condyle, with its superior aspect concavo-convex from anterior to posterior and its inferior aspect concave. This shape of the disc conforms to the shape of the adjacent articulating bones of the TMJ and is related to normal joint movements.

The disc completely divides the TMJ into two compartments or spaces. These two compartments are **synovial cavities** (sy-**no**-vee-al **kav**-i-tees), an upper synovial cavity and a lower synovial cavity. The membranes lining the inside of the joint capsule secrete **synovial fluid** that helps lubricate the joint and fills the synovial cavities.

The disc is attached to the lateral and medial poles of the mandibular condyle. The disc is not attached to the temporal bone anteriorly, except indirectly through the capsule. Posteriorly, the disc is divided into two areas. The upper division of the posterior portion of the disc is attached to the temporal bone's postglenoid process, and the lower division attaches to the neck of the condyle. The disc blends with the capsule at these points.

This posterior area of attachment of the disc to the capsule is one of the places where nerves and blood vessels enter the joint.

As a person ages, the disc can become thinner or even perforated. Recent studies suggest that disc degeneration, which may occur as a result of aging or mechanical stress, causes calcifications within the disc. At any age, the disc may become dislocated forward by injury to the posterior attachment. Both perforation and displacement can lead to clinical problems (discussed later in this chapter).

LIGAMENTS ASSOCIATED WITH THE JOINT

A *ligament* (**lig**-ah-mint) is a band of fibrous tissue connecting bones. There are three paired ligaments associated with the TMJ. These ligaments are the temporomandibular joint ligament, sphenomandibular ligament, and stylomandibular ligament (Figure 5–5).

Temporomandibular Joint Ligament

The **temporomandibular joint ligament** (tem-poh-ro-man-**dib**-you-lar) is located on the lateral side of each joint and forms a reinforcement of the capsule of the TMJ. This ligament prevents the excessive retraction or moving backward of the mandible, a situation that might lead to problems with the TMJ.

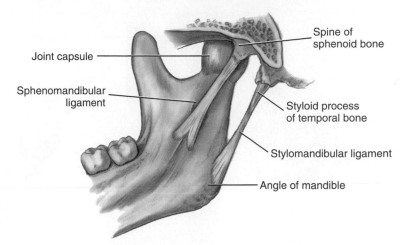

Spine of
sphenoid bone

Joint capsule

Sphenomandibular
ligament

Styloid process
of temporal bone

Stylomandibular ligament

Angle of mandible

FIGURE 5–5 ■ Internal view of the temporomandibular joint with associated ligaments.

Sphenomandibular Ligament

The **sphenomandibular ligament** (sfe-no-man-**dib**-you-lar) is not a part of the TMJ. It is located on the medial side of the mandible, some distance from the joint. This ligament runs from the angular spine of the sphenoid bone to the lingula of the mandibular foramen. It is a vestige of the embryonic lower jaw, Meckel's cartilage. The inferior alveolar nerve descends between the sphenomandibular ligament and the ramus of the mandible to gain access to the mandibular foramen.

The sphenomandibular ligament becomes accentuated and taut when the mandible is protruded. The sphenomandibular ligament is a landmark for the administration of a local anesthetic for the inferior alveolar block (see Chapter 9 for more information).

Stylomandibular Ligament

The **stylomandibular ligament** (sty-lo-man-**dib**-you-lar) is a variable ligament that is formed from a thickened cervical fascia in the area. This ligament runs from the styloid process of the temporal bone to the angle of the mandible. This ligament also becomes taut when the mandible is protruded.

▓ JAW MOVEMENTS WITH MUSCLE RELATIONSHIPS

The TMJ allows for the movement of the mandible during speech and mastication. There are two basic types of movement performed by the joint and its associated muscles: a gliding movement and a rotational movement.

The gliding movement of the TMJ occurs mainly between the disc and the articular eminence of the temporal bone in the upper synovial cavity, with the disc plus the condyle moving forward or backward down and up the articular eminence. The gliding movement allows the lower jaw to move forward or backward. Bringing the lower jaw forward involves *protrusion of the mandible* (pro-**troo**-shun). Bringing the lower jaw backward involves *retraction of the mandible* (re-**trak**-shun). Protrusion involves the bilateral contraction of the lateral pterygoid muscles. The posterior portions of both temporalis muscles are involved during retraction of the mandible.

The rotational movement of the TMJ occurs mainly between the disc and the condyle of the mandible in the lower synovial cavity. The axis of rotation of the disc plus the condyle is transverse, and the movements accomplished are depression or elevation of the mandible. *Depression of the mandible* (de-**presh**-in) is the lowering of the lower jaw. *Elevation of the mandible* (el-eh-**vay**-shun) is the raising of the lower jaw.

With these two types of movement, gliding and rotation, and with the right and left TMJs working together, the finer movements of the jaw can be accomplished. These include opening and closing the jaws and shifting the lower jaw to one side (Figure 5–6).

Opening the jaws during speech and mastication involves both depression and protrusion of

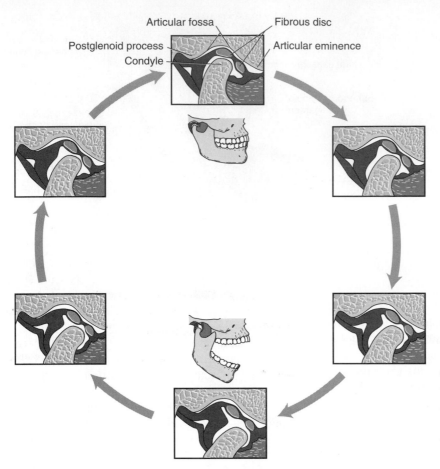

Articular fossa

Fibrous disc

Postglenoid process

Articular eminence

Condyle

FIGURE 5–6 ■ Movements of the mandible related to the temporomandibular joint to show opening and closing of the mouth. (From Bath-Balogh M. Fehrenbach MJ. *Illustrated Dental Embryology, Histology, and Anatomy*. Philadelphia, WB Saunders, 1997.)

the mandible. When the jaws close, this involves both elevation and retraction of the mandible. Thus opening and closing the jaws involve a combination of gliding and rotational movements of the TMJs in their respective joint cavities. The disc plus the condyle glide on the articular fossa in the upper synovial cavity, moving forward or backward on the articular eminence. Roughly at the same time, the condyle of the mandible rotates on the disc in the lower synovial cavity.

The muscles of mastication involved in elevating the mandible, during closing the jaws, are the bilateral masseter, temporalis, and medial pterygoid muscles (see Chapter 4 for more information). The anterior suprahyoid muscles are involved in depressing the mandible, during opening the jaws, when they bilaterally contract as the hyoid bone is stabilized by the other hyoid muscles (see Chapter 4 for more information). The inferior heads of the lateral pterygoid muscles may also be involved in depressing the mandible during opening the jaws.

Lateral deviation (de-vee-**ay**-shun) or lateral excursion of the mandible or shifting the lower jaw to one side occurs during mastication. Lateral deviation involves both the gliding and rotational movements of the opposite TMJs in their respective joint cavities. During lateral deviation, one disc plus the condyle glide forward and medially on the articular eminence in the upper synovial cavity, while the other condyle and disc remain relatively stable in position in the articular fossa. This produces a rotation around the more stable condyle.

Contraction of one of the lateral pterygoid muscles (the one on the protruding side) is involved during lateral deviation. When the mandible laterally deviates to the left, the right lateral pterygoid muscle contracts, moving the right condyle forward while the left condyle stays in position, thus causing the mandible to move to the left. The reverse situation occurs when the mandible laterally deviates to the right.

During mastication, the power stroke (when the teeth crunch the food) involves a movement from a laterally deviated position back to the midline. If the food is on the right, the mandible will be deviated to the right by the left lateral pterygoid muscle. The power stroke will return the mandible to the center, so the movement is to the left and involves a retraction of the left side. This is accomplished by the left posterior portion of the temporalis muscle. At the same time, all the closing jaw muscles on the right side contract to crush the food. The reverse situation occurs if the food is on the left.

PALPATION OF THE JOINT

To palpate the joint and its associated muscles effectively, have the patient go through all the movements of the mandible (Table 5-1). The TMJ can be palpated just anterior to the external acoustic meatus of each ear (Figure 5–7). To assess the entire joint and its associated muscles effectively, use bilateral palpation and ask the patient to open and close the mouth several times; then ask the patient to move the opened jaw left, then right, and then forward. Using digital palpation for the mandible moving at the temporomandibular joint, gently place a finger into the outer portion of the external acoustic meatus (Figure 5–8). Auscultation of the joint can also be done.

FIGURE 5–7 ■ Palpation of the patient during movements of both of the temporomandibular joints.

DISORDERS OF THE JOINT

A patient may have a disease process associated with one or both of the temporomandibular joints or a *temporomandibular disorder (TMD)* (tem-poh-ro-man-**dib**-you lar). The patient may experience chronic joint tenderness, swelling, and painful muscle spasms. Also present may be difficulties of joint movement, such as a limited or deviated mandibular opening. The dental professional plays an important role in the recognition, treatment, and maintenance of patients with this disorder.

Table 5–1 MOVEMENT OF MANDIBLE AND TMJ WITH ASSOCIATED MUSCLES

Mandibular Movements	TMJ Movements	Associated Muscles
Protrusion of mandible, moving lower jaw forward	Gliding in both upper synovial cavities	Lateral pterygoid, bilateral contraction
Retraction of mandible, moving lower jaw backward	Gliding in both upper synovial cavities	Posterior portion of temporalis, bilateral contraction
Elevation and retraction of mandible, closing jaws	Gliding in both upper synovial cavities and rotation in both lower synovial cavities	Masseter, temporalis, and medial pterygoid, bilateral contraction
Depression and protrusion of mandible, opening jaws	Gliding in both upper synovial cavities and rotation in both lower synovial cavities	Suprahyoids and inferior heads of lateral pterygoid, bilateral contraction
Lateral deviation of mandible, to shift lower jaw to opposite side	Gliding in one upper synovial cavity and rotation in opposite upper synovial cavity	Lateral pterygoid, unilateral contraction.

FIGURE 5–8 ■ Palpation of the joint by gently placing a finger into the outer portion of the external acoustic meatus.

Recognition of TMD includes palpation of the joint as the patient performs all the movements of the joint, as well as palpation of the related muscles of mastication. All signs and symptoms related to TMD, such as the amount of mandibular opening and facial pain, need to be recorded by the dental professional, as well as any parafunctional habits and related systemic diseases. The patient may have the traditional skull radiograph of the joint area, or magnetic resonance imaging (MRI) may be performed to aid in the diagnosis of TMD. MRI is a noninvasive nuclear procedure for imaging soft tissue of high fat and water content. Thus MRI can make it possible to distinguish normal tissue from diseased tissue (Figure 5–9).

There are many controversies associated with the etiology of these disorders. TMD is a heterogeneous, complex disorder involving many factors such as behavioral stressors and parafunctional habits such as clenching and bruxism. Clenching is the prolonged holding of the teeth together by the masticatory muscles. The normal condition is for the teeth to be slightly parted at rest and the muscles relaxed. Bruxism is habitual grinding of the teeth, especially at night.

Patients who clench or grind their teeth may or may not be aware of their parafunctional jaw movements. The masseter muscle may be overdeveloped in these patients, and the teeth may show abnormal wear. Clenching and bruxism are not caused by malocclusion, but both appear to be processes of the central nervous system.

Trauma to the jaw may cause TMD with the disc having adhesions to the bony surfaces, but it is not the most common etiological factor. Systemic diseases such as osteoarthritis may involve portions of the TMJ and contribute to TMD. Aging of the disc that causes wear and hardening may also be a factor in TMD, yet TMD does not become worse with age.

Most TMD cases are noted in females, with the average age at 39 years, possibly because women are more likely to seek treatment. Some researchers theorize that changes in female hormones may play

FIGURE 5–9 ■ Magnetic resonance imaging of both temporomandibular joints of a patient. A: Right side with a normal position of the disc (arrows) in relationship to the condyle (C). B: Left side with a displacement of the disc (arrows) in relationship to the condyle (C). (From Ibsen OAC, Phelan JA. *Oral Pathology for Dental Hygienists.* Philadelphia, WB Saunders, 1996.)

a role in the pathogenesis of TMD in women. More studies need to be done in this area of etiology.

Not all patients with TMD have abnormalities in the joint disc or the joint itself. Most symptoms seem to come from the muscles. Most recent studies do not support the role of TMD in directly causing headaches, neck or back pain, or instability. Headaches are usually caused by muscle tension or vascular changes. Cyclic episodes of TMD and other incidents of chronic body pain are commonly encountered in the TMD population.

Joint sounds occur because of disc derangement. The posterior portion of the disc gets caught between the condyle head and the articular eminence. Joint sounds are not a reliable indicator of TMD since they can change over time in a patient. Thus the clicking, grinding, and popping of the joint during movement that is commonly present with TMD is also found in 40–60 percent of persons without TMD.

There are also many controversies in the treatment of TMD. Most recent studies have determined that malocclusion and occlusal discrepancies are not involved in most cases of TMD. Thus occlusal adjustment, repositioning the jaw, and orthodontic treatment are not the treatments of choice for all patients with TMD, nor do these treatments seem to prevent TMD. Less than half of the patients with TMD seek treatment for their disorder.

Most patients with TMD do well over time with inexpensive and reversible treatments, including patient-based or prescription pain control, relaxation therapy, stress management, habit control, moderate home-based muscular exercises, and flat plane non-repositioning oral splints. These inexpensive and reversible treatments now have the same success as more expensive and irreversible treatments. Thus only a few TMD patients (1–2 percent) require surgery or other extensive treatment. Surgery of the TMJ can now involve arthroscopy with an endoscope and lasers.

An acute episode of TMD can occur when a patient opens the mouth too wide by causing maximal depression and protrusion of the mandible, as when yawning or receiving prolonged dental care. This causes ***subluxation*** (sub-luks-**ay**-shun) or dislocation of both joints. Subluxation happens when the head of each condyle moves too far anterior on the articular eminence. When the patient tries to close and elevate the mandible, the condylar heads cannot move posteriorly because the muscles have become spastic.

Treatment of subluxation consists of relaxing these muscles and carefully moving the mandible downward and back. The condylar heads will then be able to assume the normal posterior position in relationship to the articular eminence by the muscular action of the elevating muscles of mastication. Future care of these patients involves avoidance of extreme depression of the mandible.

IDENTIFICATION EXERCISES

Identify the structures on the following diagrams by filling in the blanks with the correct anatomical term. You can check your answers by looking back at the figure indicated in parentheses for each identification diagram.

1. (Figure 5–4)

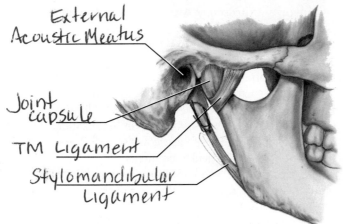

External Acoustic Meatus

Joint capsule

TM Ligament

Stylomandibular Ligament

Postglenoid process

Blood vessels

Condyle

UPPER SYNOVIAL CAVITY

Joint Disc

LOWER SYNOVIAL CAVITY

LATERAL PTERYGOID MUSCLE

2. (Figure 5–5)

JOINT CAPSULE

SPHENOMANDIBULAR LIGAMENT

SPINE OF SPHENOID

STYLOID PROCESS OF TEMPORAL BONE

STYLOMANDIBULAR LIGAMENT

ANGLE OF MANDIBLE

REVIEW QUESTIONS

1. Which of the following ligaments associated with the temporomandibular joint reinforces the joint capsule?
   A. Styloid ligament
   B. Stylomandibular ligament
   C. Temporomandibular ligament
   D. Sphenomandibular ligament

2. Which of the following landmarks is located on the mandible?
   A. Articular eminence
   B. Coronoid process
   C. Articular fossa
   D. Postglenoid process

3. Which of the following is a basic movement performed by the temporomandibular joint?
   A. Gliding movement only
   B. Rotational movement only
   C. Gliding and rotational movement
   D. No movement is performed

4. Which of the following muscles is involved in the lateral deviation of the mandible?
   A. Masseter muscle
   B. Medial pterygoid muscle
   C. Lateral pterygoid muscle
   D. Temporalis muscle
   E. Digastric muscle

5. Protrusion of the mandible primarily involves
   A. Opening the jaws
   B. Closing the jaws
   C. Bringing the lower jaw forward
   D. Bringing the lower jaw backward
   E. Shifting the lower jaw to one side

6. Which of the following movements is assisted by the temporalis muscle?
   A. Mandibular depression only
   B. Mandibular elevation only
   C. Mandibular retraction only
   D. Mandibular depression and elevation
   E. Mandibular elevation and retraction

7. Which of the following ligaments associated with the temporomandibular joint has the inferior alveolar nerve descend nearby to gain access to the mandibular foramen?
   A. Sphenomandibular ligament only
   B. Stylomandibular ligament only
   C. Temporomandibular ligament only
   D. Sphenomandibular and stylomandibular ligaments
   E. Stylomandibular and temporomandibular ligaments

8. Which of the following statements about the temporomandibular disc is false?
   A. The disc separates the TMJ into synovial cavities.
   B. The disc is attached anteriorly and posteriorly to the condyle.
   C. Gliding movements take place between the disc and the temporal bone.
   D. The inferior surface of the disc is concave.

9. Which area of the mandible articulates with the temporal bone at the temporomandibular joint?
   A. Lingula
   B. Mandibular notch
   C. Coronoid process
   D. Condyle

10. During both mandibular protrusion and retraction, the rotation of the articulating surface of the mandible against the disc in the lower synovial cavity is prevented by the
    A. Facial muscles
    B. Infrahyoid muscles
    C. Muscles of mastication
    D. Ligaments of the temporomandibular joint

11. Which structure secretes synovial fluid?
    A. Mandibular condyle
    B. Disc of the joint
    C. Inner membranes lining the capsule
    D. Lateral pterygoid muscle

12. Which list is in order, from the most anterior structure to the most posterior structure?
    A. Articular fossa, postglenoid process, articular eminence
    B. Condyle, coronoid process, mandibular notch
    C. Articular eminence, articular fossa, postglenoid process
    D. Coronoid process, condyle, mandibular notch

13. At what position does a displaced disc usually lie?
    A. Anterior to its usual position
    B. Posterior to its usual position
    C. In the articular fossa
    D. In the mandibular notch

14. The joint capsule wraps around which structure?
    A. Coronoid process
    B. Mandibular notch
    C. Condyle
    D. Zygomatic arch

15. Which situation occurs with subluxation of the joint?
    A. Head of condyle moves too far anterior on articular eminence
    B. Neck of condyle moves too far posterior on articular eminence
    C. Coronoid process moves too far anterior on articular eminence
    D. Coronoid process moves too far posterior on articular eminence

REVIEW ACTIVITIES

1. While holding a skull, locate the bony land-marks involved in the TMJ.

2. While holding a skull, move the mandible through all the movements of the TMJ, noting the location of the ligaments associated with the joint.

3. Move through the movements of your jaws while looking in a mirror that shows your face, noting the gliding and rotational movements of the TMJ and how they are related to the synovial cavities.

4. Have a patient (or peer) move the jaws through all the movements while you are palpating the TMJ, pointing out the muscles associated with each movement.

Blood Supply

CHAPTER OUTLINE

This chapter discusses the following topics:

LEARNING OBJECTIVES

After studying this chapter, the reader should be able to:

1. Define and pronounce all the key words and anatomical terms in this chapter.
2. Identify and trace the routes of the blood vessels of the head and neck on a diagram, a skull, and a patient.
3. Discuss the types of lesions that can occur with blood vessels in the head and neck region.
4. Correctly complete the identification exercises and review questions and activities for this chapter.
5. Integrate the knowledge about the head and neck blood supply into clinical practice when a vascular problem is present, especially from a local anesthetic injection or during the spread of dental infection or cancerous cells by the blood.

KEY WORDS

Anastomosis/anastomoses (ah-nas-tah-**moe**-sis, ah-nas-tah-**moe**-sees) Communication of a blood vessel with another by a connecting channel.

Arteriole (ar-**ter**-ee-ole) Smaller artery that branches off an artery and connects with a capillary.

Artery (**ar**-ter-ee) Type of blood vessel that carries blood away from the heart.

Bacteremia (bak-ter-**ee**-me-ah) Bacteria traveling within the blood system.

Capillary (**kap**-i-lare-ee) Smaller blood vessel that branches off an arteriole to supply blood directly to tissue.

Carotid pulse (kah-**rot**-id) Reliable pulse palpated from the common carotid artery.

Embolus/emboli (**em**-bol-us, **em**-bol-eye) Foreign material or thrombus traveling in the blood that can block the vessel.

Hematoma (hee-mah-**toe**-mah) Bruise that results when a blood vessel is injured and a small amount of blood escapes into the surrounding tissue and clots.

Hemorrhage (**hem**-ah-rij) Large amounts of blood that escape into the surrounding tissue without clotting when a blood vessel is seriously injured.

Plexus (**plek**-sis) Network of blood vessels, usually veins.

Thrombus/thrombi (**throm**-bus, **throm**-by) Clot that forms on the inner blood vessel wall.

Vein (vane) Type of blood vessel that travels to the heart carrying blood.

Venous sinus (**vee**-nus **sy**-nus) Blood-filled space between two layers of tissue.

Venule (**ven**-yule) Smaller vein that drains the capillaries of the tissue area and then joins larger veins.

VASCULAR SYSTEM

The vascular system of the head and neck, as is the case in the rest of the body, consists of an arterial blood supply, a capillary network, and venous drainage. The dental professional will need to be able to locate the larger blood vessels of the head and neck since these vessels may become compromised owing to a disease process or during a dental procedure, such as a local anesthetic injection. Blood vessels may also spread infection in the head and neck area (see Chapter 12 for more information). The blood vessels may also spread cancerous cells from a tumor to distant sites and at a more rapid rate than lymphatic vessels.

Blood vessels are less numerous than lymphatic vessels, yet the venous portion mainly parallels the lymphatic vessels in location (see Chapter 10 for more information). A large network of blood vessels is called a *plexus* (**plek**-sis). The head and neck area contains certain important venous plexuses. Blood vessels also may communicate with each other by an *anastomosis* (plural, *anastomoses*) (ah-nas-tah-**moe-sis**, **ah-nas-tah**-moe-sees), a connecting channel between the vessels.

An *artery* (**ar**-ter-ee) is a component of the blood system that arises from the heart carrying blood away from it. Each artery starts as a large vessel and branches into smaller vessels, each one a smaller artery or an *arteriole* (ar-**ter**-ee-ole). Each arteriole branches into even smaller vessels until it becomes a network of capillaries. Each *capillary* (**kap**-i-lare-ee) is smaller than an arteriole and is able to supply blood to a large tissue area only because there are so many of them.

A *vein* (vane) is another component of the blood system. A vein, unlike an artery, travels to the heart carrying blood. Valves in the veins are mostly absent in the head and neck area, unlike in the rest of the body. This leads to two-way flow dictated by local pressure changes, which is the reason that facial or dental infections can lead to serious complications (discussed in Chapter 12). After each smaller vein or *venule* (**ven**-yule) drains the capillaries of the tissue area, the venules coalesce to become larger veins. Veins are much larger and more numerous than arteries. Veins anastomose freely and have a greater variability in location in comparison to arteries.

There are also different kinds of venous networks found in the body. Superficial veins are found immediately below the skin. Deeper veins usually accompany larger arteries in a more protected location within the tissue. A *venous sinus* (**vee**-nus **sy**-nus) is a blood-filled space between the two layers of tissue. All these networks are connected with each other by anastomoses.

It is important to review the pathways of the arteries and veins as they exit and then enter the heart so as to understand the origins of the blood vessels of the head and neck. After the basic origins of the blood supply to the head and neck are understood, diagrams of the blood vessels overlying the skull figure are very helpful in studying this system. Relating the tissues supplied and the area's blood vessels is an additional way of understanding the location of the various blood vessels. It is important to remember that unlike innervation supplied by the nerves to the muscles, which is a one-to-one relationship, blood supply is regional. Arteries supply all structures in their vicinity, and veins receive blood from all close-by structures.

ARTERIAL BLOOD SUPPLY TO THE HEAD AND NECK

The major arteries that supply the head and neck are the common carotid and subclavian arteries. The origins from the heart to the head and neck of these two arteries are different depending on the side of the body considered. The other arteries of the head and neck are symmetrically located on each side of the body.

ORIGINS TO THE HEAD AND NECK

The origins from the heart of the common carotid and subclavian arteries that supply the head and neck are different for the right and left sides of the body (Figure 6–1). For the left side of the body, the common carotid and subclavian arteries arise directly from the aorta (**ay**-or-tah). For the right side of the body, the common carotid and subclavian arteries are both branches from the brachiocephalic artery. The

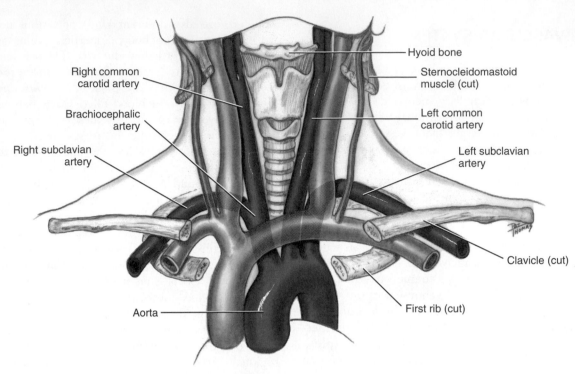

FIGURE 6–1 ■ Origins from the heart of the arterial blood supply for the head and neck highlighting the pathways of the common carotid and subclavian arteries. Note that the pathways are different in the right and left sides of the body.

brachiocephalic artery (bray-kee-o-sah-**fal**-ik) is a direct branch of the aorta.

The **common carotid artery** (**kom**-in kah-**rot**-id) is branchless and travels up the neck, lateral to the trachea and larynx, to the upper border of the thyroid cartilage (Figure 6–1). The common carotid artery travels in a sheath beneath the sternocleidomastoid muscle. This sheath also contains the internal jugular vein and the tenth cranial or vagus nerve. The common carotid artery ends by dividing into the internal and external carotid arteries at about the level of the larynx (Figure 6–2).

Just before the common carotid artery bifurcates into the internal and external carotid arteries, it exhibits a swelling called the **carotid sinus** (kah-rot-id **sy**-nus) (Figure 6–2). When the common carotid artery is palpated against the larynx, the most reliable arterial pulse of the body can be monitored. If the anterior border of the sternocleidomastoid muscle is rolled posteriorly at the level of the thyroid cartilage of the larynx ('Adam's apple'), the *carotid pulse* can be felt in the groove of tissue produced. This pulse is most reliable since the common carotid is a major artery supplying the brain and therefore in an emergency situation

(cardiopulmonary resuscitation) remains palpable when peripheral arteries such as the radial artery are not. The carotid pulse also is easily accessible during dental treatment.

The **subclavian artery** (sub-**klay**-vee-an) arises lateral to the common carotid artery (see Figure 6–1). The subclavian artery gives off branches to supply both intracranial and extracranial structures, but its major destination is the upper extremity (arm).

INTERNAL CAROTID ARTERY

The **internal carotid artery** (kah-**rot**-id) is a division that travels upward in a slightly lateral position (in relationship to the external carotid artery) after leaving the common carotid artery (see Figure 6–2). This artery is hidden by the sternocleidomastoid muscle of the neck. The internal carotid artery has no branches in the neck but continues adjacent to the internal jugular vein within the carotid sheath to the skull base, where it enters the cranium. The internal carotid artery supplies intracranial

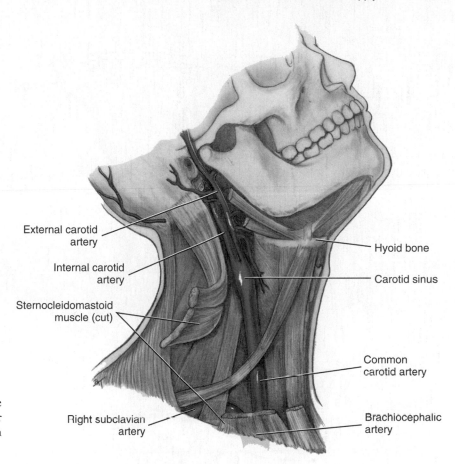

External carotid artery

Internal carotid artery

Sternocleidomastoid muscle (cut)

Right subclavian artery

Hyoid bone

Carotid sinus

Common carotid artery

Brachiocephalic artery

FIGURE 6–2 ■ Pathway of the internal carotid artery after branching off the common carotid artery.

structures and is the source of the **ophthalmic artery (of**-thal-mic), which supplies the eye, orbit, and lacrimal gland.

EXTERNAL CAROTID ARTERY

The **external carotid artery** (kah-**rot**-id) travels upward in a more medial position (to the internal carotid artery) after arising from the common carotid artery (Figure 6–3). The external carotid artery supplies the extracranial tissues of the head and neck, including the oral cavity. The external carotid artery has four sets of branches grouped according to their location to the main artery: the anterior, medial, posterior, and terminal branches (Table 6–1).

Anterior Branches of the External Carotid Artery

There are three anterior branches from the external carotid artery: the superior thyroid, lingual, and

facial arteries (Figure 6–4). The lingual and facial arteries continue to divide to serve areas of the head and neck that are of interest to dental professionals.

SUPERIOR THYROID ARTERY

The **superior thyroid artery** (thy-roid) is an anterior branch from the external carotid artery (see Figure 6–4). The superior thyroid artery has branches: the infrahyoid branch (in-frah-**hi**-oid), sternocleidomastoid branch (stir-no-klii-do-**mass**-toid), superior laryngeal artery (lah-**rin**-je-al), and superior and inferior thyroid. These branches supply the tissues inferior to the hyoid bone, including the infrahyoid muscles, sternocleidomastoid muscle, muscles of the larynx, and thyroid gland.

LINGUAL ARTERY

The **lingual artery** is an anterior branch from the external carotid artery and arises above the superior thyroid artery at the level of the hyoid bone (see Figure 6–4). The lingual artery travels anteriorly to the apex of the tongue by way of its inferior surface. The lingual artery supplies the

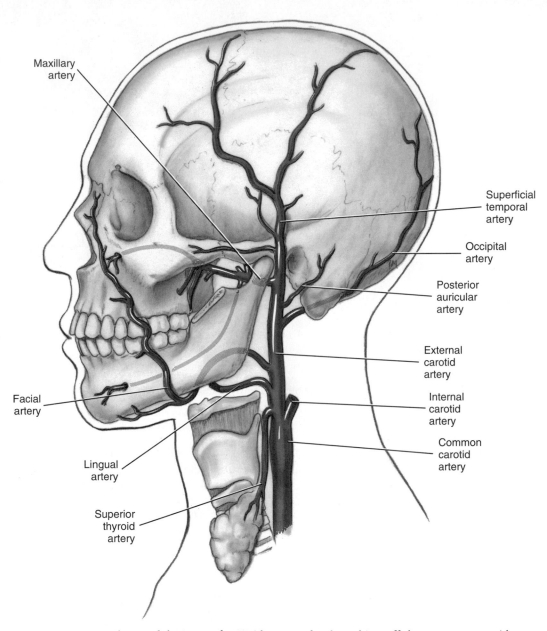

FIGURE 6–3 ■ Pathway of the external carotid artery after branching off the common carotid artery. Note that the medial branch of the external carotid artery, the ascending pharyngeal artery, cannot be seen in this view.

tissues superior to the hyoid bone, including the suprahyoid muscles and floor of the mouth by the dorsal lingual, deep lingual, sublingual, and suprahyoid branches.

The tongue is also supplied by branches of the lingual artery, including several small dorsal lingual branches to the base and body, and the deep lingual

artery, the terminal part of the lingual artery, to the apex.

The **sublingual artery** (sub-**ling**-gwal) supplies the mylohyoid muscle, sublingual salivary gland, and mucous membranes of the floor of the mouth. The small suprahyoid branch (soo-prah-**hi**-oid) supplies the suprahyoid muscles.

Table 6–1 BRANCHES OF THE EXTERNAL CAROTID ARTERY

Branches of External Carotid Artery	Position of Branches	Further Branches
Superior thyroid	Anterior	Superior and inferior thyroid, infrahyoid, superior laryngeal and sternocleidomastoid
Lingual	Anterior	Dorsal lingual, deep lingual, sublingual, and suprahyoid
Facial	Anterior	Ascending palatine, glandular, submental, inferior labial, superior labial, and angular
Ascending pharyngeal	Medial	Pharyngeal and meningeal
Occipital	Posterior	Muscular, sternocleidomastoid, auricular, and meningeal
Posterior auricular	Posterior	Auricular and stylomastoid
Superficial temporal	Terminal	Transverse facial, middle temporal, frontal, and parietal
Maxillary	Terminal	See Table 6–2

FACIAL ARTERY

The **facial artery** is the final anterior branch from the external carotid artery (Figures 6–4 and 6–5). The facial artery arises slightly superior to the lingual artery as it branches off anteriorly. Sometimes the facial and lingual arteries share a common trunk. The facial artery has a complicated path as it runs medial to the mandible, over the submandibular salivary gland, and then around the mandible's lower border to its lateral side.

From the lower border of the mandible, the facial artery runs anteriorly and superiorly near the angle of the mouth and along the side of the nose. The facial artery terminates at the medial canthus of the eye. Thus the facial artery supplies the face in the oral, buccal, zygomatic, nasal, infraorbital, and orbital regions.

The facial artery is paralleled by the facial vein in the head area, although they do not run together. In the neck, the artery is separated from the vein by the posterior belly of the digastric muscle, stylohyoid muscle, and submandibular salivary gland. The facial artery's major branches include the ascending palatine, submandibular, submental, inferior labial, superior labial, and angular arteries.

FIGURE 6–4 ■ Pathways of the lingual artery and superior thyroid artery.

Angular
artery

Superior
labial artery

Inferior
labial artery

Submental
artery

Submandibular
salivary gland

Parotid
gland (cut)

Ascending palatine artery

Facial artery

Lingual artery

External carotid artery

FIGURE 6–5 ■ Pathway of the facial artery.

The **ascending palatine artery** (ah-**send**-ing **pal**-ah-tine) is the first branch from the facial artery (see Figure 6–5). The ascending palatine artery supplies the soft palate, palatine muscles, and palatine tonsils and can be the source of the serious blood loss or hemorrhage that may occur if it is injured during a tonsillectomy (blood vessel lesions are discussed later in this chapter).

The glandular branches and **submental artery** (sub-**men**-tal) are branches from the facial artery that supply the submandibular lymph nodes, submandibular salivary gland, and mylohyoid and digastric muscles.

The **inferior labial artery** is another branch from the facial artery that supplies the lower lip tissues, including the muscles of facial expression, such as the depressor anguli oris muscle. The **superior labial artery** is also a branch from the facial artery that supplies the upper lip tissues.

The **angular artery** (**ang**-u-lar) is the termination of the facial artery and supplies the tissues along the side of the nose (see Figure 6–5).

Medial Branch of the External Carotid Artery

There is only one medial branch from the external carotid artery, the small **ascending pharyngeal artery** (ah-**send**-ing fah-**rin**-je-al), that arises close to the origin of the external carotid artery and cannot be seen in most lateral views of the head and neck. The ascending pharyngeal artery has many small branches, such as the pharyngeal branches (fah-**rin**-je-al) and meningeal branches (me-**nin**-je-al) which supply the pharyngeal walls (where they anastomose with the ascending palatine artery), soft palate, and meninges of the brain.

Posterior Branches of the External Carotid Artery

There are two posterior branches of the external carotid artery: the occipital artery and posterior auricular artery (Figure 6–6).

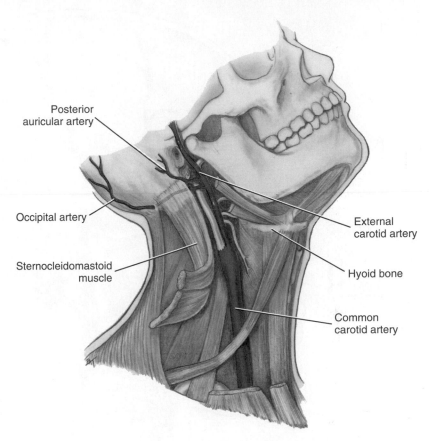

Posterior
auricular artery

Occipital artery

Sternocleidomastoid
muscle

External
carotid artery

Hyoid bone

Common
carotid artery

FIGURE 6–6 ■ Pathways of the occipital artery and posterior auricular artery.

OCCIPITAL ARTERY

The **occipital artery** (ok-**sip**-it-al), a posterior branch of the external carotid artery, arises from the external carotid artery as it passes upward behind the ascending ramus of the mandible, and travels to the posterior portion of the scalp (see Figure 6–6). The occipital artery supplies the suprahyoid and sternocleidomastoid muscles, as well as the scalp and meningeal tissues in the occipital region. The artery supplies these regions through the muscular branches, sternocleidomastoid branches (stir-no-klii-do-**mass**-toid), auricular (aw-**rik**-yule-lar), and meningeal branches (me-**nin**-je-al). At its origin, the occipital artery is closely related to the twelfth cranial or hypoglossal nerve.

POSTERIOR AURICULAR ARTERY

The small **posterior auricular artery** (aw-**rik**-yule-lar) is also a posterior branch of the external carotid artery (see Figure 6–6). The posterior auricular artery arises superior to the occipital

artery and stylohyoid muscle about the level of the tip of the styloid process. The posterior auricular artery supplies the internal ear by its auricular branch and the mastoid air cells by the **stylomastoid artery** (sty-lo-**mass**-toid).

Terminal Branches of the External Carotid Artery

There are two terminal branches of the external carotid artery, the superficial temporal artery and the maxillary artery (Figures 6–7, 6–8, and 6–9). The external carotid artery splits into these terminal branches within the parotid salivary gland. In addition, both terminal branches give rise to many important arteries in the head and neck area.

SUPERFICIAL TEMPORAL ARTERY

The **superficial temporal artery** (**tem**-poh-ral) is the smaller terminal branch of the external carotid artery (see Figure 6–7). The artery arises

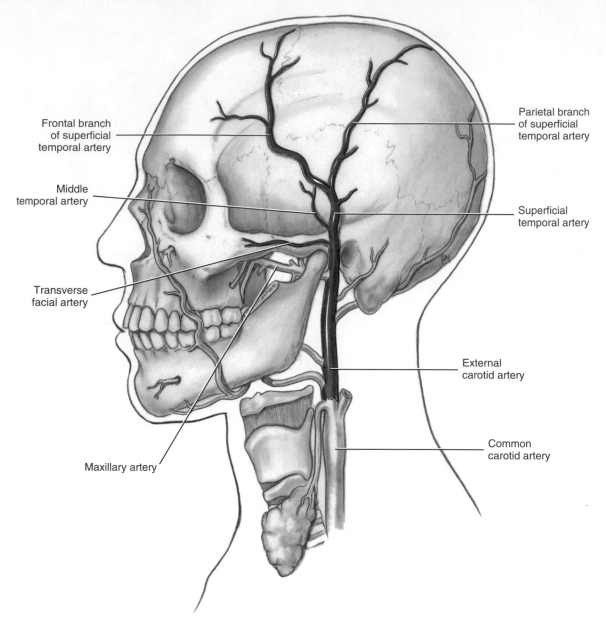

Frontal branch
of superficial
temporal artery

Parietal branch
of superficial
temporal artery

Middle
temporal artery

Superficial
temporal artery

Transverse
facial artery

External
carotid artery

Common
carotid artery

Maxillary artery

FIGURE 6–7 ■ Pathway of the superficial temporal artery.

within the parotid salivary gland. This artery can sometimes be visible in patients under the skin of the temporal region. The superficial temporal artery has several branches, including the transverse facial artery, middle temporal artery, frontal branch, and parietal branch.

The small **transverse facial artery** supplies the parotid salivary gland duct and nearby facial tissues. The equally small **middle temporal artery** (**tem**-poh-ral) supplies the temporalis muscle. The

frontal branch (**frunt**-il) and parietal branch (**pah-ry**-it-il) both supply portions of the scalp in the frontal and parietal regions.

MAXILLARY ARTERY

The **maxillary artery** (**mak**-sil-lare-ee) is the larger terminal branch of the external carotid artery (see Figures 6–8 and 6–9). The maxillary artery begins at the neck of the mandibular condyle within the parotid salivary gland. The maxillary artery runs

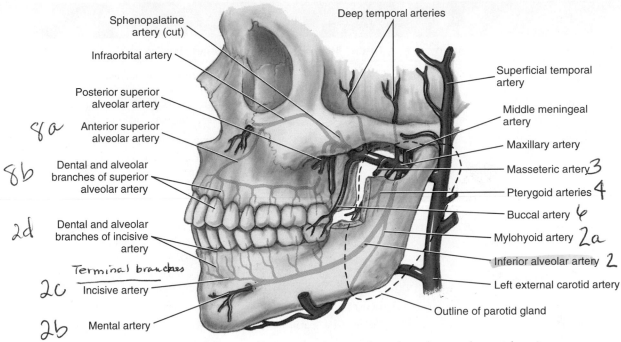

Sphenopalatine artery (cut)

Infraorbital artery

Posterior superior alveolar artery

Anterior superior alveolar artery

8a

Dental and alveolar branches of superior alveolar artery

8b

Dental and alveolar branches of incisive artery

2d

Terminal branches

Incisive artery

2c

Mental artery

2b

Deep temporal arteries

Superficial temporal artery

Middle meningeal artery

Maxillary artery

Masseteric artery 3

Pterygoid arteries 4

Buccal artery 6

Mylohyoid artery 2a

Inferior alveolar artery 2

Left external carotid artery

Outline of parotid gland

FIGURE 6–8 ■ Pathway of the maxillary artery (except those branches to the nasal cavity and palate).

between the mandible and the sphenomandibular ligament anteriorly and superiorly through the infratemporal fossa. The artery may run either superficial or deep to the lateral pterygoid muscle.

After traversing the infratemporal fossa, the maxillary artery enters the pterygopalatine fossa. The pterygopalatine fossa is behind and below the eye (see Chapter 3 for more information). Within the infratemporal and pterygopalatine fossae, the maxillary artery gives off many branches. The branches within the infratemporal fossa include the middle meningeal and inferior alveolar arteries and several arteries to muscles (Table 6–2).

The **middle meningeal artery** (meh-**nin**-je-al) supplies the meninges of the brain by way of the foramen spinosum, located on the inferior surface of the skull, as well as the skull bones (see Figure 6–8).

The **inferior alveolar artery** (al-**ve**-o-lar) also arises from the maxillary artery in the infratemporal fossa (see Figure 6–8). The artery turns inferiorly to enter the mandibular foramen and then the mandibular canal, along with the inferior alveolar nerve. The mylohyoid artery branches from the inferior alveolar artery before it enters the canal.

The **mylohyoid artery** (my-lo-**hi**-oid) arises from the inferior alveolar artery before the main artery enters the mandibular canal by way of the

mandibular foramen (see Figure 6–8). The mylohyoid artery travels in the mylohyoid groove on the inner surface of the mandible and supplies the floor of the mouth and the mylohyoid muscle.

Within the mandibular canal, the inferior alveolar artery gives off the dental and alveolar branches (see Figure 6–8). The dental branches of the inferior alveolar artery supply the pulp tissue of the mandibular posterior teeth by way of each tooth's apical foramen. The alveolar branches of the inferior alveolar artery supply the periodontium of the mandibular posterior teeth, including the gingiva. The inferior alveolar artery then branches into two arteries within the mandibular canal: the mental and incisive arteries.

The **mental artery** (**ment**-il) arises from the inferior alveolar artery and exits the mandibular canal by way of the mental foramen (see Figure 6–8). The mental foramen is located on the outer surface of the mandible, usually beneath the apices of the first and second mandibular premolar teeth. After the mental artery exits the canal, the artery supplies the tissues of the chin and anastomoses with the inferior labial artery.

The **incisive artery** (in-**sy**-ziv) branches off the inferior alveolar artery and remains in the mandibular canal to divide into dental and alveolar branches

Table 6–2   BRANCHES OF THE MAXILLARY ARTERY

Major Branches of Maxillary Artery	Further Branches	Tissues Supplied
1 Middle meningeal		Meninges of brain and bones of skull
2 Inferior alveolar	Mylohyoid, mental, and incisive	Mandibular teeth, mouth floor, and mental region
3 Deep temporal(s)		Temporalis muscle
4 Pterygoid(s)		Lateral and medial pterygoid muscles
5 Masseteric		Masseter muscle
6 Buccal		Buccinator muscle and buccal region
7 Posterior superior alveolar		Posterior maxillary teeth and maxillary sinus
8 Infraorbital	Orbital and anterior superior alveolar	Orbital region, face, and anterior maxillary teeth
9 Greater palatine	Lesser palatine(s)	Hard and soft palates
10 Sphenopalatine	Lateral nasal, septal, and nasopalatine	Nasal cavity and anterior hard palate

(see Figure 6–8). The dental branches of the incisive artery supply the pulp tissue of the mandibular anterior teeth by way of each tooth's apical foramen. The alveolar branches of the incisive artery supply the periodontium of the mandibular anterior teeth, including the gingiva, and anastomose with the alveolar branches of the incisive artery on the other side.

The maxillary artery also has branches that are located near the muscle they supply (see Figure 6–8). These arteries all accompany branches of the mandibular division of the fifth cranial or trigeminal nerve. The **deep temporal arteries** (**tem**-poh-ral) supply the anterior and posterior portions of the temporalis muscle. The **pterygoid arteries** (**the**-re-goid) supply the lateral and medial pterygoid muscles. The **masseteric artery** (mass-et-**tehr**-ik) supplies the masseter muscle. The **buccal artery** supplies the buccinator muscle and other soft tissues of the cheek.

Just as the maxillary artery leaves the infratemporal fossa and enters the pterygopalatine fossa, it gives off the **posterior superior alveolar artery** (al-**ve**-o-lar) (see Figure 6–8). This artery enters the posterior superior alveolar foramina on the maxillary tuberosity and then gives off dental branches and alveolar branches. The posterior

alveolar superior alveolar artery also anastomoses with the anterior superior alveolar artery.

The dental branches of the posterior superior alveolar artery supply the pulp tissue of the posterior maxillary teeth by way of each tooth's apical foramen. The alveolar branches of the posterior superior alveolar artery supply the periodontium of the posterior maxillary teeth, including the gingiva. Some branches also supply the maxillary sinus.

The **infraorbital artery** (in-frah-**or**-bit-al) branches from the maxillary artery in the pterygopalatine fossa and may share a common trunk with the posterior superior alveolar artery (see Figure 6–8). The infraorbital artery then enters the orbit through the inferior orbital fissure. While in the orbit, the artery travels in the infraorbital canal. Within the canal, the infraorbital artery provides orbital branches (**or**-bit-al) to the orbit and gives off the anterior superior alveolar artery.

The **anterior superior alveolar artery** (al-**ve**-o-lar) arises from the infraorbital artery and gives off dental and alveolar branches (see Figure 6–8). The anterior superior alveolar artery also anastomoses with the posterior superior alveolar artery.

The dental branches of the anterior superior alveolar artery supply the pulp tissue of the anterior maxillary teeth by way of each tooth's apical *renules ← capillaries*

↑

art

↓

veins

↓

V.C

→ ♡

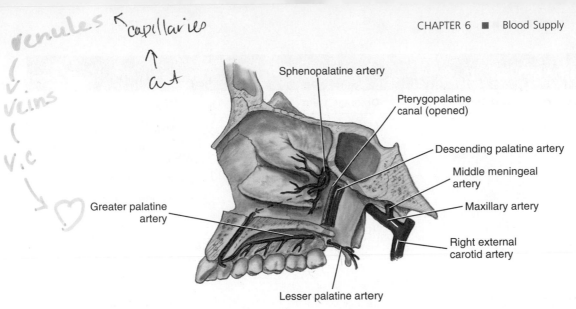

FIGURE 6–9 ■ Pathways of the greater palatine artery, lesser palatine artery, and sphenopalatine artery.

foramen. The alveolar branches of the anterior superior alveolar artery supply the periodontium of the anterior maxillary teeth, including the gingiva.

After giving off these branches in the infraorbital canal, the infraorbital artery emerges onto the face from the infraorbital foramen (see Figure 6–8). The artery's terminal branches supply parts of the infraorbital region of the face and anastomose with the facial artery.

Also in the pterygopalatine fossa, the maxillary artery gives rise to the **greater palatine artery** and **lesser palatine arteries** (**pal**-ah-tine), which travel to the palate through the pterygopalatine canal and the greater and lesser palatine foramina to supply the hard and soft palates, respectively (see Figure 6–9). The maxillary artery ends by becoming the **sphenopalatine artery** (sfe-no-**pal**-ah-tine), which supplies the nasal cavity. The sphenopalatine artery gives rise to the posterior lateral nasal branches and septal branches, including a nasopalatine branch (nay-zo-**pal**-ah-tine) that accompanies the nasopalatine nerve through the incisive foramen on the maxilla (see Figure 6–9).

▓ VENOUS DRAINAGE OF THE HEAD AND NECK

The veins of the head and neck start out as small venules and become larger as they near the base of the neck on their way to the heart. The veins of the head and upper neck are usually symmetrically located but have a greater variability in location than do the arteries, anastomosing freely. Veins are also generally larger and more numerous than arteries in the same tissue area.

The internal jugular vein drains the brain, as well as most of the other tissues of the head and neck (Table 6 3), whereas the external jugular vein drains only a small portion of the extracranial tissues. However, the two veins have many anastomoses. The beginnings of both veins are discussed initially, and then later their route to the heart.

FACIAL VEIN

The **facial vein** drains into the internal jugular vein, which is discussed later in this chapter (Figure 6–10). The facial vein begins at the medial corner of the eye with the junction of two veins from the frontal region, the **supratrochlear vein** (soo-prah-**trok**-lere) and **supraorbital vein** (soo-prah-**or**-bit-al). The supraorbital vein also anastomoses with the ophthalmic veins. The **ophthalmic veins** (of-**thal**-mic) drain the tissues of the orbit. This anastomosis provides a communication with the cavernous venous sinus, which may become fatally infected through the spread of dental infection (discussed further in this chapter and Chapter 12). This is especially significant since the facial vein, like other veins of the head, has no valves to control the direction of blood flow.

all head blood drains to internal or external jugular veins

Table 6–3 VEINS OF THE HEAD

Region or Tributaries Drained	Drainage Veins	Major Veins
Meninges of brain	Middle meningeal	Pterygoid plexus
Lateral scalp area	Superficial temporal and posterior auricular	Retromandibular and external jugular
Frontal region	Supratrochlear and supraorbital	Facial and ophthalmic
Orbital region	Ophthalmic(s)	Cavernous sinus and pterygoid plexus
Superficial temporal and maxillary veins	Retromandibular	External jugular
Upper lip area	Superior labial	Facial
Maxillary teeth	Posterior superior alveolar	Pterygoid plexus
Lower lip area	Inferior labial	Facial
Mandibular teeth and submental region	Inferior alveolar	Pterygoid plexus
Submental region	Submental	Facial
Lingual and sublingual regions	Lingual	Facial or internal jugular
Deep facial areas and posterior superior alveolar and inferior alveolar veins	Pterygoid plexus	Maxillary
Pterygoid plexus of veins	Maxillary	Retromandibular

The facial vein receives branches from the same areas of the face that are supplied by the facial artery. This vein anastomoses with the deep veins, such as the pterygoid plexus in the infratemporal fossa, and with the large retromandibular vein before joining the internal jugular vein at the level of the hyoid bone (discussed later in this chapter).

The facial vein has some important tributaries in the oral region (see Figure 6–10). The **superior labial vein** drains the upper lip. The **inferior labial vein** drains the lower lip. The **submental vein** (sub-**men**-tal) drains the tissues of the chin, as well as the submandibular region.

One excellent example of the venous variability concerns the **lingual veins.** These include the dorsal lingual veins that drain the dorsal surface of the tongue, the highly visible deep lingual veins that drain the ventral surface of the tongue, and the sublingual veins that drain the floor of the mouth. These lingual veins may join to form a single vessel or may empty into larger vessels separately. They also may drain indirectly into the facial vein or directly into the internal jugular vein.

RETROMANDIBULAR VEIN

The **retromandibular vein** (reh-tro-man-**dib**-you-lar) will form the external jugular vein from a portion of its route. The retromandibular vein is formed by the merger of the superficial temporal vein and maxillary vein (Figure 6–11). The retromandibular vein emerges from the parotid salivary gland and courses inferiorly. This vein and its beginning venules drain areas similar to those supplied by the superficial temporal and maxillary arteries.

Below the parotid gland, the retromandibular vein typically divides (Figure 6–11). The anterior division joins the facial vein, and the posterior division continues its downward course on the surface of the sternocleidomastoid muscle. After being joined by the posterior auricular vein (aw-**rik**-you-lar), which drains the lateral scalp behind the ear, this posterior division of the retromandibular veins becomes the external jugular vein. The external jugular vein is discussed later in this chapter.

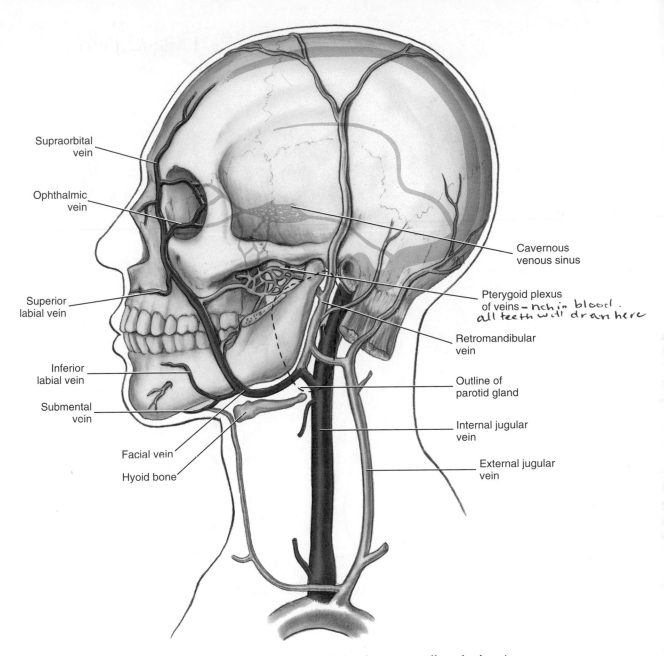

Supraorbital vein

Ophthalmic vein

Superior labial vein

Inferior labial vein

Submental vein

Facial vein

Hyoid bone

Cavernous venous sinus

Pterygoid plexus of veins — *rich in blood.* *all teeth will drain here*

Retromandibular vein

Outline of parotid gland

Internal jugular vein

External jugular vein

FIGURE 6–10 ■ Pathways of the internal jugular vein and facial vein, as well as the location of the cavernous venous sinus.

Superficial Temporal Vein

The **superficial temporal vein** (tem-poh-ral) drains the lateral scalp and is superficially located (see Figure 6–11). The superficial temporal vein goes on to drain into and form the retromandibular vein, along with the deeper maxillary vein.

Maxillary Vein

The **maxillary vein** (mak-sil-lare-ee) is deeper than the superficial temporal vein and begins in the infratemporal fossa by collecting blood from the pterygoid plexus, near the maxillary artery (see Figure 6–11). Through the pterygoid plexus,

Superficial temporal vein

Middle meningeal vein

Pterygoid plexus of veins

Posterior superior alveolar veins

Alveolar and dental branches of posterior superior alveolar vein

Alveolar and dental branches of inferior alveolar vein

Mental branch of inferior alveolar vein

Inferior alveolar vein

Facial vein

Anterior jugular vein

Maxillary vein

Retromandibular vein

Posterior auricular vein

Sternocleidomastoid muscle (cut)

External jugular vein

Internal jugular vein

FIGURE 6–11 ■ Pathways of the retromandibular vein and external jugular vein, including the anterior jugular vein.

the maxillary vein receives the middle meningeal, posterior superior alveolar, inferior alveolar, and other veins, such as those from the nose and palate (those areas served by the maxillary artery). After receiving these veins, the maxillary vein merges with the superficial temporal vein to drain into and form the retromandibular vein.

PTERYGOID PLEXUS OF VEINS

The **pterygoid plexus of veins** (the-ri-goid) is a collection of small anastomosing vessels located around the pterygoid muscles and surrounding the maxillary artery on each side of the face in the infratemporal fossa (see Figure 6–11). This plexus anastomoses with both the facial and retromandibular veins. The pterygoid plexus protects the maxillary artery from being compressed during mastication. By either filling or emptying, the pterygoid plexus can accommodate changes in volume of the infratemporal fossa that occur when the mandible moves.

The pterygoid plexus drains the veins from the deep portions of the face and then drains into the maxillary vein. The **middle meningeal vein** (meh-**nin**-je-al) also drains the blood from the meninges of the brain into the pterygoid plexus of veins.

Some portions of the pterygoid plexus of veins are near the maxillary tuberosity, reflecting the drainage of dental tissues into the plexus. Thus there is a possibility of piercing the pterygoid plexus when a posterior superior alveolar anesthetic block is performed if there is overinsertion of the needle (see Chapter 9 for more information). When the pterygoid plexus of veins is pierced, a small amount of the blood escapes and enters the tissues, causing tissue tenderness, swelling, and the discoloration of a hematoma (discussed later in this chapter).

A spread of infection along the needle tract deep into the tissues can also occur when the posterior superior alveolar anesthetic block is incorrectly administered (see Chapter 12 for more information). The pterygoid plexus of veins may also be involved in the spread of infection to the cavernous venous sinus (discussed later in this chapter and in Chapter 12).

POSTERIOR SUPERIOR ALVEOLAR VEIN

The pterygoid plexus of veins also drains the **posterior superior alveolar vein** (al-**ve**-o-lar), which is formed by the merging of its dental and alveolar branches (see Figure 6–11). The dental branches of the posterior superior alveolar vein drain the pulp tissue of the maxillary teeth by way of each tooth's apical foramen. The alveolar branches of the posterior alveolar vein drain the periodontium of the maxillary teeth, including the gingiva.

INFERIOR ALVEOLAR VEIN

The **inferior alveolar vein** (al-**ve**-o-lar) forms from the merging of its dental branches, alveolar branches, and mental branches in the lower arch, where they also drain into the pterygoid plexus (see Figure 6–11). The dental branches of the inferior alveolar vein drain the pulp tissue of the mandibular teeth by way of each tooth's apical foramen. The alveolar branches of the inferior alveolar vein drain the periodontium of the mandibular teeth, including the gingiva.

The mental branches of the inferior alveolar vein (**ment**-il) enter the mental foramen after draining the chin area, on the outer surface of the mandible, where they anastomose with branches of the facial vein. The mental foramen is on the surface of the mandible, usually between the apices of the mandibular first and second premolars.

VENOUS SINUSES

There are **venous sinuses** located in the meninges of the brain. Specifically, these sinuses are within the dura mater of the brain, a dense connective tissue that lines the inside of the cranium. These dural sinuses are channels by which blood is conveyed from the cerebral veins into the veins of the neck, particularly the internal jugular vein.

The venous sinus most important to dental professionals is the **cavernous venous sinus** (**kav**-er-nus) that is located on each side of the body of the sphenoid bone (see Figure 6–10). Each cavernous venous sinus communicates with the one on the opposite side and also with the pterygoid plexus of veins and superior ophthalmic vein, which anastomoses with the facial vein. The cavernous venous sinus may be involved with the spread of infection from the teeth or periodontium, which can lead to fatal results (discussed further in Chapter 12).

INTERNAL JUGULAR VEIN

The **internal jugular vein** (**jug**-you-lar) drains most of the tissues of the head and neck (Figures 6–10 and 6–12). As mentioned before, the internal jugular vein, unlike many veins in other parts of the body, does not have any one-way valves, nor does any head and neck vein (with the minor exception of the external jugular vein, discussed later). Not having any valves to prevent the flow of blood backward, this vein may become involved with the spread of infection (discussed in Chapter 12).

The internal jugular vein originates in the cranial cavity and leaves the skull through the jugular foramen. It receives many tributaries, including the veins from the lingual, sublingual, and pharyngeal areas, as well as the facial vein. The internal jugular vein

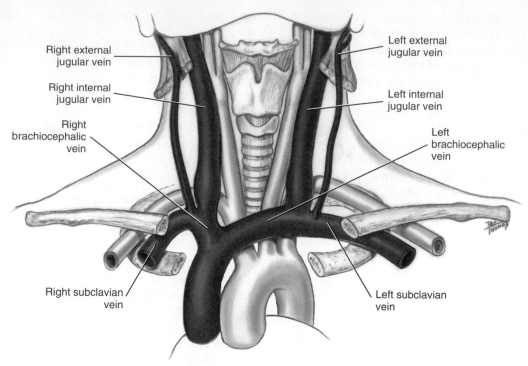

Right external jugular vein

Right internal jugular vein

Right brachiocephalic vein

Right subclavian vein

Left external jugular vein

Left internal jugular vein

Left brachiocephalic vein

Left subclavian vein

FIGURE 6–12 ■ Pathways to the heart from the head and neck, including the external and internal jugular veins, subclavian vein, brachiocephalic veins, and superior vena cava.

runs with the common carotid artery and vagus nerve in the carotid sheath. The internal jugular vein descends in the neck to merge with the subclavian vein.

EXTERNAL JUGULAR VEIN

As mentioned before, the posterior division of the retromandibular vein becomes the **external jugular vein** (jug-you-lar). The external jugular vein continues the descent down the neck, terminating in the subclavian vein (see Figures 6–11 and 6–12). Alone among the veins of the head and neck, the external jugular vein has valves near its entry into the subclavian vein. Usually the external jugular vein is visible as it crosses the sternocleidomastoid muscle; to increase its visibility, it can be distended by gentle supraclavicular digital pressure to block outflow.

The **anterior jugular vein** drains into the external jugular vein (or directly into the subclavian vein) before it joins the subclavian vein (see Figure 6–11). The anterior jugular vein begins below the chin, communicating with veins in the area, and descends near the midline, within the superficial fascia, receiving branches from the superficial cervical structures. Only one anterior jugular vein may be present, but usually two veins are present, anastomosing with each other through a jugular venous arch.

PATHWAYS TO THE HEART FROM THE HEAD AND NECK

On each side of the body, the external jugular vein joins the subclavian vein from the arm, and then the internal jugular vein merges with the **subclavian vein** (sub-**klay**-vee-an) to form the **brachiocephalic vein** (bray-kee-oo-sah-**fal**-ik) (see Figure 6–12). The brachiocephalic veins unite to form the **superior vena cava** (**vee**-na **kay**-va) and then travel to the heart. Because the superior vena cava is on the right side of the heart, the brachiocephalic veins are asymmetrical. The right brachiocephalic vein is short and vertical, and the left brachiocephalic vein is long and horizontal.

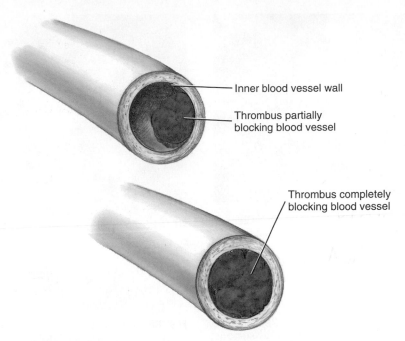

FIGURE 6–13 ■ Diagrams of a thrombus formed on the inner blood vessel wall and partially and completely blocking the blood vessel.

⬛ BLOOD VESSEL LESIONS

Blood vessels may become compromised in certain disease processes, such as high blood pressure, infection, trauma, or endocrine pathology. These disease processes may lead to blood vessel lesions. One of these lesions is a clot or *thrombus* (plural, *thrombi*) (**throm**-bus, **throm**-by) that forms on the inner vessel wall (Figure 6–13).

A thrombus may dislodge from the inner vessel wall and travel as an *embolus* (plural, *emboli*) (**em**-bol-us, **em**-bol-eye) (Figure 6–14). Both of these blood vessel lesions can cause occlusion of the vessel, where the blood flow is blocked either partially or fully. Bacteria traveling in the blood can also cause a *bacteremia* (bak-ter-**ee**-me-ah). A transient bacteremia can occur with dental treatment and is very serious in certain medically compromised patients (discussed further in Chapter 12).

This occlusion of the blood vessel can hamper blood circulation and cause further complications, such as a stroke (cerebrovascular accident), a heart attack (myocardial infarction), or tissue destruction (gangrene), depending on the lesion's location. These thrombi may also be infected and spread infection by way of embolus formation to such areas as the cavernous venous sinus (see Chapter 12 for more information). A dental professional needs to keep the possibility of blood vessel lesions in mind when treating a patient with blood vessel disease or dentally related infections.

When a blood vessel is seriously traumatized, large amounts of the blood can escape into

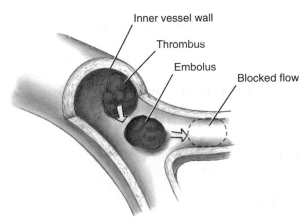

FIGURE 6–14 ■ Diagram of a dislodged thrombus forming an embolus and then traveling in a blood vessel and creating a blocked flow of blood.

FIGURE 6–15 ■ Two extraoral hematomas formed in a patient after administration of a local anesthetic injection in the area of the pterygoid plexus on the left side and an injection near the infraorbital foramen on the right side. (Courtesy of Dr. Mark Egbert.)

FIGURE 6–16 ■ An intraoral hematoma in the tissues on the medial surface of the mandibular ramus after an inferior alveolar nerve block.

the surrounding tissue without clotting, causing a *hemorrhage* (**hem**-ah-rij). This is a serious, life-threatening blood vessel lesion. Other blood vessel lesions can involve tumorous or abnormal developmental growth of blood vessel tissues. A dental professional needs to be aware of the patient's health history with regard to these serious blood vessel diseases.

Blood vessels may also undergo localized trauma that results temporarily in a bruise. A bruise or *hematoma* (hee-mah-**toe**-mah) results when a blood vessel is injured and a small amount of the blood escapes into the surrounding tissue and then clots (Figures 6–15 and 6–16). This escaped blood causes tissue tenderness, swelling, and discoloration that will last until the blood is broken down by the body.

A hematoma may result during a local anesthetic injection, especially when giving a posterior superior alveolar block near the pterygoid plexus of veins (see Chapter 9 for more infor-mation) or other blocks, such as an infraorbital block or inferior alveolar block. Thus a dental professional needs to be aware of the location of the blood vessels to prevent their injury during dental treatment.

IDENTIFICATION EXERCISES

Identify the structures on the following diagrams by filling in the blanks with the correct anatomical term. You can check your answers by looking back at the figure indicated in parentheses for each identification diagram.

1. (Figure 6–1)

R   L

Right Common Carotid

Brachiocephalic A

Right Subclavian A

Aorta

Hyoid Bone

Cut S C M

Left Common Carotid A

Left Subclavian A

Clavicle (Cut)

First Rib (Cut)

2. (Figure 6–3)

Maxillary Artery

Facial Artery

Lingual Artery

Superior Thyroid Artery

Superior Temporal

Occipital

Posterior Auricular

External Carotid

Internal Carotid

Common Carotid

3. (Figure 6–4)

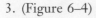

Lingual Artery

External Carotid

Facial Artery

Apex of Tongue

Internal Carotid

Sublingual Artery

Hyoid Bone

4. (Figure 6–5)

Angular Artery

Superior Labial A.

Parotid gland

Inferior Labial A.

Ascending palatine A.

Facial A.

Lingual A.

External Carotid

Submental A.

Submand. Salivary Gland

5. (Figure 6–7)

frontal branch of
superficial temporal A.

Middle temporal A.

Transverse facial A.

Maxillary A.

Parietal Branch of
Superficial temporal A.

Superficial temporal A.

External Carotid A.

Common Carotid A.

foramen rotundum
ovale
spinosum

SCM

✳ Infer. Alveolar Artery
provides all blood to mand
teeth & tissue

6. (Figure 6–8)

Sphenopalatine A.
Infra orbital A
Post. Sup. Alveolar A.
Ant. Sup Alveolar A.
Dental and alveolar
branches of Superior
Alveolar A.
Dental and Alveolar
branches of Incisive A.
Incisive A.
Mental A.

Deep temporal arteries

Superficial temporal A.

Middle menegial A. . .
~~Masseteric~~ A. Maxillary A.
5 ~~Pterygoid~~ A. Massateric A.
4 ~~Buccal~~ A Pterygoid A.
6 ~~Mylohyoid~~ A. Buccal A
~~Inferior alveolar~~ A. Mylohy.
Inferior alveolar A.
Left external carotid A
Outline of parotid gland

7. (Figure 6–9)

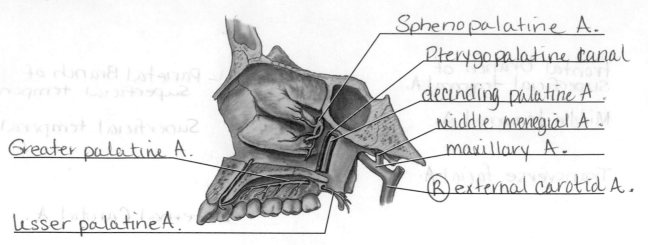

Sphenopalatine A.
Pterygopalatine canal
decending palatine A.
middle menegial A.
maxillary A.
ⓑ external carotid A.

Greater palatine A.

Lesser palatine A.

8. (Figure 6–10) VEINS

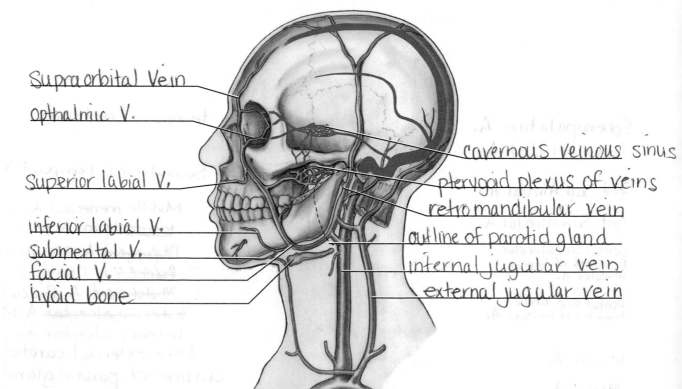

Supraorbital Vein
opthalmic V.

Superior labial V.

inferior labial V.
submental V.
facial V.
hyoid bone

cavernous veinous sinus
pterygoid plexus of veins
retromandibular vein
outline of parotid gland
internal jugular vein
external jugular vein

9. (Figure 6–11)   VEINS

superficial temporal V.
middle meningeal V.
pterygoid plexus / V.
post. sup. alveolar V.

alv./dental branches
post. sup. alveolar V.
alv./dental branches
inf. alveolar V.
mental branch of inf.
alveolar V.
inferior alveolar V.
facial V.
anterior jugular V.

maxillary V.
retromandibular V.
posterior auricular V.
SCM
external jugular V.
internal jugular V.

10. (Figure 6–12)

right external jugular V.
right internal jugular V.
right brachiocephalic V.

left external jugular V.
left internal jugular V.
left brachiocephalic V.

right subclavian V.

left subclavian V.

REVIEW QUESTIONS

1. The posterior superior alveolar artery and its branches supply the
   A. Maxillary posterior teeth and periodontium
   B. Mandibular posterior teeth and periodontium
   C. Sternocleidomastoid muscle and thyroid gland
   D. Temporalis muscle and parotid salivary gland

2. Which of the following statements concerning the pterygoid plexus is correct?
   A. Is located around the infrahyoid muscles
   B. Protects the superficial temporal artery
   C. Drains the maxillary and mandibular dental tissues
   D. Contains valves to prevent backflow of blood

3. Which of the following veins results from the merger of the superficial temporal vein and maxillary vein?
   A. Facial vein
   B. Retromandibular vein
   C. Internal jugular vein
   D. External jugular vein
   E. Brachiocephalic vein

4. Which of the following arteries arises from the inferior alveolar artery before the artery enters the mandibular canal?
   A. Mylohyoid artery
   B. Incisive artery
   C. Mental artery
   D. Posterior superior alveolar artery
   E. Submental artery

5. Which of the following artery and foramen pairs below is matched correctly?
   A. Buccal artery-infraorbital foramen
   B. Middle meningeal artery-foramen spinosum
   C. Incisive artery-mental foramen
   D. Inferior labial artery-mandibular foramen
   E. Submental artery-mental foramen

6. Which of the following arteries listed below supply the mucous membranes and glands of the hard and soft palates?
   A. Greater and lesser palatine arteries
   B. Posterior superior alveolar artery
   C. Anterior superior alveolar artery
   D. Infraorbital artery

7. Which of the following blood vessel lesions may result when a clot on the inner blood vessel wall becomes dislodged and travels in the vessel?
   A. Hematoma
   B. Venous sinus
   C. Embolus
   D. Hemorrhage

8. Which of the following statements concerning the maxillary artery is correct?
   A. Arises from the internal carotid artery
   B. Enters the pterygopalatine fossa and forms terminal branches
   C. Arises from the zygomaticofacial foramen to emerge on the face
   D. Has mandibular, maxillary, nasal, palatine, and occipital branches

9. A venous sinus of the vascular system is a:
   A. Network of blood vessels
   B. Clot on the inner vessel wall
   C. Blood-filled space between two tissue layers
   D. Smaller vein or venule

10. Which of the following is a branch from the facial artery?
    A. Superior labial artery
    B. Ascending pharyngeal artery
    C. Posterior auricular artery
    D. Transverse facial artery

11. Which of the following structures are smaller vessels that branch off an arteriole to supply blood directly to tissue?
    A. Artery
    B. Capillary
    C. Vein
    D. Venule

12. The carotid pulse can be palpated at the level of the:
    A. Thyroid cartilage
    B. Hyoid bone
    C. Angle of the mandible
    D. Supraclavicular fossa

13. The tongue is supplied mainly by a branch from the:
    A. Internal carotid artery
    B. External carotid artery
    C. Sublingual artery
    D. Facial artery

14. Which of the following can sometimes be visible under the skin of the temporal region?
    A. Maxillary artery
    B. Transverse facial artery
    C. Middle temporal artery
    D. Superficial temporal artery

15. Which of the following arteries anastomoses with the anterior superior alveolar artery?
    A. Mylohoid artery
    B. Posterior superior alveolar artery
    C. Facial artery
    D. Maxillary artery

✓ posterior superior alveolar artery + its branches supply the Maxillary posterior + periodtium.
✓ Pterygoid plexus is located around the infrahyoid muscels.
✓ Superficial temporal vein + maxillary vein = retromandibular vein
✓ Mylohyoid artery arises from the inferior alveolar artery before it enters the mandibular canal.
✓ embolus = blood clot
✓ greater and lesser palatine arteries supply the mucous membranes + glands of the hard + soft palates.
✓ maxillary artery enters the pterygopalatine fossa + forms terminal branches
✓ A blood filled space between 2 tissue layers is a venous sinus of the vascular system.
✓ Superior labial artery is a branch from the facial artery
✓ A capillary is smaller vessels that branch off an arteriole + supplys blood directly to tissue.
✓ The carotid pulse can be palpated at the thyroid cartilage
✓ The tongue is supplied mainly by a branch from the external carotid artery
✓ Superficial temporal artery is visible under the skin
✓ The posterior superior alveolar artery ANASTOMOSES with the anterior superior alveolar artery

REVIEW ACTIVITIES

1. Make a drawing that shows how an artery relates to a vein (with the heart between) and how it forms arterioles and capillaries.

2. Create a flow chart of the flow of blood from the heart to the lingual artery in the tongue.

3. List the various branches of the maxillary artery and put a star near those that supply the teeth.

4. Looking in a mirror, trace the pathway of the facial vein.

5. Create a flow chart of the flow of blood in the veins from the maxillary canine to the heart.

Glandular Tissue

CHAPTER OUTLINE

This chapter discusses the following topics:

I. Glandular Tissue
II. Lacrimal Glands
III. Salivary Glands
   A. Major Salivary Glands
   B. Minor Salivary Glands
IV. Thyroid Gland
V. Parathyroid Glands
VI. Thymus Gland

LEARNING OBJECTIVES

After reading and studying this chapter, the reader should be able to:

1. Define and pronounce all the key words and anatomical terms in this chapter.
2. Locate and identify all the glandular tissue and associated structures in the head and neck region on a diagram, a skull, and a patient.
3. Correctly complete the identification exercises and review questions and activities for this chapter.
4. Integrate the knowledge about the head and neck glands during clinical practice when these glands may be involved in a disease process.

KEY WORDS

Duct (dukt) Passageway to carry the secretion from the exocrine gland to the location where it will be used.

Endocrine gland (**en**-dah-krin) Type of gland without a duct, with the secretion being poured directly into the blood, which then carries the secretion to the region in which it is to be used.

Exocrine gland (**ek**-sah-krin) Type of gland with an associated duct that serves as a passageway for the

secretion so it can be emptied directly into the location where the secretion is to be used.

Gland (gland) Structure that produces a chemical secretion necessary for normal body functioning.

Goiter (**goit**-er) Enlarged thyroid gland due to a disease process.

GLANDULAR TISSUE

The glandular tissue in the head and neck area includes the lacrimal, salivary, thyroid, parathyroid, and thymus glands. A dental professional needs to be able to locate and identify these glands and their innervation, lymphatic drainage, and blood supply (Table 7–1). This information will help the dental professional determine if the glands are involved in a disease process and the extent of that involvement.

A *gland* (gland) is a structure that produces a chemical secretion necessary for normal body functioning. An *exocrine gland* (**ek**-sah-krin) is a gland having a duct associated with it. A *duct* (dukt) is a passageway that allows the secretion to be emptied directly into the location where the secretion is to be used. An *endocrine gland* (**en**-dah-krin) is a ductless gland, with the secretion being poured directly into the blood, which then carries the secretion to the region in which it is to be used. Motor nerves associated with both types of

Table 7–1   GLANDULAR TISSUE: LOCATION, INNERVATION, LYMPHATIC DRAINAGE, AND BLOOD SUPPLY

Glandular Tissue	Location	Innervation	Lymphatics	Blood Supply
Lacrimal gland with nasolacrimal duct	Lacrimal fossa of frontal bone	Greater petrosal and lacrimal nerves	Superficial parotid	Lacrimal and ophthalmic arteries
Parotid gland with parotid duct	Parotid space posterior to the mandibular ramus, anterior and inferior to ear	Ninth and fifth cranial nerves	Deep parotid nodes	Branches of external carotid artery
Submandibular gland with submandibular duct	Submandibular space: inferior and posterior to the body of mandible	Chorda tympani and seventh cranial nerve	Submandibular nodes	Facial and lingual arteries
Sublingual gland with sublingual duct(s)	Sublingual space: floor of mouth, medial to body of mandible	Chorda tympani and seventh cranial nerve	Submandibular nodes	Sublingual and submental arteries
Minor salivary glands with ducts	Buccal, labial, and lingual mucosa, soft and hard palate, floor of mouth, and base of circumvallate lingual papillae	Seventh cranial nerve	Various nodes, depending on location	Various arteries, depending on location
Thyroid gland	Inferior to hyoid bone, junction of larynx and trachea	Cervical ganglion	Superior deep cervical nodes	Superior and inferior thyroid arteries
Parathyroid gland	Close to or within thyroid	Cervical ganglion	Superior deep cervical nodes	Inferior thyroid artery
Thymus gland	In thorax, inferior to hyoid bone, deep to sternum and superficial and lateral to trachea	Tenth cranial and cervical nerves	Within substance of gland	Inferior thyroid and internal thoracic arteries

glands help regulate the flow of the secretion, and sensory nerves are also present.

LACRIMAL GLANDS

The **lacrimal glands** (lak-ri-mal) are paired exocrine glands that secrete **lacrimal fluid** or tears. Lacrimal fluid is a watery fluid that lubricates the conjunctiva lining the inside of the eyelids and the front of the eyeball. The fluid leaves the gland through 8–12 fine tubules. After passing over the eyeball, the lacrimal fluid is drained through a small hole in each eyelid, ending in the nasolacrimal sac (nay-so-**lak**-rim-al), a thin-walled structure behind the medial canthus. From the **nasolacrimal sac,** the

lacrimal fluid continues into the **nasolacrimal duct**, ultimately draining into the inferior nasal meatus. This connection explains why crying leads to a runny nose.

LOCATION. Each lacrimal gland is located in the lacrimal fossa of the frontal bone (see Chapter 3 and Figure 2–4). The lacrimal fossa is located just inside the lateral portion of the supraorbital ridge inside the orbit. The nasolacrimal duct is formed at the junction of the lacrimal and maxillary bones.

INNERVATION. The lacrimal glands are innervated by parasympathetic fibers from the greater petrosal nerve, a branch of the facial or seventh cranial nerve. These preganglionic fibers synapse at the pterygopalatine ganglion, and postganglionic fibers reach the gland through branches of the trigeminal nerve. The lacrimal nerve serves as an afferent nerve for the lacrimal gland.

LYMPHATICS. The lacrimal glands drain into the superior parotid lymph nodes.

BLOOD SUPPLY. The lacrimal glands are supplied by the lacrimal artery, a branch of the ophthalmic artery of the internal carotid artery.

SALIVARY GLANDS

The **salivary glands** (sal-i-ver-ee) produce **saliva** (sah-**li**-vah) that lubricates and cleanses the oral cavity and helps in digestion. These glands are controlled by the autonomic nervous system. There are major salivary glands and minor salivary glands as defined by their size. Both the major and minor salivary glands are exocrine glands and thus have ducts associated with them. These ducts help drain the saliva directly into the oral cavity where the saliva is used.

The salivary glands may become enlarged, tender, and possibly firmer due to various disease processes. The salivary glands may also become involved in salivary stone (sialolith) formation, blocking the drainage of saliva from the duct and causing gland enlargement and tenderness (Figures 7–1 and 7–2). Certain medications and disease processes may result in decreased or increased production of saliva by these glands.

MAJOR SALIVARY GLANDS

The **major salivary glands** are large paired glands and have named ducts associated with them. There are three major salivary glands: the parotid, submandibular, and sublingual glands.

Parotid Salivary Gland

The **parotid salivary gland** (pah-**rot**-id) is the largest encapsulated major salivary gland but provides only 25 percent of the total salivary volume. The saliva from the parotid is a purely serous type of secretion, a watery protein fluid. The parotid gland is divided into two lobes, a superficial lobe and a deep lobe. The duct associated with the parotid gland is the **parotid duct** or Stensen's duct. This long duct emerges from the anterior

FIGURE 7–1 ■ Mucocele of a minor salivary gland due to severance of the duct from trauma (lip bite) and then blockage of saliva.

border of the gland, superficial to the masseter muscle. The duct pierces the buccinator muscle. The duct then opens up into the oral cavity upon the inner surface of the cheek, usually opposite the second maxillary molar. The **parotid papilla** (pah-**pil**-ah) is a small elevation of tissue that

FIGURE 7–2 ■ Ranula of the submandibular salivary gland due to blockage of saliva resulting from stone formation.

marks the opening of the parotid duct on the inner surface of the cheek.

The parotid salivary gland becomes enlarged and tender when the patient has mumps. This enlargement and tenderness usually involves the gland bilaterally, first one side and then the other side. Mumps is a viral infection of the parotid gland that is being prevented by a childhood vaccination. The parotid gland can also be involved in tumorous growth that can also change the consistency of the gland and cause facial paralysis on the involved side (the facial nerve travels through the gland).

LOCATION. The parotid gland occupies the parotid fascial space, an area posterior to the mandibular ramus, anterior and inferior to the ear (Figure 7–3 and Figure 7–7). The gland extends irregularly from the zygomatic arch to the angle of the mandible. This gland is effectively palpated bilaterally. Start in front of each ear and move to the cheek area and then down to the angle of the mandible (Figure 7–4).

INNERVATION. The parotid gland is innervated by the motor or efferent (parasympathetic) nerves of the otic ganglion of the ninth cranial or glossopharyngeal nerve, as well as by the afferent nerves from the auriculotemporal branch of the fifth cranial

FIGURE 7–4 ■ Palpating the parotid salivary gland by starting in front of each ear and then moving to the cheek area and then down to the angle of the mandible.

or trigeminal nerve. The seventh cranial or facial nerve and its branches travel through the parotid gland between its lobes but are not involved in its innervation.

LYMPHATICS. The parotid gland drains into the deep parotid lymph nodes.

FIGURE 7–3 ■ The parotid salivary gland and associated structures.

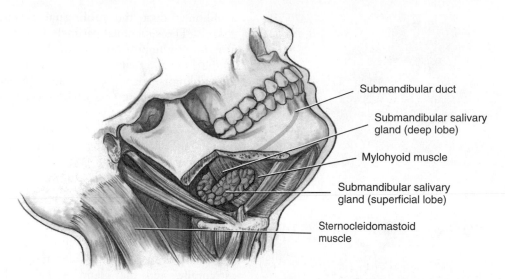

FIGURE 7–5 ■ The submandibular salivary gland and associated structures.

BLOOD SUPPLY. The parotid gland is supplied by branches of the external carotid artery.

Submandibular Salivary Gland

The **submandibular salivary gland** (sub-man-**dib**-you-lar) is the second largest encapsulated major salivary gland, yet provides 60–65 percent of total salivary volume. The saliva from the submandibular gland is a mixed secretion of both serous and mucous types, having both thick carbohydrate and watery protein fluids. The duct associated with the submandibular gland is the submandibular duct or Wharton's duct. This long duct travels along the anterior floor of the mouth. The duct then opens into the oral cavity at the **sublingual caruncle** (sub-**ling**-gwal **kar**-unk-el), a small papilla near the midline of the mouth floor on each side of the lingual frenum. The duct's tortuous travel for a considerable upward distance in its course may be the reason the submandibular gland is the most common salivary gland to be involved in salivary stone formation.

LOCATION. The submandibular gland occupies the submandibular fossa in the submandibular fascial space, mainly the posterior portion (Figure 7–5). Most of the gland is a lobe superficial to the mylohyoid muscle, but a small deep lobe wraps around the posterior border of the muscle. The duct arises from this deep lobe and stays on the inside of the mylohyoid muscle.

The duct lies very close to the large lingual nerve, a branch of the fifth cranial or trigeminal nerve, which is sometimes injured in surgery performed to remove salivary stones from the duct. The submandibular gland is posterior to the sublingual salivary gland. The submandibular gland is effectively palpated inferior and posterior to the body of the mandible bilaterally. Start by moving inward from the lower border of the mandible near its angle as the patient lowers the head (Figure 7–6 and 7–7).

INNERVATION. The submandibular gland is innervated by the efferent (parasympathetic) fibers of the chorda tympani and the submandibular ganglion of the seventh cranial or facial nerve.

LYMPHATICS. The submandibular gland drains into the submandibular lymph nodes.

BLOOD SUPPLY. The submandibular gland is supplied by branches of the facial and lingual arteries.

Sublingual Salivary Gland

The **sublingual salivary gland** (sub-**ling**-gwal) is the smallest, most diffuse, and only unencapsulated major salivary gland, providing only 10 percent of the total salivary volume. The saliva from the sublingual gland is a mix of both mucous and serous secretions, having both thick carbohydrate and watery protein fluids, with the mucous component predominating. The short ducts associated with the sublingual gland sometimes combine to

FIGURE 7–6 ■ Palpating the submandibular salivary gland by palpating inward from the lower border of the mandible near its angle as the patient lowers the head.

form the **sublingual duct** or Bartholin's duct. The sublingual duct then opens directly into the oral cavity through the same opening as the sub-

mandibular duct, the **sublingual caruncle (kar-unk-el)**. The sublingual caruncle is a small papilla near the midline of the mouth floor on each side of the lingual frenum. The other small ducts of the sublingual gland open along the **sublingual fold**, a fold of tissue on each side of the mouth floor.

LOCATION. The sublingual gland is located in the sublingual fossa in the sublingual fascial space at the floor of the mouth (Figure 7–7). This gland is superior to the mylohyoid muscle and medial to the body of the mandible. The sublingual gland is also anterior to the submandibular gland. The gland is effectively palpated on the floor of the mouth posterior to each mandibular canine. One hand is placed intraorally and one is placed extraorally, and the gland is palpated between (Figure 7–8).

INNERVATION. The sublingual gland is innervated by the efferent (parasympathetic) fibers of the chorda tympani and the submandibular ganglion of the seventh cranial or facial nerve.

LYMPHATICS. The sublingual gland drains into the submandibular lymph nodes.

BLOOD SUPPLY. The sublingual gland is supplied by the sublingual and submental arteries.

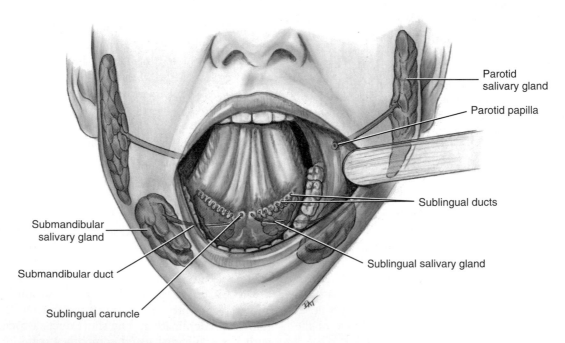

Parotid salivary gland

Parotid papilla

Sublingual ducts

Sublingual salivary gland

Submandibular salivary gland

Submandibular duct

Sublingual caruncle

FIGURE 7–7 ■ The salivary glands and associated structures.

FIGURE 7–8 ■ Palpating the sublingual salivary gland by palpating the floor of the mouth behind each mandibular canine with one hand placed intraorally and one hand placed extraorally.

MINOR SALIVARY GLANDS

The **minor salivary glands** are smaller than the major salivary glands but are more numerous. The minor salivary glands are also exocrine glands, but their unnamed ducts are shorter than those of the major salivary glands.

LOCATION. These minor salivary glands are scattered in the tissues of the buccal, labial, and lingual mucosa, the soft palate, the lateral portions of the hard palate, and the floor of the mouth. There are also minor salivary glands, **von Ebner's glands** (**eeb**-ners), in the connective tissue layers associated with the large circumvallate lingual papillae, on the posterior portion of the tongue's dorsal surface (see Chapter 1). Most minor salivary glands secrete a mainly mucous saliva, a thicker carbohydrate fluid, with some serous components of a watery protein nature. The exception is von Ebner's glands, which secrete only a serous saliva of a watery protein nature.

INNERVATION. The minor salivary glands are innervated by the seventh cranial or facial nerve.

LYMPHATICS AND BLOOD SUPPLY. The minor salivary glands drain into various lymph nodes and are supplied by various arteries depending on the area where they are located.

THYROID GLAND

The **thyroid gland** (**thy**-roid) is the largest endocrine gland. Since it is ductless, the thyroid gland produces and secretes **thyroxine** (thy-**rok**-sin) directly into the blood. Thyroxine is a hormone that stimulates the metabolic rate. The gland consists of two lateral lobes. The right and left lobes are connected anteriorly by an isthmus. In a healthy patient, the gland is not visible yet can be palpated as a soft mass. In a healthy state, the gland is mobile when swallowing occurs. Thus when the patient swallows, the gland moves up, as does the whole larynx.

During a disease process involving the thyroid gland, the gland may become enlarged and possibly may be visible during an extraoral examination. This enlarged thyroid gland is called a *goiter* (**goit**-er). A goiter may be firmer and tender when palpated and may contain hard masses. The diseased gland may lose its mobility and not move up when the patient swallows. The thyroid gland may also be partially or fully removed surgically for various disease processes. The patient should be referred to a physician if there are any undiagnosed changes in the thyroid gland. It is also important to find out whether the patient had the thymus gland irradiated as an infant. This outdated procedure can cause thyroid cancer (discussed later in this chapter).

LOCATION. The thyroid gland is located in the anterior and lateral regions of the neck. The gland is inferior to the thyroid cartilage, at the junction between the larynx and trachea (Figure 7–9A). The thyroid gland is effectively palpated by placing one hand on one side of the trachea and gently displacing the thyroid tissue to the other side of the neck while the other hand palpates the displaced gland tissue (Figure 7–10). Then compare the two lobes of the thyroid using bimanual or manual palpation and visual inspection. Many clinicians find that having the patient swallow water helps the examination, as well as having the patient flex the neck slightly to the side being examined. Finally, ask the patient to swallow to check for mobility of the gland.

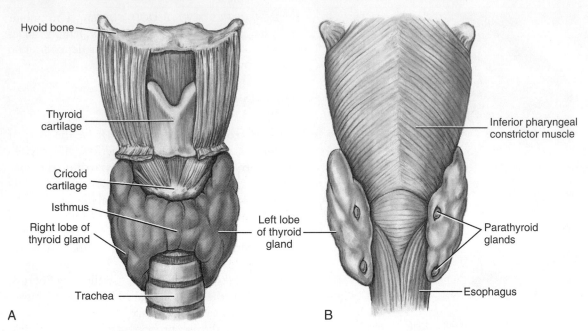

Hyoid bone

Thyroid cartilage

Cricoid cartilage

Isthmus

Right lobe of thyroid gland

Trachea

Inferior pharyngeal constrictor muscle

Parathyroid glands

Left lobe of thyroid gland

Esophagus

A   B

FIGURE 7–9 ■ A: Anterior view of the thyroid gland and associated structures. B: Posterior view of the parathyroid glands and associated structures.

INNERVATION. The thyroid gland is innervated by sympathetic nerves through the cervical ganglia.

FIGURE 7–10 ■ Palpating the thyroid gland by placing one hand on one side of the trachea and gently displacing the thyroid tissue to the other side of the neck, while the other hand palpates the displaced gland tissue.

LYMPHATICS. The thyroid gland drains into the superior deep cervical lymph nodes.

BLOOD SUPPLY. The thyroid gland is supplied by the superior and inferior thyroid arteries.

PARATHYROID GLANDS

The **parathyroid glands** (par-ah-**thy**-roid) typically consist of four small endocrine glands, two on each side. Since the parathyroid glands are ductless, they produce and secrete **parathyroid hormone** directly into the blood to regulate calcium and phosphorus levels. The parathyroid glands are not visible or palpable during an extraoral examination of a patient. However, the parathyroid glands may alter the thyroid gland if they are involved in a disease process.

LOCATION. The parathyroid glands are usually close to or even inside the thyroid gland on its posterior surface (Figure 7–9B).

INNERVATION. The parathyroid glands are innervated by the same nerves that innervate the thyroid gland, sympathetic nerves through the cervical ganglia.

LYMPHATICS. The parathyroid glands drain into the superior deep cervical lymph nodes.

BLOOD SUPPLY. The parathyroid glands are supplied primarily by the inferior thyroid arteries.

▓ THYMUS GLAND

The **thymus gland** (**thy**-mus) is an endocrine gland and therefore is ductless. The thymus gland is a part of the immune system that fights disease processes. The **T-cell lymphocytes**, white blood cells of the immune system, mature in the gland in response to stimulation by thymus hormones. The gland grows in size from birth to puberty while performing this task. After puberty, the gland stops growing and starts to shrink.

By adulthood, the gland has almost disappeared, making it mainly a temporary structure. The adult gland consists of two lateral lobes in close contact at the midline. The thymus gland is not easily palpated, but its involvement in various disease processes may alter the treatment of the patient.

Older patients may have had radiation therapy to the thymus in childhood to shrink the gland so as to prevent sudden infant death. It is now known that the large thymus of a child is not related to suffocation and sudden infant death. The radiation levels used on these patients in the past may result in thyroid cancer.

LOCATION. The thymus gland is located in the thorax and the anterior region of the base of the neck, inferior to the thyroid gland (Figure 7–11). The gland is deep to the sternum and the sternohyoid and sternothyroid muscles. The gland is also superficial and lateral to the trachea.

INNERVATION. The thymus gland's innervation consists of branches of the tenth cranial or vagus nerve and cervical nerves.

LYMPHATICS. The thymus gland's lymphatics arise within the substance of the gland and terminate in the internal jugular vein.

BLOOD SUPPLY. The thymus gland is supplied by the inferior thyroid and internal thoracic arteries.

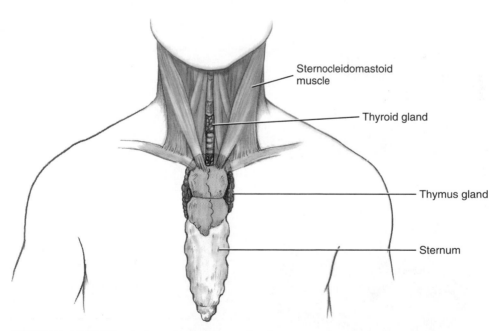

FIGURE 7–11 ■ The thymus gland and associated structures.

IDENTIFICATION EXERCISES

Identify the structures on the following diagrams by filling in the blanks with the correct anatomical term. You can check your answers by looking back at the figure indicated in parentheses for each identification diagram.

1. (Figure 7–3)

2. (Figure 7–5)

3. (Figure 7–7)

4. (Figure 7-9A)

REVIEW QUESTIONS

1. The sublingual salivary gland is located
   A. Anterior to the submandibular gland
   B. Inferior to the mylohyoid muscle
   C. Lateral to the body of the mandible
   D. In the mandibular vestibule area

2. Which of the following glands has both a superficial and deep lobe?
   A. Thymus gland
   B. Parotid gland
   C. Thyroid gland
   D. Sublingual gland
   E. Lacrimal gland

3. Which of the following nerves innervates both the submandibular and sublingual salivary glands?
   A. Trigeminal nerve
   B. Chorda tympani
   C. Hypoglossal nerve
   D. Vagus nerve

4. Which of the following nerves travels through the parotid salivary gland but is not involved in its innervation?
   A. Trigeminal nerve
   B. Facial nerve
   C. Vagus nerve
   D. Glossopharyngeal nerve

5. Which of the following glands shrinks as a person matures?
   A. Thymus gland
   B. Parotid gland
   C. Thyroid gland
   D. Sublingual gland
   E. Submandibular gland

6. Which gland has a duct that usually opens on the inner surface of the cheek, opposite the second maxillary molar?
   A. Thymus gland
   B. Parotid gland
   C. Thyroid gland
   D. Sublingual gland
   E. Submandibular gland

7. Which oral landmark marks the opening of the submandibular duct?
   A. Parotid raphe
   B. Lingual frenum
   C. Parotid papilla
   D. Sublingual caruncle
   E. Nasolacrimal duct

8. The thyroid gland is located
   A. Anterior to the larynx
   B. Superior to the hyoid bone
   C. Posterior to the surrounding pharynx
   D. In the posterior and medial neck region

9. Which of the following blood vessels supplies the parotid salivary gland?
   A. Facial artery
   B. Lingual artery
   C. Internal carotid artery
   D. External carotid artery

10. As endocrine glands, the parathyroid glands are known to
    A. Have one primary duct
    B. Have multiple secondary ducts
    C. Drain directly into blood vessels
    D. Drain directly into the thyroid gland

11. The lacrimal gland drains into the
    A. Lacrimal fossa
    B. Inferior nasal meatus
    C. Parotid salivary gland
    D. Internal carotid artery

12. Which of the following can block the drainage of saliva from the duct?
    A. Excessive amounts of secretion
    B. Stone formation
    C. Lacrimal gland drainage
    D. Inflammation of blood vessels

13. Which of the following statements concerning minor salivary glands is correct?
    A. Minor glands are smaller and less numerous than the major glands.
    B. Minor glands secrete only mucous saliva.

C. Minor glands have longer ducts than major glands.

D. Minor glands are located in the buccal, labial, and lingual mucosa.

14. In a healthy patient, the thyroid gland

A. Consists of two lobes that are connected by an isthmus

B. Does not move with the thyroid cartilage when swallowing

C. Secretes thyroxine, which slows down the metabolic rate

D. Is clearly visible and easily palpated

15. When examining the thyroid gland

A. Ask the patient to swallow

B. Ask the patient to cough

C. Palpate the tissue directly over the trachea

D. Move the gland superiorly and then inferiorly

REVIEW ACTIVITIES

1. Create a flow chart showing the movement of the lacrimal fluid from the lacrimal gland to the inferior nasal meatus.

2. Palpate on yourself (or a peer) the various major salivary glands of the face and neck while looking in a mirror.

3. List the areas of the oral cavity that contain minor salivary glands in their tissues.

4. Palpate the thyroid gland on yourself (or a peer) while looking in a mirror; swallow.

5. List the innervation and lymphatic supply of the thyroid gland.

Nervous System

CHAPTER OUTLINE

This chapter discusses the following topics:

I. Nervous System
   A. Central Nervous System
   B. Peripheral Nervous System
   C. Cranial Nerves
II. Nerves to the Oral Cavity and Associated Structures
   A. Trigeminal Nerve
   B. Facial Nerve
III. Nerve Lesions of the Head and Neck

LEARNING OBJECTIVES

After studying this chapter, the reader should be able to:

1. Define and pronounce all the key words and anatomical terms in this chapter.
2. Describe the components of the nervous system and outline the actions of nerves.
3. Discuss in general the major divisions of the central and peripheral nervous systems.
4. Identify and trace the routes of the cranial nerves from the skull on a series of diagrams.
5. Briefly discuss the general function of each of the cranial nerves.
6. Identify and trace the routes of the nerves to the oral cavity and associated structures of the head and neck on a diagram, a skull, and a patient.
7. Describe the tissues innervated by each of the nerves of the head and neck.
8. Discuss certain nerve lesions associated with the head and neck region.
9. Correctly complete the identification exercises and review questions and activities of this chapter.
10. Integrate the knowledge about the head and neck nerves into the functioning of the region's muscles, joints, and glands, the concepts of pain management with local anesthesia, and also the related nervous system disorders.

KEY WORDS

Action potential (po-**ten**-shal) Rapid depolarization of the cell membrane that results in propagation of the nerve impulse along the membrane.

Afferent nerve (**af**-er-ent) Sensory nerve that carries information from the periphery of the body to the brain or spinal cord.

Bell's palsy (belz **pawl**-ze) Type of unilateral facial paralysis involving the facial nerve.

Efferent nerve (**ef**-er-ent) Motor nerve that carries information away from the brain or spinal cord to the periphery of the body.

Facial paralysis (pah-**ral**-i-sis) Loss of action of the facial muscles.

Ganglion/ganglia (**gang**-gle-in, **gang**-gle-ah) Accumulation of neuron cell bodies outside the central nervous system.

Innervation (in-er-**vay**-shin) Supply of nerves to tissues or organs.

Nerve (nurv) Bundle of neural processes outside the central nervous system; part of the peripheral nervous system.

(continued)

Neuron (**noor**-on) Cellular component of the nervous system that is individually composed of a cell body and neural processes.

Neurotransmitter (**nu**-ro-**tranz**-mitt-er) Chemical agent from the neuron that is discharged with the arrival of the action potential, diffuses across the synapse, and binds to receptors on another cell's membrane.

Resting potential (po-**ten**-shal) Charge difference between the fluid outside and inside a cell that results in differences in the distribution of ions.

Synapse (**sin**-aps) Junction between two neurons or between a neuron and an effector organ, where neural impulses are transmitted by electrical or chemical means.

Trigeminal neuralgia (try-**jem**-i-nal noor-**al**-je-ah) Type of lesion of the trigeminal nerve involving facial pain.

▓ NERVOUS SYSTEM

The **nervous system** causes muscles to contract, resulting in facial expressions and joint movements such as those involved in mastication and speech. The system stimulates glands to secrete and also regulates many other systems of the body, such as the blood system. The nervous system also allows for sensation to be perceived, such as pain and touch.

Knowledge of the nervous system and its components is important to the dental professional since this system allows for the function of the muscles, temporomandibular joint, and glands of the head and neck (see Chapters 4, 5, and 7 for more information). A thorough understanding of certain nerves is important in pain management that involves local anesthesia during dental treatment (see Chapter 9 for more information). Finally, there are certain related nervous system disorders of the head and neck that need to be known by the dental professional (discussed later in this chapter).

The nervous system has two main divisions, the central nervous system and the peripheral nervous system (Figure 8–1). These two portions of the nervous system are constantly interacting. The *neuron* (**noor**-on) is the cellular component of the nervous system and is composed of a cell body and neural processes. A *nerve* (nurv) is a bundle of neural processes outside the central nervous system and in the peripheral nervous system. A *synapse* (**sin**-aps) is the junction between two neurons or between a neuron and an effector organ, where neural impulses are transmitted.

In order to function, most tissues and organs have *innervation* (in-er-**vay**-shin), a supply of nerves to the part. A nerve allows information to be carried to and from the brain, which is the central informational center. An accumulation of neuron cell bodies outside the central nervous system is termed a *ganglion* (plural *ganglia*) (**gang**-gle-on, **gang**-gle-ah).

There are two types of nerves, afferent and efferent (Figure 8–1). An *afferent nerve* (**af**-er-ent) or *sensory nerve* carries information from the periphery of the body to the brain (or spinal cord). Thus an afferent nerve carries sensory information such as taste, pain, and proprioception to the brain. Proprioception is information concerning the movement and position of the body. This information is sent on to the brain to be analyzed, acted upon, associated with other information, and stored as memory.

An *efferent nerve* (**ef**-er-ent) or *motor nerve* carries information away from the brain (or spinal cord) to the periphery of the body. Thus an efferent nerve carries information to the muscles in order to activate them, often in response to information received by way of the afferent nerves. One motor neuron with its branching process may control hundreds of muscle fibers.

The plasma membrane of a neuron, like all other cells, has an unequal distribution of ions and electrical charges between the two sides of the membrane. The fluid outside of the membrane has a positive charge; the fluid inside has a negative charge. This charge difference is a *resting potential* (po-**ten**-shal) and is measured in millivolts. Resting potential results in part from differences in the distribution of positively charged ions (sodium and potassium) and negatively charged ions in the cytoplasm and the extracellular fluid. Sodium ions are more heavily concentrated outside the membrane, while potassium ions are more heavily concentrated inside the membrane. This imbalance is maintained by the active transport of ions against their concentration gradients by the sodium-potassium pump.

The rapid depolarization of the cell membrane, called the *action potential* (po-**ten**-shal), results in the propagation of the nerve impulse along the

CENTRAL NERVOUS SYSTEM

Cerebrum (cerebral hemispheres brainstem)

Brainstem

Cerebellum

Spinal cord

PERIPHERAL NERVOUS SYSTEM

Nerve ganglion

Nerve

Afferent nerve from skin

Efferent nerve to muscle

NEURON

Action potential (impulse propagation)

Muscle fiber

Neurotransmitter

SYNAPSE

FIGURE 8–1 ■ An overview of the nervous system with its two main divisions: the central nervous and peripheral nervous systems.

membrane (Figure 8–1). An action potential is a temporary reversal of the electrical potential along the membrane for brief period (less than a millisecond). Sodium gates suddenly open in the membrane to allow sodium ions to pour in, bringing their positive charge. At the height of the membrane potential reversal, sodium gates close and potassium channels open to allow potassium ions to pass to the outside of the membrane, reestablishing the resting potential. The changed ionic distributions must be reset by the continuously running sodium-potassium pump.

The action potential begins at one spot on the membrane, but spreads to adjacent areas of the membrane, propagating the impulse along the length of the cell membrane. After passage of the action potential, there is a brief period, the refractory period, during which the membrane cannot be stimulated. This prevents the impulse from being transmitted backward along the membrane. By means of the action potential, nerve impulses travel the length of the neuron.

To have the impulse cross the synapse to another cell requires the actions of chemical agents or *neurotransmitters* (**nu**-ro-**tranz**-mitt-er) from the neuron, which are discharged with the arrival of the action potential.

Released neurotransmitters diffuse across the synapse and bind to receptors on the membrane of the other cell. Neurotransmitters cause ion channels to open or close in the second cell, prompting changes in the excitability of that cell's membrane. Excitatory neurotransmitters, such as acetylcholine and norepinephrine (in most organs), make it more likely that an action potential will be triggered in the second cell. Inhibitory neurotransmitters, such as dopamine and serotonin, make an action potential in the second cell less likely. Neurotransmitters are either destroyed by specific enzymes, diffuse away, or are reabsorbed by the neuron.

Neurotransmitters tend to be small molecules; some are even hormones. Some neurological diseases, for example Parkinson's disease and Huntington's chorea, are associated with imbalances of neurotransmitters. Some of the symptoms of Parkinson's disease, for example rigidity, are due to a dopamine deficiency. Some symptoms of Huntington's chorea are thought to be caused by loss of a different inhibitory neurotransmitter. Alzheimer's disease is accompanied by a loss of acetylcholine-producing neurons, which may explain the memory problems that result. In addition, depression can be linked to low levels of excitatory neurotransmitters, and drug therapy for depression alters those levels. Among the drugs that affect neurotransmitter function is cocaine, which blocks the uptake of norepinephrine while stimulating the uptake of dopamine.

Special neurotransmitters involved with the sensation of pain in the central nervous system are endorphins, natural opioids that produce elation and reduction of pain, as do nonnatural neurotransmitting chemicals such as opium and heroin. Many local anesthetics such as lidocaine, as used in dentistry, mimic inhibitory neurotransmitters by decreasing sensory neurons' ability to generate an action potential, thus producing anesthesia.

CENTRAL NERVOUS SYSTEM

One of the major divisions of the nervous system, the **central nervous system (CNS),** is composed of the brain and spinal cord. The CNS is surrounded by bone, either the skull or vertebrae,

FIGURE 8–2 ■ A ventral view of the gross brain showing the cerebellum, cerebral hemisphere, and diencephalon, with the brainstem highlighted.

with fluid and tissue serving as further protection. The major regions of the **brain** include the cerebrum, the cerebellum, the brainstem, and the diencephalon (Figure 8–2).

The **cerebrum** (ser-**e**-brum) is the largest portion of the brain and consists of two cerebral hemispheres (Figure 8–2). The cerebrum coordinates sensory data and motor functions and governs many aspects of intelligence and reasoning, learning and memory. The **cerebellum** (ser-e-**bel**-um) is the second largest portion of the brain, after the cerebrum. It functions to produce muscle coordination and maintains normal muscle tone and posture, as well as coordinating balance.

The **brainstem** has a number of portions, including the medulla, the pons, and the midbrain (Figure 8–3). The **medulla** (me-**dul**-ah) is closest to the spinal cord, and is involved with the regulation of heartbeat, breathing, vasoconstriction (blood pressure), and reflex centers for vomiting, coughing, sneezing, swallowing, and hiccupping. The cell bodies of the motor neurons for the tongue are located in the medulla. The **pons** (ponz) connects the medulla with the cerebellum and with higher brain centers. Cell bodies for cranial nerves V and VII are found in the pons. The **midbrain** includes relay stations for hearing, vision, and motor pathways.

FIGURE 8–3 ■ A lateral sagittal section of the gross brain showing the brainstem highlighted with its midbrain, medulla, and pons, and the diencephalon with its thalamus and hypothalamus, as well as the spinal cord, cerebellum, and cerebral hemisphere.

Superior to the brainstem, the **diencephalon** (di-en-**sef**-a-lon) consists primarily of the thalamus and hypothalamus (Figure 8–3). The **thalamus** (**thal**-a-mus) serves as a central relay point for incoming nerve impulses and the **hypothalamus** (**hi**-po-**thal**-a-mus) regulates homeostasis. It has regulatory areas for thirst, hunger, body temperature, water balance, and blood pressure, and links the nervous system to the endocrine system.

The **spinal cord** (**spi**-nal) runs along the dorsal side of the body and links the brain to the rest of the body (Figure 8–3). The spinal cord in adults is encased in a series of bony vertebrae that make up the vertebral column. The gray matter of the spinal cord consists mostly of unmyelinated cell bodies and dendrites. The surrounding white matter is made up of tracts of axons, insulated in sheaths of myelin, a combination of lipids and proteins. Some tracts are ascending (carrying messages to the brain), others are descending (carrying messages from the brain). The spinal cord is also involved in reflexes that do not immediately involve the brain.

PERIPHERAL NERVOUS SYSTEM

The other major division of the nervous system, the **peripheral nervous system (PNS),** is made up of all the nerves stretching between the CNS and the receptors, muscles, and glands of the body. The PNS is further divided into the sensory or **afferent nervous system** (af-er-ent), which carries information from receptors to the brain or spinal cord, and the motor or **efferent nervous system** (ef-er-ent), which carries information from the brain or spinal cord to muscles or glands. A nerve cell leading from the eye to the brain and carrying visual information is part of the afferent nervous system. A nerve cell leading from the brain to muscles controlling the eye's movement is a portion of the efferent nervous system. The motor system of the PNS is further subdivided into the somatic nervous system and autonomic nervous system.

vous System

...matic nervous system (SNS) is a portion ...he peripheral nervous system and includes all ...rves controlling the muscular system and external sensory receptors. External sense organs (including skin) are receptors. Muscle fibers and gland cells are effectors. Sensory input from the PNS is processed by the CNS, and responses are sent by the PNS from the CNS to the organs of the body. The motor neurons of the somatic system are distinct from those of the autonomic system. Inhibitory signals cannot be sent through the motor neurons of the somatic system.

Autonomic Nervous System

The **autonomic nervous system** (awt-o-**nom**-ik) **(ANS)** is the other portion of the peripheral nervous system. This system operates without conscious control as the caretaker of the body. Autonomic fibers are efferent nerves and they always occur in two-nerve chains. The first nerve carries autonomic fibers to a ganglion where they end near the cell bodies of the second nerve. The ANS itself has two portions: the sympathetic system and the parasympathetic system. Most tissues and organ systems are supplied by both portions of the ANS. However, the sympathetic and parasympathetic systems generally work in opposition to each other: one stimulates an organ while the other inhibits it.

The **sympathetic nervous system** (sim-pah-**thet**-ik) is involved in 'fight-or-flight responses' such as the shutdown of salivary gland secretion. Thus such a response by the sympathetic system leads to a dry mouth (xerostomia). Sympathetic nerves arise in the spinal cord and relay in ganglia arranged like a chain running up the neck close to the vertebral column on both sides. Therefore, all the sympathetic neurons in the head have already relayed in a ganglion. Sympathetic fibers reach the cranial tissues they supply by traveling with the arteries.

The **parasympathetic nervous system** (pare-ah-sim-pah-**thet**-ik) is involved in 'rest-or-digest' responses such as the stimulation of salivary gland secretions. Thus such a response by the parasympathetic system leads to salivary flow to aid in digestion.

Parasympathetic fibers associated with the glands of the head and neck region are carried in various cranial nerves and are briefly described here as well as in greater detail later in this chapter. Their ganglia are located in the head, and therefore parasympathetic neurons in this region may be either preganglionic neurons (before relaying in the ganglion) or postganglionic neurons (after relaying in the ganglion).

The principal parasympathetic outflow for glands in the head and neck is carried in the seventh and ninth cranial nerves. The seventh cranial or facial nerve has two branches involved in glandular secretion. The greater petrosal nerve is associated with the pterygopalatine ganglion and the lacrimal gland is the major target organ. The chorda tympani nerve is associated with the submandibular ganglion, and the target organs are the submandibular and sublingual salivary glands. The lesser petrosal nerve, a branch of the ninth cranial or glossopharyngeal nerve, is associated with the otic ganglion, and the target organ is the parotid salivary gland.

CRANIAL NERVES

The **cranial nerves** (**kray**-nee-al) are an important portion of the peripheral nervous system. There are 12 paired cranial nerves, and all are connected to the brain at its base and pass through the skull by way of fissures or foramina (Figures 8–4 and 8–5, Table 8–1) (see Chapter 3).

Some cranial nerves are either afferent or efferent, and others have both types of neural processes. A general background of all 12 cranial nerves is discussed in this chapter (Figure 8–4 and Table 8–1). Roman numerals and anatomical terms are used to designate the cranial nerves.

Cranial Nerve I

The first cranial nerve, cranial nerve I or the **olfactory nerve** (ol-**fak**-ter-ee), transmits smell from the nasal mucosa to the brain and thus functions as an afferent nerve. The olfactory nerve enters the skull through the perforations in the cribriform plate of the ethmoid bone to join the olfactory bulb in the brain.

Cranial Nerve II

The second cranial nerve, cranial nerve II or **optic nerve** (**op**-tik), transmits sight from the retina of

FIGURE 8–4 ■ Inferior view of the brain showing cranial nerves and the organs and tissues they innervate.

the eye to the brain and thus functions as an afferent nerve. The optic nerve enters the skull through the optic canal of the sphenoid bone on its way from the retina. In the skull, the right and left optic nerves join at the optic chiasma, where many of the fibers cross to the opposite side before continuing into the brain as the optic tracts.

Cranial Nerve III

The third cranial nerve, cranial nerve III or **oculomotor nerve** (ok-yule-oh-**mote**-er), serves as an efferent nerve to some of the eye muscles that move the eyeball. The oculomotor nerve also carries preganglionic parasympathetic

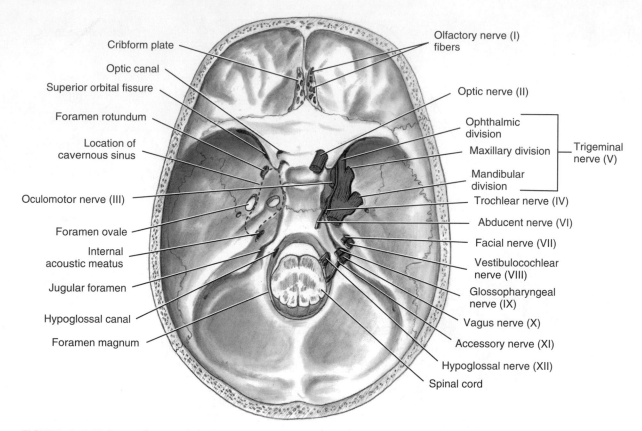

Cribform plate
Optic canal
Superior orbital fissure
Foramen rotundum
Location of
cavernous sinus
Oculomotor nerve (III)
Foramen ovale
Internal
acoustic meatus
Jugular foramen
Hypoglossal canal
Foramen magnum

Olfactory nerve (I)
fibers
Optic nerve (II)
Ophthalmic
division
Maxillary division
Mandibular
division
Trigeminal
nerve (V)
Trochlear nerve (IV)
Abducent nerve (VI)
Facial nerve (VII)
Vestibulocochlear
nerve (VIII)
Glossopharyngeal
nerve (IX)
Vagus nerve (X)
Accessory nerve (XI)
Hypoglossal nerve (XII)
Spinal cord

FIGURE 8–5 ■ Internal view of the base of the skull showing cranial nerves exiting or entering the skull.

fibers to the ciliary ganglion near the eyeball. The postganglionic fibers innervate small muscles inside the eyeball. The oculomotor nerve lies in the lateral wall of the cavernous sinus and exits the skull through the superior orbital fissure of the sphenoid bone on its way to the orbit.

Cranial Nerve IV

The very small fourth cranial nerve, cranial nerve IV or **trochlear nerve** (**trok**-lere), also serves as an efferent nerve for one eye muscle, as well as proprioception, similar to the oculomotor nerve but without any parasympathetic fibers. Similar to the oculomotor nerve, the trochlear nerve runs in the lateral wall of the cavernous sinus and exits the skull through the superior orbital fissure of the sphenoid bone on its way to the orbit.

Cranial Nerve V

The fifth cranial nerve, cranial nerve V or **trigeminal nerve** (try-**jem**-i-nal), has both an efferent component for the muscles of mastication, as well as some other cranial muscles, and an afferent component for the teeth, tongue, and oral cavity, as well as most of the skin of the face and head. Although the trigeminal has no preganglionic parasympathetic fibers, many postganglionic parasympathetic fibers travel along with its branches.

The trigeminal nerve is the largest cranial nerve and has two roots, sensory and motor roots (see Figure 8–4). The **sensory root of the trigeminal nerve** has three divisions: the ophthalmic, maxillary, and mandibular divisions. The ophthalmic division provides sensation to the upper face and scalp. The maxillary and mandibular divisions provide sensation to the middle and lower face, respectively.

| Table 8–1 | THE TWELVE CRANIAL NERVES AND THE NERVE TYPE AND TISSUES INNERVATED |

Nerve	Nerve Type and Tissues Innervated
I: Olfactory	Afferent: nasal mucosa
II: Optic	Afferent: retina of the eye
III: Oculomotor	Efferent: eye muscles
IV: Trochlear	Efferent: eye muscles
V: Trigeminal	Efferent: muscles of mastication and other cranial muscles Afferent: face and head skin, teeth, oral cavity, and tongue (general sensation)
VI: Abducens	Efferent: eye muscles
VII: Facial	Efferent: muscles of facial expression, other cranial muscles, and lacrimal, submandibular, sublingual, and minor glands (parasympathetic) Afferent: skin around ear and tongue (taste sensation)
VIII: Vestibulocochlear	Afferent: inner ear
IX: Glossopharyngeal	Efferent: stylopharyngeus muscle and parotid gland (parasympathetic) Afferent: skin around ear and tongue (taste and general sensation)
X: Vagus	Efferent: muscles of soft palate, pharynx, and larynx and thorax and abdominal organs (parasympathetic) Afferent: skin around ear and epiglottis (taste sensation)
XI: Accessory	Efferent: muscles of neck, soft palate, and pharynx
XII: Hypoglossal	Efferent: tongue muscles

Each division of the sensory root of the nerve enters the skull in a different location in the sphenoid bone. The ophthalmic division enters through the superior orbital fissure. The maxillary division enters by way of the foramen rotundum. The mandibular division passes through the skull by way of the foramen ovale.

The **motor root of the trigeminal nerve** accompanies the mandibular division of the sensory root and also exits the skull through the foramen ovale of the sphenoid bone.

The trigeminal nerve is the most important cranial nerve to the dental professional since it innervates many relevant tissues of the head and neck (Table 8–2). The trigeminal nerve is discussed in greater detail later in this chapter.

Cranial Nerve VI

The sixth cranial nerve, cranial nerve VI or abducent nerve, **abducens** (ab-**doo**-senz), serves as an efferent nerve to one of the muscles that moves the eyeball, similar to the oculomotor and trochlear nerves. Similar to both of those cranial nerves, the abducens exits the skull through the superior orbital fissure of the sphenoid bone on its way to the orbit.

However, the abducens has a somewhat different intracranial course. Rather than lying in the wall of the cavernous sinus, the nerve runs through the sinus, close to the internal carotid artery, and is often the first nerve affected by infection of the sinus (see Chapter 12 for more information).

Cranial Nerve VII

The seventh cranial nerve, cranial nerve VII or **facial nerve,** carries both efferent and afferent components. The facial nerve carries an efferent component for the muscles of facial expression and for the preganglionic parasympathetic innervation of the lacrimal gland (relaying in the pterygopalatine ganglion) and sub-mandibular and sublingual salivary glands (relaying in the submandibular ganglion). The afferent component serves a tiny patch of skin behind the ear, taste sensation, and the body of the tongue.

The facial nerve leaves the cranial cavity by passing through the internal acoustic meatus, which leads to the facial canal inside the temporal bone. Finally, the facial nerve exits the skull by way of the stylomastoid foramen of the temporal bone. The facial nerve is also important to dental professionals since it innervates many relevant tissues of the head

Table 8–2 TISSUES OF THE HEAD AND NECK AND THEIR ASSOCIATED NERVES AND TYPE

Head and Neck Tissues	Nerves and Type
Maxillary anterior lingual gingiva and anterior hard palate	Nasopalatine of V_2: afferent
Maxillary posterior lingual gingiva and posterior hard palate	Greater palatine of V_2: afferent
Soft palate and palatine tonsillar tissue	Lesser palatine of V_2, glossopharyngeal; afferent Branches of V_3, accessory, and vagus: efferent
Maxillary anterior teeth, maxillary anterior facial gingiva, and anterior labial mucosa	ASA of V_2: afferent
Maxillary posterior teeth, maxillary posterior buccal gingiva, posterior labial mucosa, and maxillary sinus	MSA and PSA of V_2: afferent
Mandibular teeth and facial gingiva of mandibular anterior teeth and premolars	IA of V_3: afferent
Mandibular buccal gingiva and buccal mucosa	Buccal of V_3: afferent
Mandibular labial mucosa	Mental of V_3: afferent
Floor of mouth and mandibular lingual gingiva	Lingual of V_3: afferent
Tongue muscles	Hypoglossal: efferent
Tongue general sensation	Body, lingual of V_3: afferent Base, glossopharyngeal: afferent
Tongue taste sensation	Body, chorda tympani of facial: afferent Base, glossopharyngeal: afferent
Parotid gland	Lesser petrosal of glossopharyngeal: efferent (parasympathetic)
Submandibular and sublingual glands	Chorda tympani of facial: efferent (parasympathetic)
Muscles of facial expression	Branches of facial: efferent
Muscles of mastication	Medial pterygoid, deep temporal, masseteric, and lateral pterygoid of V_3: efferent
Trapezius and sternocleidomastoid muscles	Accessory: efferent

ASA = anterior superior alveolar; MSA = middle superior alveolar; PSA = posterior superior alveolar; IA = inferior alveolar.

and neck (see Table 8–2). The facial nerve is discussed in greater detail later in this chapter.

Cranial Nerve VIII

The eighth cranial nerve, cranial nerve VIII or **vestibulocochlear nerve** (ves-tib-you-lo-**kok**-lere), serves as an afferent nerve for hearing and balance.

This nerve conveys signals from the inner ear to the brain. The inner ear is located within the temporal bone. The vestibulocochlear nerve enters the cranial cavity through the internal acoustic meatus of the temporal bone.

The nerve supplies the two major parts of the inner ear. The first part, the cochlea, serves the function of hearing and is supplied by the cochlear

part of the vestibulocochlear nerve. The second part, the semicircular canals, serves the function of balance and is supplied by the vestibular part of the semicircular canals.

Cranial Nerve IX

The ninth cranial nerve, cranial nerve IX or **glossopharyngeal nerve** (gloss-oh-fah-**rin**-je-al), carries an efferent component for a pharyngeal muscle, the stylopharyngeus muscle, and preganglionic gland parasympathetic innervation for the parotid salivary gland (relaying the otic ganglion). The nerve also carries an afferent component for the pharynx and for taste and general sensation from the base of the tongue.

The glossopharyngeal nerve passes through the skull by way of the jugular foramen, between the occipital and temporal bones. The tympanic branch, with sensory fibers for the middle ear and preganglionic parasympathetic fibers for the parotid gland, arises here and reenters the skull.

After supplying the ear, parasympathetic fibers leave the skull through the foramen ovale of the sphenoid bone as the **lesser petrosal nerve** (peh-**troh**-sil). These preganglionic fibers then end in the **otic ganglion** (**ot**-ik). The otic ganglion is located near the medial surface of the mandibular division of the trigeminal or fifth cranial nerve, just inferior to the foramen ovale.

Lower branches of the glossopharyngeal nerve supply the carotid artery, pharynx, and base of the tongue (afferent component), as well as the stylopharyngeus muscle. This nerve is important to dental professionals since it innervates many relevant tissues of the head and neck (see Table 8–2).

Cranial Nerve X

The tenth cranial nerve, cranial nerve X or **vagus nerve** (**vay**-gus), carries a large efferent component for the muscles of the soft palate, pharynx, and larynx and for parasympathetic fibers to many organs in the thorax and abdomen, including the thymus gland, heart, and stomach. The nerve carries a smaller afferent component for a small amount of skin around the ear and for taste sensation for the epiglottis.

The vagus nerve passes through the skull by way of the jugular foramen, between the occipital and temporal bones. This nerve is important to dental professionals since it innervates many relevant tissues of the head and neck (see Table 8–2).

Cranial Nerve XI

The eleventh cranial nerve, cranial nerve XI or **accessory nerve** (ak-**ses**-o-re), functions as an efferent nerve for the trapezius and sternocleidomastoid muscles, as well as for muscles of the soft palate and pharynx. This nerve is only partly a cranial nerve and consists of two roots, one arising from the brain and one from the spinal cord. The accessory nerve exits the skull through the jugular foramen, between the occipital and temporal bones. This nerve is important to dental

professionals since it innervates many relevant tissues of the head and neck (see Table 8–2).

Cranial Nerve XII

The twelfth cranial nerve, cranial nerve XII or **hypoglossal nerve** (hi-poh-**gloss**-al), functions as an efferent nerve for the intrinsic and extrinsic muscles of the tongue. The hypoglossal nerve exits the skull through the hypoglossal canal in the occipital bone. This nerve is important to dental professionals since it innervates the tongue (see Table 8–2).

NERVES TO THE ORAL CAVITY AND ASSOCIATED STRUCTURES

The dental professional must understand the basic components of the nervous system, as well as the location of the major nerves of the head and neck. Knowledge of the nervous system is important because it adds to the general background of certain disease processes of the head and neck muscles (discussed later in this chapter), temporomandibular joint, and salivary glands.

The management of dentally related pain using local anesthetics is an important tool in dentistry. The dental professional involved in the injection of local anesthetics in the head and neck area must have an increased level of knowledge of the nervous system (see Chapter 9 for more information).

Two cranial nerves that affect the head and neck tissues, the trigeminal and facial nerves, are discussed in greater detail, with the stronger emphasis on the trigeminal nerve.

TRIGEMINAL NERVE

The dental professional must have a thorough knowledge of the **trigeminal nerve** (try-**jem**-i-nal) or cranial nerve V. Each trigeminal nerve is a short nerve trunk composed of two closely adapted roots (Figure 8–6). These roots of the trigeminal nerve consist of a thicker sensory root and thinner motor root.

Within the skull, a bulge can be noted in the **sensory root of the trigeminal nerve.** This bulge is the **trigeminal ganglion** (semilunar or

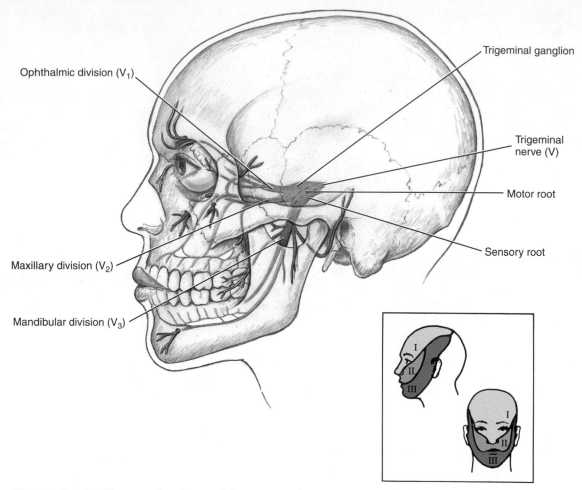

Ophthalmic division (V₁)

Trigeminal ganglion

Trigeminal nerve (V)

Motor root

Sensory root

Maxillary division (V₂)

Mandibular division (V₃)

FIGURE 8–6 ■ The general pathway of the trigeminal or fifth cranial nerve and its motor and sensory roots and three divisions (inset shows the pattern of innervation for each division).

gasserian ganglion), which is located on the anterior surface of the petrous portion of the temporal bone. Anterior to the trigeminal ganglion, the sensory root arises from three divisions that pass into the skull by way of different fissures or foramina.

As mentioned before and detailed later, these divisions of the sensory root of the trigeminal nerve are the ophthalmic, maxillary, and mandibular divisions. The ophthalmic and maxillary divisions of the sensory root carry only afferent nerves. In contrast, the mandibular division of the sensory root runs together with the motor root and thus carries both afferent and efferent nerves.

The **motor root of the trigeminal nerve** supplies the efferent nerves for the muscles of mastication. The motor root exits the skull at the

foramen ovale of the sphenoid bone and then travels with the mandibular division of the sensory root of the trigeminal nerve.

Ophthalmic Division of the Trigeminal Nerve (Ophthalmic Nerve)

The first and smallest division of the sensory root is the ophthalmic division of the trigeminal nerve, the **ophthalmic nerve** (of-**thal**-mik) or V₁ (Figure 8–7). The ophthalmic nerve serves as an afferent nerve for the conjunctiva, cornea, eyeball, orbit, forehead, and ethmoid and frontal sinuses, plus a portion of the dura mater.

The ophthalmic nerve carries this sensory information toward the brain by way of the superior

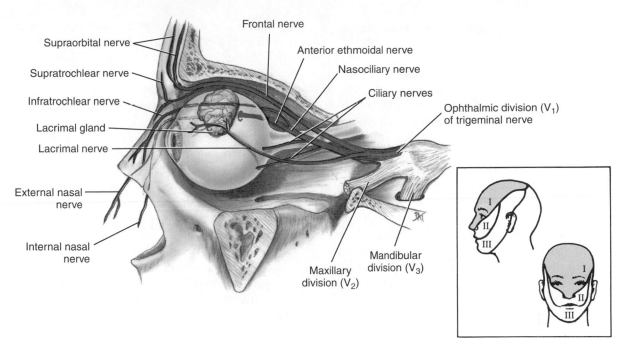

FIGURE 8–7 ■ Lateral view of the cut-away orbit with the pathway of the ophthalmic division of the trigeminal nerve highlighted.

orbital fissure of the sphenoid bone. Other nerves that traverse this fissure include cranial nerves III, IV, and VI. The ophthalmic nerve arises from three major nerves: the frontal, lacrimal, and nasociliary nerves.

FRONTAL NERVE

The **frontal nerve** (**frunt**-il) is an afferent nerve located in the orbit and is composed of a merger of the **supraorbital nerve** (soo-prah-**or**-bit-al) from the forehead and anterior scalp and the **supratrochlear nerve** (soo-prah-**trok**-lere) from the bridge of the nose and medial parts of the upper eyelid and forehead. The frontal nerve courses along the roof of the orbit toward the superior orbital fissure of the sphenoid bone where it is joined by the lacrimal and nasociliary nerves to form the ophthalmic nerve or V_1.

LACRIMAL NERVE

The **lacrimal nerve** (**lak**-ri-mal) serves as an afferent nerve for the lateral part of the upper eyelid, conjunctiva, and lacrimal gland. The nerve also delivers the postganglionic parasympathetic nerves to the lacrimal gland. These nerves are responsible for the production of lacrimal fluid or

tears. The lacrimal nerve runs posteriorly along the lateral roof of the orbit and then joins the frontal and nasociliary nerves near the superior orbital fissure of the sphenoid bone to form the ophthalmic nerve or V_1.

NASOCILIARY NERVE

Several afferent nerve branches converge to form the **nasociliary nerve** (nay-zo-**sil**-ee-a-re). These branches include the **infratrochlear nerve** (in-frah-**trok**-lere) from the skin of the medial part of the eyelids and the side of the nose, **ciliary nerves** (**sil**-ee-a-re) to and from the eyeball, and **anterior ethmoidal nerve** (eth-**moy**-dal) from the nasal cavity and paranasal sinuses. The anterior ethmoidal nerve is formed by the **external nasal nerve** (**nay**-zil) from the skin of the ala and apex of the nose and the **internal nasal nerves** from the anterior part of the nasal septum and lateral wall of the nasal cavity.

The nasociliary nerve is an afferent nerve that runs within the orbit, superior to cranial nerve II, the optic nerve, to join the frontal and lacrimal nerves near the superior orbital fissure of the sphenoid bone to form the ophthalmic nerve or V_1.

Maxillary Division of the Trigeminal Nerve (Maxillary Nerve)

The second division from the sensory root is the maxillary division of the trigeminal nerve, the **maxillary nerve** (**mak**-sil-ar-ee) or V_2 (Figure 8–8). The afferent nerve branches of the maxillary nerve carry sensory information for the maxilla and overlying skin, maxillary sinuses, nasal cavity, palate, and nasopharynx and a portion of the dura mater.

The maxillary nerve is a nerve trunk formed in the pterygopalatine fossa by the convergence of many nerves. The largest contributor is the infraorbital nerve. Tributaries of the infraorbital nerve or maxillary nerve trunk include the zygomatic, anterior, middle and posterior superior alveolar, greater and lesser palatine, and nasopalatine nerves.

After all these branches come together in the pterygopalatine fossa to form the maxillary nerve and thus V_2 of the trigeminal nerve, the maxillary nerve enters the skull through the foramen rotundum of the sphenoid bone (see Figure 3–61). Small afferent meningeal branches (me-**nin**-je-al) from portions of the dura mater join the maxillary division as it enters the trigeminal ganglion.

Another ganglion, the **pterygopalatine ganglion** (teh-ri-go-**pal**-ah-tine), lies just below the maxillary nerve in the pterygopalatine fossa. This ganglion serves as a relay station for parasympathetic nerves that arise in the facial nerve (described later). Fibers from the ganglion (postganglionic) are then distributed to the various tissues, such as the minor salivary glands, by the nerves of the maxillary division.

Because the pterygopalatine ganglion lies between the maxillary nerve and its tributaries from the palate, the sensory fibers actually pass through the ganglion. However, unlike the

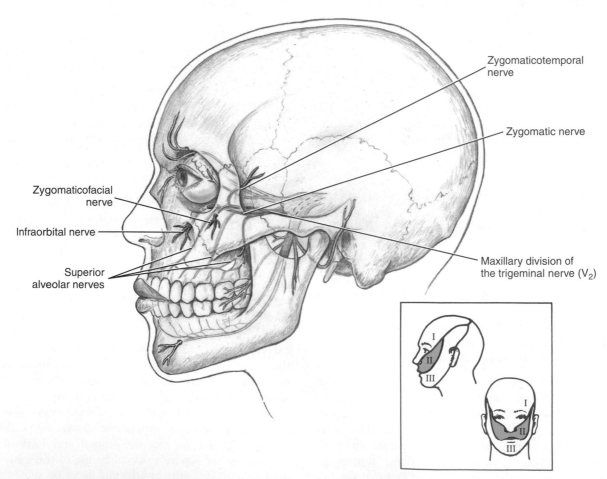

Zygomaticotemporal nerve

Zygomatic nerve

Zygomaticofacial nerve

Infraorbital nerve

Superior alveolar nerves

Maxillary division of the trigeminal nerve (V_2)

FIGURE 8–8 ■ The pathway of the maxillary division of the trigeminal nerve highlighted.

parasympathetic fibers, the sensory fibers do not synapse in the ganglion.

ZYGOMATIC NERVE

The **zygomatic nerve** (zy-go-**mat**-ik) is an afferent nerve composed of the merger of the zygomaticofacial nerve and the zygomaticotemporal nerve in the orbit (see Figure 8–8). This nerve also conveys the postganglionic parasympathetic fibers for the lacrimal gland to the lacrimal nerve. The zygomatic nerve courses posteriorly along the lateral orbit floor, enters the pterygopalatine fossa through the inferior orbital fissure, between the sphenoid bone and maxilla, and finally joins the maxillary nerve.

The rather small **zygomaticofacial nerve** (zy-go-mat-i-ko-**fay**-shal) serves as an afferent nerve for the skin of the cheek. This nerve pierces the frontal process of the zygomatic bone and enters the orbit through its lateral wall. The zygomaticofacial nerve then turns posteriorly to join with the zygomaticotemporal nerve.

The other nerve, the **zygomaticotemporal nerve** (zy-go-mat-i-ko-**tem**-poh-ral) serves as an afferent nerve for the skin of the temporal region, pierces the temporal surface of the zygomatic bone, and traverses the lateral wall of the orbit to join the zygomaticofacial nerve, forming the zygomatic nerve.

INFRAORBITAL NERVE

The **infraorbital nerve** (in-frah-**or**-bit-al) or **IO nerve** is an afferent nerve formed from the merger of cutaneous branches from the upper lip, medial portion of the cheek, lower eyelid, and side of the nose (Figure 8–9). The IO nerve then passes into the infraorbital foramen of the maxilla and travels posteriorly through the infraorbital canal, along with the infraorbital blood vessels, where it is joined by the anterior superior alveolar nerve.

From the infraorbital canal and groove, the IO nerve passes into the pterygopalatine fossa through the inferior orbital fissure. After it leaves the infraorbital groove and within the pterygopalatine fossa, the IO nerve receives the posterior superior alveolar (PSA) nerve.

ANTERIOR SUPERIOR ALVEOLAR NERVE

The **anterior superior alveolar nerve** (al-ve-o-lar) or **ASA nerve** serves as an afferent nerve of sensation (including pain) for the maxillary central incisors, lateral incisors, and canine, as well as their associated tissues.

The anterior superior alveolar nerve originates from dental branches in the pulp tissue of these teeth that exit through the apical foramina (see Figure 8–9). The nerve also receives interdental branches from the surrounding periodontium, forming a dental plexus or nerve network in the maxilla for the region. The ASA nerve also innervates the overlying facial gingiva. The ASA nerve then ascends along the anterior wall of the maxillary sinus to join the infraorbital nerve in the infraorbital canal.

Many times the anterior superior alveolar nerve crosses over the midline to the opposite side in a patient. This is important to consider when giving a local anesthetic injection for the maxillary anterior teeth or associated tissues (see Chapter 9).

MIDDLE SUPERIOR ALVEOLAR NERVE

The **middle superior alveolar nerve** (al-**ve**-o-lar) or **MSA nerve** serves as an afferent nerve of sensation (including pain), typically for the maxillary premolar teeth and mesial buccal root of the maxillary first molar and their associated periodontium and overlying buccal gingiva.

The middle superior alveolar nerve originates from dental branches in the pulp tissue that exit the teeth through the apical foramina, as well as interdental and interradicular branches from the periodontium (see Figure 8–9). The MSA nerve, like the PSA and ASA nerves, forms the dental plexus or nerve network in the maxilla. The MSA nerve then ascends to join the infraorbital nerve by running in the lateral wall of the maxillary sinus.

The middle superior alveolar nerve is not present in all patients. If this nerve is not present, the area is innervated by both the ASA and PSA nerves, but mainly by the ASA nerve. If the MSA nerve is present, there is communication between the MSA nerve and both the ASA and PSA nerves. These considerations are important when giving local anesthetic injections to the maxillary teeth (see Chapter 9).

POSTERIOR SUPERIOR ALVEOLAR NERVE

The **posterior superior alveolar nerve** (al-**ve**-o-lar) or **PSA nerve** joins the infraorbital nerve (or the maxillary nerve directly) in the pterygopalatine fossa (see Figure 8–9). The PSA nerve serves as an afferent nerve of sensation (including pain) for most portions of the maxillary molar teeth and their periodontium and buccal gingiva, as well as the maxillary sinus.

Zygomatic nerve

Infraorbital nerve

Anterior superior
alveolar nerve

Dental plexus

Inferior orbital fissure

Ophthalmic nerve

Maxillary nerve

Ptygopalatine
ganglion

Mandibular nerve

Greater and lesser
palatine nerves

Posterior superior
alveolar nerve

Middle superior alveolar nerve

FIGURE 8–9 ■ Lateral view of the skull (a portion of the lateral wall of the orbit removed) with the branches of the maxillary nerve highlighted.

Some branches of the posterior superior alveolar nerve remain external to the posterior surface of the maxilla. These branches provide afferent innervation for the buccal gingiva overlying the maxillary molars.

Other afferent nerve branches of the posterior superior alveolar nerve originate from dental branches in the pulp tissue of each of the maxillary molar teeth that exit the teeth by way of the apical foramina. These dental branches are joined by interdental and interradicular branches from the periodontium, forming a dental plexus or nerve network in the maxilla for the region.

All these internal branches of the PSA nerve exit from several posterior superior alveolar foramina on the maxillary tuberosity of the maxilla. The posterior superior alveolar arteries (from the maxillary artery) enter the maxillary tuberosity through these same foramina.

Both the external and internal branches of the posterior superior alveolar nerve then ascend together along the maxillary tuberosity, which forms the posterolateral wall of the maxillary sinus, to join the IO nerve or maxillary nerve.

The PSA nerve typically provides afferent innervation for the maxillary second and third molars and the palatal and distal buccal root of the maxillary first molar, as well as the mucous membranes of the maxillary sinus.

GREATER AND LESSER PALATINE NERVES

Both palatine nerves join with the maxillary nerve from the palate (Figure 8–10). The **greater palatine nerve** (**pal**-ah-tine) or **GP nerve** or anterior palatine nerve is located between the mucoperiosteum and bone of the anterior hard palate. This nerve serves as an afferent nerve for the posterior hard palate and posterior lingual gingiva. There is communication with the terminal fibers of the nasopalatine nerve in the hard palate area, lingual to the maxillary canines.

Posteriorly, the greater palatine nerve enters the greater palatine foramen in the palatine bone near the maxillary second or third molar to travel in the pterygopalatine canal, along with the greater palatine blood vessels.

The **lesser palatine nerve** (**pal**-ah-tine) or posterior palatine nerve serves as an afferent

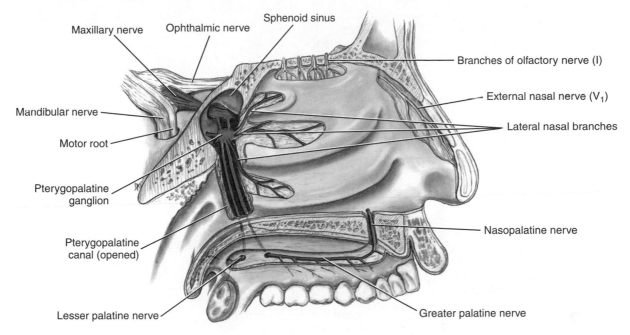

FIGURE 8–10 ■ Medial view of the lateral nasal wall and opened pterygopalatine canal highlighting the maxillary nerve and its palatine branches. The nasal septum has been removed, thus severing the nasopalatine nerve.

nerve for the soft palate and palatine tonsillar tissues. The lesser palatine nerve enters the lesser palatine foramen in the palatine bone near its junction with the pterygoid process of the sphenoid bone, along with the lesser palatine blood vessels (see Figure 8–10). The lesser palatine nerve then joins the greater palatine nerve in the pterygopalatine canal.

Both palatine nerves ascend through the pterygopalatine canal, toward the maxillary nerve in the pterygopalatine fossa. On the way, the palatine nerves are joined by lateral nasal branches (**nay**-zil), which are afferent nerves from the posterior nasal cavity.

NASOPALATINE NERVE

The **nasopalatine nerve** (nay-zo-**pal**-ah-tine) or **NP nerve** originates in the mucosa of the anterior hard palate, lingual to the maxillary anterior teeth (see Figure 8–10). The right and left nasopalatine nerves enter the incisive canal by way of the incisive foramen, thus exiting the oral cavity. The nerve then travels along the nasal septum. The nasopalatine nerve serves as an afferent nerve for the anterior hard palate and the lingual gingiva of the maxillary anterior teeth, as

well as the nasal septal tissues. There is also communication with the greater palatine nerve in the area lingual to the maxillary canines.

Mandibular Division of the Trigeminal Nerve (Mandibular Nerve)

The mandibular division of the trigeminal nerve, the **mandibular nerve** (man-**dib**-you-lar) or V_3, is a short main trunk formed by the merger of a smaller anterior trunk and a larger posterior trunk in the infratemporal fossa before the nerve passes through the foramen ovale of the sphenoid bone (Figure 8–11). The mandibular nerve then joins with the ophthalmic and maxillary nerves to form the trigeminal ganglion of the trigeminal nerve. The mandibular nerve is the largest of the three divisions that form the trigeminal nerve.

A few small branches arise from the V_3 trunk before its separation into the anterior and posterior trunks (see Figure 8–14). These branches from the undivided mandibular division include the meningeal branches (me-**nin**-je-al), which are afferent nerves for portions of the dura mater. Also from the undivided mandibular division are

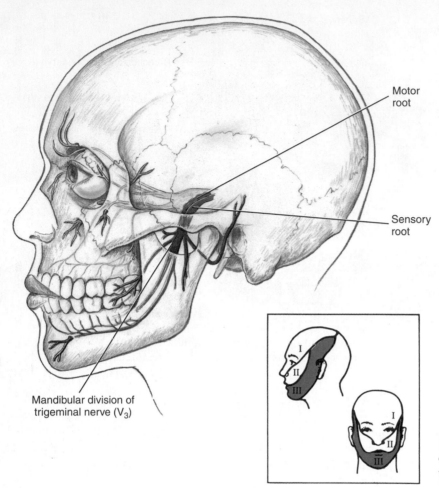

Motor
root

Sensory
root

Mandibular division of
trigeminal nerve (V₃)

FIGURE 8–11 ■ The pathway of the mandibular division of the trigeminal nerve highlighted.

muscular branches, which are efferent nerves for the medial pterygoid, tensor tympani, and tensor veli palatini muscles.

The anterior trunk of the mandibular division is formed by the merger of the buccal nerve and additional muscular nerve branches (Figure 8–12). The posterior trunk of the mandibular division is formed by the merger of the auriculotemporal, lingual, and inferior alveolar nerves (Figure 8–13).

BUCCAL NERVE

The **buccal nerve** or long buccal nerve serves as an afferent nerve for the skin of the cheek, buccal mucous membranes, and buccal gingiva of the mandibular posterior teeth. The nerve is located on the surface of the buccinator muscle (see Figure 8–12). The buccal nerve then travels posteriorly in the cheek, deep to the masseter muscle.

At the level of the occlusal plane of the last mandibular molar, the nerve crosses in front of the anterior border of the ramus and goes between the two heads of the lateral pterygoid muscle to join the anterior trunk of V_3. It is important not to confuse this nerve with the nerve to the buccinator muscle, an efferent nerve branch from the facial nerve.

MUSCULAR BRANCHES

There are several muscular branches that are part of the anterior trunk of the V_3 (see Figure 8–12). They arise from the motor root of the trigeminal nerve. The **deep temporal nerves** (**tem**-poh-ral), usually two in number, anterior and posterior, are efferent nerves that pass between the sphenoid bone and the superior border of the lateral pterygoid muscle and turn

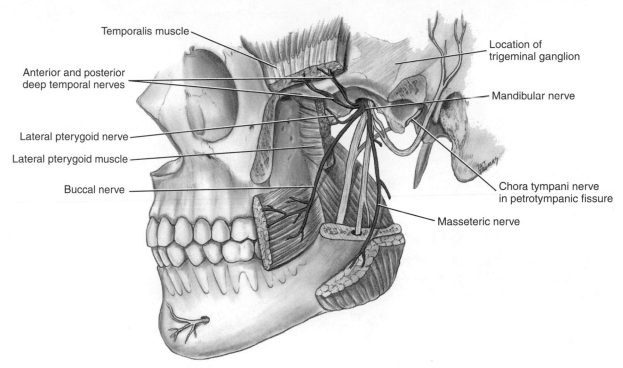

Temporalis muscle

Anterior and posterior
deep temporal nerves

Lateral pterygoid nerve

Lateral pterygoid muscle

Buccal nerve

Location of
trigeminal ganglion

Mandibular nerve

Chora tympani nerve
in petrotympanic fissure

Masseteric nerve

FIGURE 8–12 ■ The pathway of the anterior trunk of the mandibular division of the trigeminal nerve highlighted.

around the infratemporal crest of the sphenoid bone to end in the deep surface of the temporal muscle that they innervate. The posterior temporal nerve may arise in common with the masseteric nerve, and the anterior temporal nerve may be associated at its origin with the buccal nerve.

The **masseteric nerve** (mass-et-**tehr**-ik) is also an efferent nerve that passes between the sphenoid bone and the superior border of the lateral pterygoid muscle. The nerve then accompanies the masseteric blood vessels through the mandibular notch to innervate the masseter muscle. A small sensory branch also goes to the temporomandibular joint. The **lateral pterygoid nerve** (**teh**-ri-goid), after a short course, enters the deep surface of the lateral pterygoid muscle between the muscle's two heads of origin and serves as an efferent nerve for that muscle.

AURICULOTEMPORAL NERVE

The nerve known as the **auriculotemporal nerve** (aw-rik-yule-lo-**tem**-poh-ral) travels with the superficial temporal artery and vein and serves

as an afferent nerve for the external ear and scalp (Figure 8–13 and 8–14). The nerve also carries postganglionic parasympathetic nerve fibers to the parotid salivary gland. It is important to note that these parasympathetic fibers arise from the lesser petrosal branch of the glossopharyngeal nerve or ninth cranial nerve, joining the auriculotemporal nerve only after relaying in the otic ganglion near the foramen ovale.

There is also communication of the auriculotemporal nerve with the facial nerve near the ear. The nerve courses deep to the lateral pterygoid muscle and neck of the mandible, then splits to encircle the middle meningeal artery, and finally joins the posterior trunk of V_3.

LINGUAL NERVE

The **lingual nerve** is formed from afferent branches from the body of the tongue that travel along the lateral surface of the tongue (see Figures 8-13 and 8-14). The nerve then passes posteriorly, passing from the medial to the lateral side of the duct of the submandibular salivary gland by going under the duct.

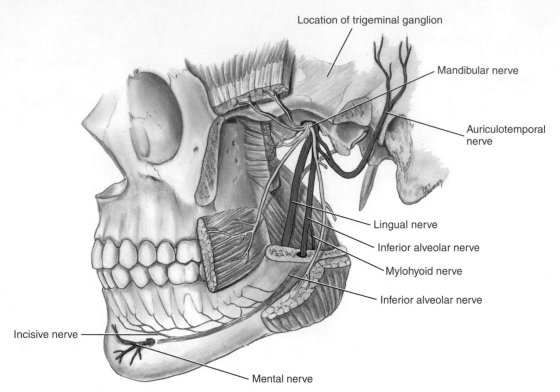

Location of trigeminal ganglion

Mandibular nerve

Auriculotemporal nerve

Lingual nerve

Inferior alveolar nerve

Mylohyoid nerve

Inferior alveolar nerve

Incisive nerve

Mental nerve

FIGURE 8–13 ■ The pathway of the posterior trunk of the mandibular division of the trigeminal nerve highlighted.

The lingual nerve communicates with the **submandibular ganglion** (sub-man-**dib**-you-lar) located superior to the deep lobe of the submandibular salivary gland (Figure 8–15). The submandibular ganglion is part of the parasympathetic system. Parasympathetic efferent innervation for the sublingual and submandibular salivary glands arises from the facial nerve (specifically, a branch of the facial nerve, the chorda tympani, which is discussed later in this chapter) but travels along with the lingual nerve.

At the base of the tongue, the lingual nerve ascends and runs between the medial pterygoid muscle and the mandible, anterior and slightly medial to the inferior alveolar nerve. Thus the lingual nerve is anesthetized when giving an inferior alveolar anesthetic nerve block. When the nerve is only a short distance posterior to the roots of the last mandibular molar tooth, it is covered only by a thin layer of oral mucosa and thus its location is sometimes visible clinically. Thus the lingual nerve is often endangered by dental procedures in this region, such as the extraction of mandibular third molars.

The lingual nerve then continues to travel upward to join the posterior trunk of V_3. Thus the lingual nerve serves as an afferent nerve for general sensation for the body of the tongue, floor of the mouth, and lingual gingiva of the mandibular teeth.

INFERIOR ALVEOLAR NERVE

The **inferior alveolar nerve** (al-**ve**-o-lar) or **IA nerve** is an afferent nerve formed from the merger of the mental and incisive nerves (see Figure 8–13). The mental and incisive nerves are discussed later in this section.

After forming, the inferior alveolar nerve continues to travel posteriorly through the mandibular canal, along with the inferior alveolar artery and vein. The nerve is joined by dental branches and interdental and interradicular branches from the mandibular posterior teeth, forming a dental plexus or nerve network in the region. The inferior alveolar nerve then exits the mandible through the mandibular foramen, where it is joined by the mylohyoid nerve (discussed later). The mandibular foramen is a central opening on the internal surface of the ramus.

Middle meningeal nerve
Motor root of trigeminal nerve
Greater petrosal nerve
Ophthalmic nerve
Maxillary nerve
Ear ossicles
Otic ganglion
Pterygopalatine ganglion
Facial nerve
Nerve to tensor veli palatini muscle
Nerve to medial pterygoid muscle
Auriculotemporal nerve
Chorda tympani nerve
Ingferior alveolar nerve
Lingual nerve
Branches to tongue
Mylohyoid nerve
Submandibular ganglion
Submandibular duct
Sublingual salivary gland
Submandibular salivary gland
Mylohoid muscle

FIGURE 8–14 ■ Medial view of the mandible with the motor and sensory branches of the mandibular nerve highlighted.

The inferior alveolar nerve then travels lateral to the medial pterygoid muscle, between the sphenomandibular ligament and ramus of the mandible within the pterygomandibular space. This is posterior and slightly lateral to the lingual nerve. The inferior alveolar nerve then joins the posterior trunk of V_3 (see Figures 8–13 and 8–14). The inferior alveolar nerve carries afferent innervation for the mandibular teeth.

In some cases, there are two nerves present on the same side, creating bifid inferior alveolar nerves. This situation can occur unilaterally or bilaterally and can be detected on a radiograph by the presence of a double mandibular canal. As discussed in Chapter 3, there can be more than one mandibular foramen, usually inferiorly placed, either unilaterally or bilaterally, along with the bifid inferior alveolar nerves. These considerations must be kept in mind when administering a local anesthetic for the mandibular arch (see Chapter 9).

MENTAL NERVE

The **mental nerve** (**ment**-il) is composed of external branches that serve as an afferent nerve for the chin, lower lip, and labial mucosa near the mandibular anterior teeth (see Figure 8–13). The mental nerve then enters the mental foramen on the anterior-lateral surface of the mandible, usually between the apices of the first and second mandibular premolars, and merges with the incisive nerve to form the inferior alveolar nerve in the mandibular canal.

INCISIVE NERVE

The **incisive nerve** (in-**sy**-ziv) is an afferent nerve composed of dental branches from the anterior mandibular teeth that originate in the pulp tissue, exit the teeth through the apical foramina, and join with interdental branches from the surrounding periodontium, forming a dental plexus in the region (see Figure 8–13). The incisive nerve then merges with the mental nerve, just posterior

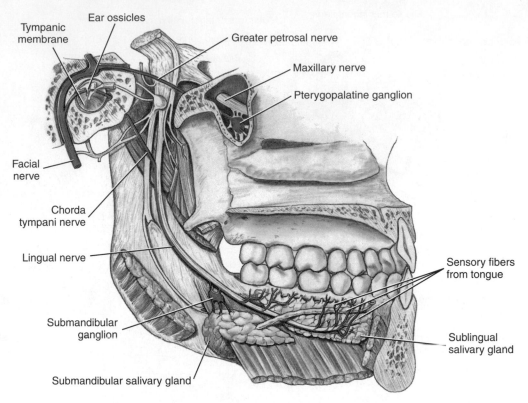

FIGURE 8–15 ■ The pathway of the trunk of the facial nerve, greater petrosal nerve, and chorda tympani nerve (note relationship with lingual nerve) highlighted.

to the mental foramen, to form the inferior alveolar nerve in the mandibular canal. The incisive nerve serves as an afferent nerve for the anterior mandibular teeth.

There is sometimes crossover from the opposite incisive nerve, which is an important consideration when using a local anesthetic in the area of the mandibular anterior teeth (see Chapter 9).

MYLOHYOID NERVE

The **mylohyoid nerve** (my-lo-**hi**-oid) is a small branch of the inferior alveolar nerve after the IA nerve exits the mandibular foramen (see Figures 8–13 and 8–14). This nerve pierces the sphenomandibular ligament and runs inferiorly and anteriorly in the mylohyoid groove and then onto the lower surface of the mylohyoid muscle. The mylohyoid nerve serves as an efferent nerve to the mylohyoid muscle and anterior belly of the digastric muscle (the posterior belly of the digastric muscle is innervated by a branch from the facial nerve).

FACIAL NERVE

The dental professional must also have an understanding of the **facial nerve** or cranial nerve VII. The facial nerve carries both efferent and afferent nerves. The facial nerve emerges from the brain and enters the internal acoustic meatus in the petrous portion of the temporal bone. Within the bone, the nerve gives off a small efferent branch to the muscle in the middle ear (stapedius) and two larger branches, the greater petrosal and chorda tympani nerves, both of which carry parasympathetic fibers (see Figure 8–15).

The main trunk of the nerve emerges from the skull through the stylomastoid foramen of the temporal bone and gives off two branches, the posterior auricular nerve and a branch to the posterior belly of the digastric and stylohyoid muscles (Figure 8–16). The facial nerve then passes into the parotid salivary gland and divides into numerous branches to supply the muscles of facial expression, but not the parotid gland itself. It is important to

FIGURE 8–16 ■ The pathway of the branches of the facial nerve to the muscles of facial expression highlighted.

avoid anesthesia of this nerve at this location when giving an inferior alveolar nerve block (see Chapter 9) because it may result in transient facial paralysis (discussed later in this chapter).

Greater Petrosal Nerve

The **greater petrosal nerve** (peh-**troh**-sil) is a branch off the facial nerve before it exits the skull (see Figure 8–15). The greater petrosal nerve carries efferent nerve fibers; preganglionic parasympathetic fibers to the **pterygopalatine ganglion** (teh-ri-go-**pal**-ah-tine) in the pterygopalatine fossa.

The postganglionic fibers arising in the pterygopalatine ganglion then join with branches of the maxillary division of the trigeminal nerve to be carried to the lacrimal gland (via the zygomatic and lacrimal nerves), nasal cavity, and minor salivary glands of the hard and soft palate. The greater petrosal nerve also carries afferent nerve fibers for taste sensation in the palate.

Chorda Tympani Nerve

This small branch of the facial nerve, the **chorda tympani nerve** (**kor**-dah **tim**-pan-ee), is a parasympathetic efferent nerve for the submandibular and sublingual salivary glands and also serves as an afferent nerve for taste sensation for the body of the tongue.

After branching off the facial nerve within the petrous portion of the temporal bone, the chorda tympani nerve crosses the medial surface of the tympanic membrane (eardrum) (see Figure 8–15), which thereby exits the skull by the **petrotympanic fissure** (pe-troh-tim-**pan**-ik), located immediately posterior to the temporomandibular joint (see Figures 8–13 and 8–14). The chorda tympani nerve then travels with the lingual nerve along the floor of the mouth in the same nerve bundle.

In the submandibular triangle, the chorda tympani nerve, appearing as part of the lingual nerve, has communication with the submandibular ganglion. The **submandibular ganglion** (sub-man-**dib**-you-lar) is located superior to the deep lobe of the submandibular salivary gland, for which it supplies parasympathetic efferent innervation (see Figure 8–15).

Posterior Auricular, Stylohyoid, and Posterior Digastric Nerves

The **posterior auricular nerve** (aw-**rik**-you-lar), **stylohyoid nerve** (sty-lo-**hi**-oid), and **posterior digastric nerve** (di-**gas**-trik) are branches of the facial nerve after it exits the stylomastoid foramen. All are efferent nerves. The posterior auricular nerve supplies the occipital belly of the epicranial muscle (see Figure 8–16). The other two nerves supply the stylohyoid muscle and the posterior belly of the digastric muscle, respectively.

Branches to the Muscles of Facial Expression

Additional efferent nerve branches of the facial nerve originate in the parotid salivary gland and pass to the muscles they innervate (see Figure 8–16). These branches to the muscles of facial expression are the temporal, zygomatic, buccal, (marginal) mandibular, and cervical branches. However, these branches are rarely seen as five independent nerves. They may vary in number and connect irregularly. For convenience, they are described as five simple branches.

The temporal branch(es) (**tem**-poh-ral) supplies the muscles anterior to the ear, frontal belly of the epicranial muscle, superior portion of the orbicularis oculi muscle, and corrugator supercilii muscle.

The zygomatic branch(es) (zy-go-**mat**-ik) supplies the inferior portion of the orbicularis oculi muscle and zygomatic major and minor muscles. The buccal branch(es) supplies the muscles of the upper lip and nose and buccinator, risorius, and orbicularis oris muscles. The zygomatic and buccal branches are usually closely associated, exchanging many fibers.

The (marginal) mandibular branch (man-**dib**-you-lar) supplies the muscles of the lower lip and mentalis muscle. The mandibular branch should not be confused with the mandibular nerve or V$_3$.

The cervical branch (**ser**-vi-kal) runs inferior to the mandible to supply the platysma muscle.

▦ NERVE LESIONS OF THE HEAD AND NECK

A dental professional needs to have a background concerning certain lesions of the head and neck that pertain to the nervous system before treating patients. These lesions are facial paralysis, Bell's palsy, and trigeminal neuralgia.

Facial paralysis (pah-**ral**-i-sis) is a loss of muscular action of the muscles of facial expression (see Chapter 4 and Figure 4–6). This lesion can occur secondarily to a brain injury by way of a stroke (cerebrovascular accident), with other muscles of the head and neck also affected. The lesion can also occur by directly injuring the nerve that supplies the efferent nerves to the muscles of facial expression, the seventh cranial or facial nerve. Facial paralysis can be unilateral or bilateral depending on the nature of the nerve damage. These injuries are common because the facial nerve branches are superficially located and vulnerable to trauma.

The injury to the facial nerve can occur secondarily through injury to the parotid salivary gland or surrounding region. If cancer (malignant neoplasm) occurs in the parotid salivary gland, the facial nerve can be injured since it travels through the gland. During facial surgery or due to a laceration (deep wound) to the parotid gland region, the facial nerve within the tissues can be affected. Transient facial paralysis can occur due to injection into the gland during an incorrectly administered inferior alveolar local anesthetic block (see Chapter 9).

The affected facial muscles lose tone on the involved side (see Chapter 4). Clinically, the patient with facial paralysis has a drooping eyebrow, eyelid, and labial commissure, with a dribbling of saliva. There is also an inability to show normal expression, close the eye, or whistle. As a result, there can be infection in the involved eye. Speech and mastication are difficult.

Bell's palsy (**pawl**-ze) involves unilateral facial paralysis with no known cause, except that there is a loss of excitability of the involved facial nerve. All or just some of the branches of the facial nerve are affected. The onset of this paralysis is abrupt. One theory of its cause is that the facial nerve becomes inflamed within the temporal bone.

Bell's palsy may undergo remission or may become chronic depending on the amount of loss of facial nerve excitability. There is no specific treatment, but injections of anti-inflammatory medications or physical therapy may be helpful.

Trigeminal neuralgia (try-**jem**-i-nal noor-**al**-jeah) also has no known cause but involves the afferent nerves of the fifth cranial or trigeminal nerve. It usually involves the maxillary or mandibular nerve branches but not the ophthalmic branch. One theory is that this lesion is caused by pressure on the sensory root of the trigeminal ganglion by area blood vessels.

Clinically, the patient feels excruciating short-term pain when facial trigger zones are touched or when speaking or masticating. These trigger zones vary with the patient but can include areas around the eyes or the ala of the nose. The right side of the face is affected more commonly than the left. The pattern of pain follows the pattern of the trigeminal nerve branch involved.

Treatment for trigeminal neuralgia can include peripheral neurectomy by surgical or ultrasonic means in which the sensory root of the trigeminal nerve is sectioned, cutting off innervation to the tissues. Alcohol injection of the trigeminal nerve has also been used to cause necrosis of the nerve, as have systemic anticonvulsant drugs, with varying degrees of success.

IDENTIFICATION EXERCISES

Identify the structures on the following diagrams by filling in the blanks with the correct anatomical term. You can check your answers by looking back at the figure indicated in parentheses for each identification diagram.

1. (Figure 8–5)

CRIBIFORM PLATE
OPTIC CANAL
S. ORBITAL FISSURE
FORAMEN ROTUNDUM
Cavernous Sinus

Occulomotor Nerve
Foramen Ovale
Int. Acoustic Meatus
Jugular Foramen
Hypoglossal Canal
Foramen Magnum,

2. (Figure 8–6)

3. (Figure 8–9)

4. (Figure 8–12)

5. (Figure 8–13)

6. (Figure 8–14)

REVIEW QUESTIONS

1. The brainstem consists of which structures?
   A. Cerebrum, cerebellum, pons, and medulla
   B. Medulla, cerebrum, midbrain, and pons
   C. Medulla, pons, and midbrain
   D. Midbrain, ganglia, and nerves

2. The central nervous system consists of which structures?
   A. Spinal cord and peripheral nervous system
   B. Brain and spinal cord
   C. Autonomic and somatic nervous systems
   D. Brain and autonomic nervous system

3. Which of the following is a correct statement concerning neurotransmitters?
   A. They are discharged with the arrival of the action potential
   B. They bind to red blood cells so as to prompt transmission of impulses
   C. Inhibitory ones initiate an action potential in an adjacent cell
   D. They are destroyed by specific white blood cells while still active

4. To which portion of the nervous system does a nerve cell belong if it leads from the eye to the brain and carries visual information?
   A. Central nervous system
   B. Medulla and pons
   C. Afferent nervous system
   D. Efferent nervous system

5. An efferent nerve carries information:
   A. From the periphery of the body to the brain (or spinal cord)
   B. Such as taste or pain to the spinal cord
   C. Such as proprioception to the brain
   D. Away from the brain (or spinal cord) to the periphery of the body

6. The posterior superior alveolar nerve and its branches supply the:
   A. Frontal sinus
   B. Maxillary posterior teeth
   C. Parotid salivary gland
   D. Temporalis muscle

7. Through which of the following foramina does the facial nerve pass through the skull?
   A. Foramen rotundum
   B. Foramen ovale
   C. Jugular foramen
   D. Stylomastoid foramen

8. Which of the following cranial nerves is involved in Bell's palsy?
   A. Trigeminal nerve
   B. Facial nerve
   C. Glossopharyngeal nerve
   D. Vagus nerve

9. Which of the following nerve and muscle pairs is correctly matched?
   A. Long buccal nerve, buccinator muscle
   B. Accessory nerve, platysma muscle
   C. Hypoglossal nerve, intrinsic tongue muscles
   D. Auriculotemporal nerve, temporalis muscle

10. Which of the following nerve and tissue pairs are correctly matched?
    A. Facial nerve, parotid salivary gland
    B. Chorda tympani, sublingual salivary gland
    C. Vagus nerve, temporomandibular joint
    D. Lingual nerve, base of tongue

11. Which of the following cranial nerves has fibers that cross to the opposite side in the skull before continuing into the brain?
    A. Facial nerve
    B. Optic nerve
    C. Trochlear nerve
    D. Vestibulocochlear nerve

12. Which of the following cranial nerves carries taste sensation for the base of the tongue?
    A. Trigeminal nerve
    B. Facial nerve
    C. Vagus nerve
    D. Glossopharyngeal nerve

13. In which of the following areas is the trigeminal ganglion located?
A. Superior to the deep lobe of the submandibular salivary gland
B. Anterior surface of the petrous portion of the temporal bone
C. Posterior surface of the maxillary tuberosity of the maxilla
D. Anterior to the infraorbital foramen of the maxilla

14. Sensory information is supplied for the soft palate by the:
A. Greater palatine nerve
B. Lesser palatine nerve
C. Nasopalatine nerve
D. Posterior alveolar nerve

15. The posterior belly of the digastric muscle is innervated by branches from the:
A. Facial nerve
B. Mylohyoid nerve
C. Buccal nerve
D. Maxillary nerve

16. Which of the following nerves may show crossover from the opposite side in a patient?
A. Posterior superior alveolar nerve
B. Anterior superior alveolar nerve
C. Posterior auricular nerve
D. Buccal nerve

17. Which of the following nerves is part of the ophthalmic division of the trigeminal nerve?
A. Nasociliary nerve
B. Maxillary nerve
C. Zygomaticotemporal nerve
D. Zygomaticofacial nerve

18. Which of the following anatomical names is also used for cranial nerve X?
A. Hypoglossal nerve
B. Vagus nerve
C. Glossopharyngeal nerve
D. Accessory nerve

19. Which of the following nerves is located in the mandibular canal?
A. Lingual nerve
B. Mylohyoid nerve
C. Inferior alveolar nerve
D. Masseteric nerve

20. Which of the following nerves exits the foramen ovale of the sphenoid bone?
A. Chorda tympani of the facial nerve
B. Greater petrosal nerve of the facial nerve
C. Ophthalmic division of the trigeminal nerve
D. Motor root of the trigeminal nerve

CTSSG   ASA   EMT   On Old Oly

NICE BANDANA

Parf Parafunctional Habits for Bitesplint

Veiwins hops

REVIEW ACTIVITIES

1. List each cranial nerve and then state its nerve type and the tissues innervated.

2. Creat a flow chart of pain sensation felt in the mandibular third molar as it is sent to the brain.

3. Trace the branches of the mandibular division of the trigeminal nerve while looking in a mirror or standing in front of a peer or patient.

4. Trace the branches of the maxillary division of the trigeminal nerve on a skull.

5. Create a flow chart of pain sensation as it is felt in a maxillary anterior tooth as it is sent to the brain.

Anatomy of Local Anesthesia

CHAPTER OUTLINE

This chapter discusses the following topics:

I. Anatomical Considerations for Local Anesthesia
II. Maxillary Nerve Anesthesia
   A. Posterior Superior Alveolar Block
   B. Middle Superior Alveolar Block
   C. Anterior Superior Alveolar Block
   D. Infraorbital Block
   E. Greater Palatine Block
   F. Nasopalatine Block
III. Mandibular Nerve Anesthesia
   A. Inferior Alveolar Block
   B. Buccal Block
   C. Mental Block
   D. Incisive Block
   E. Gow-Gates Mandibular Nerve Block

LEARNING OBJECTIVES

After studying this chapter, the reader should be able to:

1. Define and pronounce all the key words and anatomical terms in this chapter.
2. List the tissues anesthetized by each type of injection and describe the target areas.
3. Locate and identify the anatomical structures used to determine the local anesthetic needle's penetration site for each type of injection on a skull and a patient.
4. Demonstrate the correct placement of the local anesthetic needle for each type of injection on a skull and a patient.
5. Identify the correct depth and tissues penetrated by the local anesthetic needle for each type of injection.
6. Discuss the complications of local anesthesia of the oral cavity associated with anatomical considerations for each type of injection.
7. Correctly complete the identification exercises and review questions and activities for this chapter.
8. Integrate the knowledge about the nerves into the administration of local anesthesia and control of pain during dental procedures.

KEY WORDS

Local infiltration (in-fil-**tray**-shun) Type of injection that anesthetizes a small area, one or two teeth and associated structures when the anesthetic solution is deposited near terminal nerve endings.

Nerve block Type of injection that anesthetizes a larger area than the local infiltration because the anesthetic solution is deposited near large nerve trunks.

ANATOMICAL CONSIDERATIONS FOR LOCAL ANESTHESIA

The management of pain through local anesthesia by dental professionals requires a thorough knowledge of the anatomy of the skull, fifth cranial nerve, and related tissues. This text discusses the anatomical considerations for local anesthesia. Dental professionals will also want to refer to a current textbook on local anesthesia for more information on this topic.

The skull bones involved in the local anesthetic administration are the maxilla, palatine bone, and mandible (see Chapter 3 for review). Soft tissues of the face and oral cavity may serve the dental professional as initial landmarks to visualize and palpate for local anesthesia (see Chapter 2). However, there are many variations in soft tissue topographical anatomy among patients. Thus to increase the reliability of anesthesia, the dental professional must learn to rely mainly on the visualization and palpation of hard tissues for landmarks while injecting patients.

The dental professional must also know the location of certain adjacent soft tissue structures, such as major blood vessels and glandular tissue, so as to avoid inadvertently injecting these structures (see Chapters 6 and 7 for review). If certain soft tissue structures are accidentally injected with anesthetic solution, complications may occur. Infections also may be spread to deeper tissues by needle-tract contamination (see Chapter 12 for more information).

The fifth cranial nerve or trigeminal nerve provides the sensory information for the teeth and associated tissues (see Chapter 8 for review). Thus branches of the trigeminal nerve are those anesthetized prior to most dental procedures. Knowledge of the location of these nerve branches in relationship to the facial skull bones, as well as soft tissues, also increases the reliability of each injection.

There are two types of local anesthetic injections commonly used in dentistry: the local infiltration and nerve block. The type of injection used for a given dental procedure is determined by the type and length of the procedure.

The *local infiltration* (in-fil-**tray**-shun) anesthetizes a small area, one or two teeth and associated tissues, by injection near their apices. For this type of local anesthetic injection, the anesthetic solution is deposited near terminal nerve endings. This localized desposition has varying degrees of success depending on the anatomy of the region. This text does not discuss local infiltration in detail except for a discussion of the anterior superior alveolar block, which some clinicians feel is a local infiltration.

The *nerve block* affects a larger area than the local infiltration. With a nerve block, the anesthetic solution is deposited near large nerve trunks. All the injections, such as the posterior alveolar block, discussed in this chapter are considered by most clinicians to be nerve block injections.

Dental procedures can usually commence within 3–5 minutes after the correct administration of local anesthesia. If failure or incomplete anesthesia occurs, reassess the injection technique and consider the need for reinjection using an alternative technique or other injections. Never reinject with the same technique or in the same area unless careful consideration is given as to why failure or incomplete anesthesia has occurred.

The dental professional also needs to keep in mind the total number of injections and dosage of anesthetic solution needed to complete the planned dental procedures. This will help prevent systemic complications of local anesthesia that may occur when a patient receives more than the maximum safe dosage (see other texts for specific recommendations). It is also important never to inject through an area with abscess, cellulitis, or osteomyelitis so as to prevent the spread of dental infection (see Chapter 12). Also, the effectiveness of local anesthetic agents is greatly reduced when administered in areas of infection.

MAXILLARY NERVE ANESTHESIA

The maxillary nerve and its branches can be anesthetized in a number of ways depending on the tissues requiring anesthesia (Figure 9–1, Chart 9–1). Most anesthesia of the maxilla is more successful than that of the mandible because the bone over the facial surface of the maxillary teeth is less dense than that of the mandible over similar teeth (see Chapter 3). There is also less variation in the anatomy of the maxillary and palatine bones and associated nerves with respect to local anesthetic

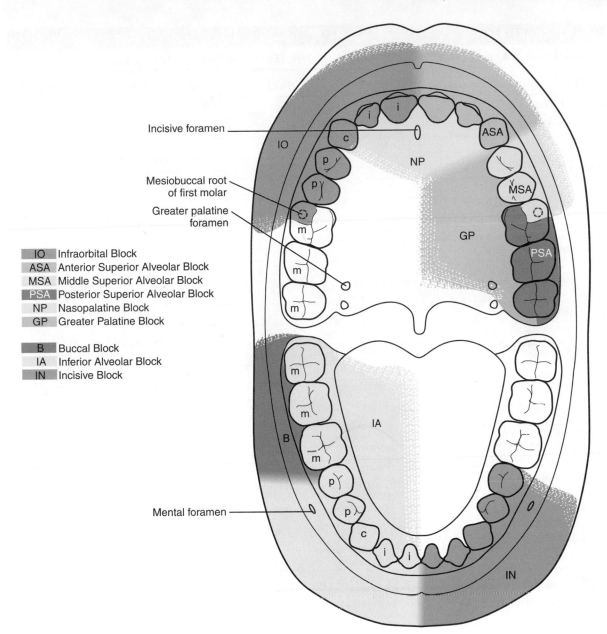

FIGURE 9–1 ■ A diagram of the types of local anesthetic blocks of oral tissues innervated by branches of the maxillary nerve and mandibular nerve.

landmarks as compared with similar mandibular structures.

Pulpal anesthesia is achieved through anesthesia of each nerve's dental branches as they extend into the pulp tissue by way of each tooth's apical foramen. The hard and soft tissues of the periodontium are anesthetized by way of each nerve's interdental and interradicular branches.

The posterior superior alveolar block is generally recommended for anesthesia of the maxillary molar teeth and associated buccal tissues in one quadrant. The middle superior alveolar block is generally recommended for anesthesia of the maxillary premolars and associated buccal tissues in one quadrant. Generally, the anterior superior alveolar block is recommended for anesthesia

CHART 9–1

SUMMARY OF MAXILLARY LOCAL ANESTHESIA OF THE TEETH AND ASSOCIATED TISSUES

Maxillary Tooth and Tissues	PSA Block	MSA Block	IO Block	NP Block	GP Block
Central Incisor					
Facial/pulpal			X		
Lingual				X	
Lateral Incisor					
Facial/pulpal			X		
Lingual				X	
Canine					
Facial/pulpal			X		
Lingual				X	
First Premolar					
Buccal/pulpal		X	X		
Lingual					X
Second Premolar					
Buccal/pulpal		X	X		
Lingual					X
First Molar					
Buccal/pulpal	X				
Lingual					X
Second Molar					
Buccal/pulpal	X				
Lingual					X
Third Molar					
Buccal/pulpal	X				
Lingual					X

The anesthesia is not included for the mesobuccal root of the first molar or for anatomical variants. PSA = posterior superior alveolar, MSA = middle superior alveolar, IO = infraorbital, NP = nasopalatine, GP = greater palatine.

of the maxillary canine and incisors and their associated facial tissues in one quadrant. The infraorbital block is generally recommended for anesthesia of the maxillary anterior and premolar teeth and associated facial tissues in one quadrant.

Palatal anesthesia involves anesthesia of the soft and hard tissues of the periodontium of the palatal area, such as the gingiva, periodontal ligament, and alveolar bone. Palatal anesthesia does not provide any pulpal anesthesia to the maxillary teeth or associated facial or buccal tissues. The greater palatine block is generally recommended for anesthesia of

the palatal tissues distal to the maxillary canine in one quadrant. The nasopalatine block is generally recommended for anesthesia of the palatal tissues between the right and left maxillary canines.

POSTERIOR SUPERIOR ALVEOLAR BLOCK

The **posterior superior alveolar block** (al-ve-o-lar) or **PSA block** is used to achieve pulpal anesthesia in the maxillary third, second, and first molars in most patients. Thus the PSA block is indicated when the dental procedure involves two or more maxillary molars or their associated buccal tissues. This block also is useful for restorative procedures on these teeth.

In some patients, the mesiobuccal root of the maxillary first molar is not innervated by the posterior superior alveolar nerve, but by the middle superior alveolar nerve. Therefore a second injection to anesthetize the middle superior alveolar nerve may be needed to achieve pulpal anesthesia of all the roots of the maxillary first molar.

The PSA block also anesthetizes the buccal periodontium overlying the maxillary third, second, and first molars, including the associated gingiva, periodontal ligament, and alveolar bone. This buccal tissue anesthesia is useful for periodontal treatment of these teeth. If anesthesia of the lingual tissues is desired, such as with extraction, the greater palatine block also may be needed.

Target Area and Injection Site for PSA Block

The target area for the PSA block is the PSA nerve as it enters the maxilla through the posterior superior alveolar foramina on the maxilla's infratemporal surface (Figures 9–2 and 9–3). This area is posterosuperior and medial on the maxillary tuberosity.

The injection site for the PSA block is into the tissues at the height of the mucobuccal fold at the apex of the maxillary second molar, distal to the zygomatic process of the maxilla (Figures 9–4 and 9–5). The patient is supine, with the mouth partially open and the mandible extended toward the side of the injection. Retract the patient's cheek with your finger and pull the tissues at the injection site until they are taut. The needle is inserted into the mucobuccal fold tissues to the desired depth in a distal and medial direction to the tooth and maxilla without touching the maxillary bone in order to reduce trauma (Figure 9–6). In order to achieve visibility of the area, retract the alveolar mucosa about 1 cm distal to the zygomatic process so that the distal portion of the maxillary tuberosity is exposed. A concavity in the mucobuccal fold distal to the maxillary tuberosity will be present.

A certain angulation of the needle to the injection site needs to be maintained. The angulation of the needle should be upward or superiorly at a 45-degree angle to the occlusal plane, inward or medially at a 45-degree angle to the occlusal plane, and backward or posteriorly at a 45-degree angle to the long axis of the second maxillary

FIGURE 9–2 ■ Target area for the PSA block is the PSA nerve located at the posterior superior alveolar foramina on the infratemporal surface of the maxilla, posterosuperior and medial to the maxillary tuberosity. Area anesthetized is highlighted.

FIGURE 9–4 ■ Dissection showing needle piercing for a PSA block. 10. Posterior surface of maxilla; 11. lateral pterygoid; 12. medical pterygoid; 13. buccal nerve; 14. maxillary artery; 15. posterior superior alveolar nerve and vessels; 16. parotid duct; 17. buccinator; 18. lingual nerve; 19. inferior alveolar nerve; 20. inferior alveolar artery. (From McMinn RMH, Hutchings RT, Logan B. *Color Atlas of Head and Neck Anatomy*, 2nd ed. St. Louis, Mosby, 1994.)

FIGURE 9–3 ■ Deep dissection of the face of the right infratemporal fossa with the zyogomatic arch and mandible removed showing the nerves and other structures in the area. 1. Deep temporal nerve; 2. deep temporal artery; 3. upper head of lateral pterygoid; 4. maxillary nerve; 5. posterior superior alveolar nerve; 6. posterior superior alveolar artery; 7. infratemporal surface of maxilla; 8. buccinator; 9. buccal nerve; 10. medial pterygoid; 11. lingual nerve; 12. inferior alveolar nerve; 13. inferior alveolar artery; 14. nerve to mylohyoid; 15. lower head of lateral pterygoid; 16. maxillary artery; 17. masseteric nerve; 18. articular disc and head of mandible; 19. capsule. (From McMinn RMH, Hutchings RT, Logan B. *Color Atlas of Head and Neck Anatomy*, 2nd ed. St. Louis, Mosby, 1994.)

molar. Try to do all three planes in one movement after initial trials so that it is a smooth one- to two-action movement.

The syringe should be extended to the same-side labial commissure, pressing downward on the lower lip to maintain the angulation. If bone is contacted too early or resistance is felt, the angle of the needle toward the midline is too great (more than a 45-degree angle), so move the syringe barrel closer to the occlusal plane, thereby reducing the angle (to less than 45 degrees).

The desired depth of needle insertion for the PSA block depends on the size of the maxilla. In an adult of average size, the penetration is 16 mm. In small adults and children, it is important not to advance the needle more than a depth of 10–14 mm. This conservative insertion technique may also be used in all adults so as to reduce possible complications (discussed next in this chapter).

Symptoms and Possible Complications of PSA Block

There are usually no symptoms resulting from soft tissue anesthesia with a PSA block. Thus the patient frequently has difficulty determining the

FIGURE 9–5 ■ The injection site for the PSA block is probed at the height of the mucobuccal fold at the apex of the maxillary second molar.

extent of anesthesia since a lip or the tongue is not anesthetized. Instead, the patient will state that the teeth in the area feel dull when gently tapped, and there will be an absence of discomfort during dental procedures. It may be necessary to inform the patient of this before starting the procedure so as to allay fears that the anesthetic has not worked.

Complications can occur if the needle is advanced too far distally into the tissues during a PSA block (Figure 9–7). The needle may pene-

trate the pterygoid plexus of veins and the maxillary artery if overinserted, possibly causing a hematoma in the infratemporal fossa (see Chapter 6 for more information). This results in a bluish-reddish extraoral swelling of hemorrhaging blood in the tissues on the side of the face a few minutes after the injection, progressing over time inferiorly and anteriorly toward the lower anterior region of the cheek. If the needle is contaminated, there may be a spread of infection to the

FIGURE 9–6 ■ Needle penetration of the mucobuccal fold tissues for the PSA block is demonstrated at the apex of the maxillary second molar. Injection site is highlighted.

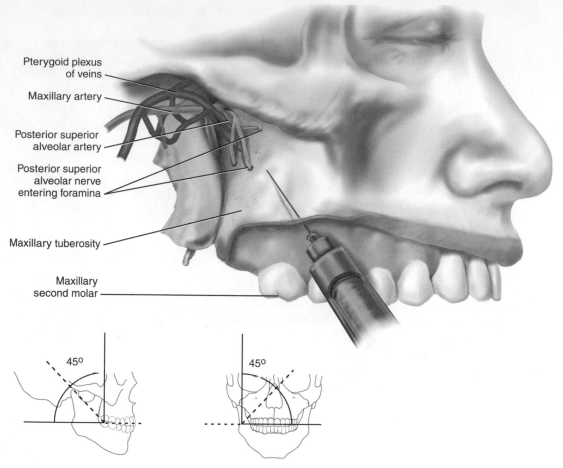

Pterygoid plexus of veins

Maxillary artery

Posterior superior alveolar artery

Posterior superior alveolar nerve entering foramina

Maxillary tuberosity

Maxillary second molar

45°

45°

FIGURE 9–7 ■ Correct insertion of the needle during a PSA block. If the needle is overinserted, it can penetrate the pterygoid plexus of the veins and maxillary artery, which may lead to complications such as a hematoma.

FIGURE 9–8 ■ Target area for the MSA block is the MSA nerve located at the apex of the maxillary second premolar. Area anesthetized is highlighted.

cavernous venous sinus (see Chapter 12). Aspiration should always be attempted in all injections in order to avoid injection into blood vessels, and strict aseptic protocol should be observed.

Inadvertent and harmless anesthesia of branches of the mandibular nerve may occur with a PSA block since they are located lateral to the PSA nerve. This may result in varying degrees of lingual anesthesia and anesthesia of the lower lip.

MIDDLE SUPERIOR ALVEOLAR BLOCK

The **middle superior alveolar block** (al-**ve**-o-lar) or **MSA block** has limited clinical usefulness since the middle superior alveolar nerve is not present in all patients. However, when the more useful infraorbital block fails to achieve pulpal anesthesia distal to the maxillary canine, the MSA block is indicated for dental procedures on the maxillary premolars and mesiobuccal root of the maxillary first molar, such as with restorative procedures.

The MSA block is also used when the dental procedure involves only the maxillary premolars or their associated buccal tissues. Where the MSA nerve is absent, the area is innervated by the anterior superior alveolar nerve and can be anesthetized using the same MSA block technique.

FIGURE 9–9 ■ Coronal section of maxilla and cheek through the permanent maxillary first premolar tooth, showing the needle piercing for MSA block (needle to the reader's left) and NP block (needle to the reader's right). 1. Lip; 2. buccal fold of mucous membrane; 3. alveolar process of maxilla; 4. apex of tooth; 5. pulp cavity; 6. gingival margin; 7. mucoperiosteum of hard palate. (From McMinn RMH, Hutchings RT, Logan B. *Color Atlas of Head and Neck Anatomy*, 2nd ed. St. Louis, Mosby, 1994.)

Thus the MSA block anesthetizes the pulp tissue of the maxillary first and second premolars and possibly the mesiobuccal root of the maxillary first molar and the associated buccal periodontal tissues, including the gingiva, periodontal ligament, and alveolar bone. The buccal tissue anesthesia is useful for periodontal treatment of these teeth. If lingual tissue anesthesia of these

FIGURE 9–10 ■ The injection site for the MSA block is probed at the height of the mucobuccal fold at the apex of the maxillary second premolar.

FIGURE 9–11 ■ Needle penetration of the mucobuccal fold tissues for the MSA block is demonstrated at the apex of the maxillary second premolar. Injection site is highlighted.

teeth is desired, as with an extraction or periodontal treatment, the greater palatine block may also be needed.

Target Area and Injection Site for MSA Block

The target area for the MSA block is the MSA nerve at the apex of the maxillary second premolar (Figures 9–8 and 9–9). Thus the injection site is the tissues at the height of the mucobuccal fold at the apex of the maxillary second premolar (Figure 9–10). The patient is supine, with the mouth partially open and the mandible extended toward the side of the injection. Stretch the patient's upper lip to make the tissues at the injection site taut. The needle is inserted into the mucobuccal fold tissues until its tip is located well above the apex of the maxillary second premolar without touching the bone in order to reduce trauma (Figure 9–11).

Symptoms and Possible Complications of MSA Block

Symptoms of anesthesia with the MSA block include harmless tingling or numbness of the upper lip and absence of discomfort during dental procedures. Overinsertion with complications such as a hematoma is rare with the MSA block.

ANTERIOR SUPERIOR ALVEOLAR BLOCK

The **anterior superior alveolar block** (al-ve-o-lar) or **ASA block** is considered by some to be a local infiltration. An ASA block is commonly used in conjunction with an MSA block instead of using an IO block. There is communication between the ASA nerve and the MSA and PSA nerves. In addition, many times the ASA nerve crosses over the midline to the opposite side in a patient and this may need to be taken into account when using local anesthesia in this area.

The ASA block is used when the dental procedure involves only the maxillary canine and incisors and their associated facial tissues. The ASA block anesthetizes the pulp tissue of these teeth as well as the associated facial periodontal tissues, including the gingiva, periodontal ligament, and alveolar bone. The facial tissue anesthesia is useful for periodontal treatment. If lingual tissue anesthesia of these teeth is desired, as with an extraction or periodontal treatment, a nasopalatine block may also be needed.

Target Area and Injection Site for ASA Block

The largest area for the ASA block is the ASA nerve at the apex of the maxillary canine (Figure 9–12). The injection site is the tissues at the

FIGURE 9–12 ■ Target area for the ASA block is the ASA nerve located at the apex of the maxillary canine. The area anesthetized is highlighted.

FIGURE 9–13 ■ The injection site for the ASA block is probed at the height of the mucobuccal fold at the apex of the maxillary canine.

FIGURE 9–14 ■ Needle penetration of the mucobuccal fold tissues for the ASA block is demonstrated at the apex of the maxillary canine. Injection site is highlighted.

height of the mucobuccal fold at the apex of the maxially canine, just anterior to and parallel with the canine eminence. Note that a slight depression or canine fossa is located anterior to the canine eminence (Figure 9–13). The patient is supine, with the mouth partially open and the mandible moved to the side of the injection. Stretch the patient's upper lip to make the tissues at the injection site taut. The needle is inserted into the mucobuccal fold tissues until its tip is located well above the apex of the maxillary canine, without touching the bone so as to reduce trauma (Figure 9–14). This is approximately 10 degrees off an imaginary line drawn parallel to the long axis of the canine tooth.

Symptoms and Possible Complications of ASA Block

Symptoms of the ASA block include harmless tingling or numbness of the upper lip and an absence of discomfort during dental procedures. Over-insertion with complications, such as a hematoma, is rare with ASA block.

INFRAORBITAL BLOCK

The **infraorbital block** (in-frah-**or**-bit-al) or **IO block** is a useful nerve block since it anesthetizes both the middle and anterior superior alveolar nerves. The IO block is used for anesthesia of the maxillary premolars, maxillary canine, and maxillary incisors. The IO block is indicated when the dental procedures involve more than two maxillary premolars or anterior teeth and the overlying facial periodontium, including the gingiva, periodontal ligament, and alveolar bone.

Thus the IO nerve injection is useful for restorative procedures since it gives pulpal anesthesia of these teeth and also for periodontal treatment since it gives facial tissue anesthesia. If lingual tissue anesthesia is needed, such as with an extraction or periodontal treatment, a nasopalatine block may also be needed.

In many patients, the ASA nerve crosses over the midline from the opposite side, so bilateral injections of the IO block or local infiltration

FIGURE 9–15 ■ Target area for the IO block is the ASA and MSA nerve located at the infraorbital foramen. Note the position of the infraorbital rim. Area anesthetized is highlighted.

over the opposite maxillary central incisor may be indicated. The maxillary central incisor may be additionally innervated by branches from the palatally located nasopalatine nerve, which may need to be anesthetized as well (discussed later).

Target Area and Injection Site for IO Block

The target area for the IO block is the ASA and MSA nerves as they ascend to join the infraorbital nerve after the infraorbital nerve enters the infraorbital foramen (Figure 9–15). Branches of the infraorbital nerve to the lower eyelid, side of the nose, and upper lip are also inadvertently anesthetized.

To locate the infraorbital foramen, palpate extraorally the patient's infraorbital rim and then move slightly downward about 10 mm, applying

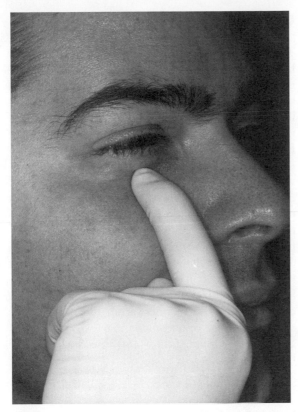

FIGURE 9–16 ■ Palpation of the depression created by the infraorbital foramen for the IO block is demonstrated by moving slightly downward on the face from the infraorbital rim.

pressure until the depression created by the infraorbital foramen is located (Figure 9–16). The patient may feel a dull aching sensation when pressure is applied to the nerves in the region. The infraorbital foramen is about 1–4 mm medial to the pupil of the eye if the patient looks straight forward.

The injection site for the IO block is the tissues at the height of the muccobuccal fold at the apex of the maxillary first premolar. A preinjection approximation of the depth of needle penetration for the IO block can be made by placing one finger on the infraorbital foramen and the other one on the injection site and estimating the distance between them (Figure 9–17). The approximate depth of needle penetration for the IO block will be 16 mm for an adult of average height, although the depth of penetration may vary. In a patient with a high or deep

mucobuccal fold or low infraorbital foramen, less tissue penetration will be required than in a patient with a shallow mucobuccal fold or high infraorbital foramen.

The patient is supine, with the mouth partially open and the mandible extended toward the side of the injection. After locating the infraorbital foramen and maintaining your finger on the site, retract the patient's upper lip with a finger of your other hand and pull the tissues at the injection site taut (gauze may help in retracting the lip). The needle is inserted for the IO block into the mucobuccal fold tissues while keeping the finger of the other hand on the infraorbital foramen during the injection to help keep the syringe toward the foramen (Figure 9–18). The needle is advanced while keeping it parallel with the long axis of the tooth to avoid premature contact with the maxillary bone. The point

FIGURE 9–17 ■ The injection site for the IO block is probed at the height of the mucobuccal fold at the apex of the maxillary first premolar. The palpation over the infraorbital foramen is maintained.

FIGURE 9–18 ■ Needle penetration of the mucobuccal fold tissues for the IO block is demonstrated at the apex of the maxillary first premolar. The palpation over the infraorbital foramen is maintained. Injection site is highlighted.

of contact of the needle with the maxillary bone should be the upper rim of the infraorbital foramen. Keeping the needle in contact with the bone at the roof of the infraorbital foramen prevents overinsertion and possible puncture of the orbit.

Symptoms and Possible Complications of IO Block

Symptoms of the IO block include harmless tingling and numbness of the eyelid, side of the nose, and upper lip since there is inadvertent anesthesia of the branches of the infraorbital nerve. Additionally, there is numbness in the teeth and associated tissue along the distribution of the ASA and MSA nerves and absence of discomfort during dental procedures. Rarely the complication of a hematoma may develop across the lower eyelid and the tissues between it and the infraorbital foramen (see Chapter 6 for more information and Figure 6–15).

GREATER PALATINE BLOCK

The **greater palatine block** (pal-ah-tine) or **GP block** is used during dental procedures that involve more than two maxillary posterior teeth or palatal soft tissues distal to the maxillary canine. This maxillary block anesthetizes the posterior portion of the hard palate, anteriorly as far as the maxillary first premolar and medially to the midline.

Since the greater palatine block does not provide pulpal anesthesia of the area teeth, the use of the ASA, PSA, and MSA blocks or the IO block may also be indicated during restorative or extraction procedures. The greater palatine block is useful for periodontal treatment of the involved teeth due to its lingual tissue anesthesia. However, soft tissue anesthesia in the palatal area of the maxillary first premolar may prove inadequate because of overlapping nerve fibers from the nasopalatine nerve. This lack of anesthesia may be corrected by additional administration of the nasopalatine block.

FIGURE 9–19 ■ Target area for the greater palatine block is the greater palatine nerve located at the greater palatine foramen, which is at the junction of the maxillary alveolar process and the hard palate, at the apex of the maxillary second or third molar. Area anesthetized is highlighted.

FIGURE 9–20 ■ Dissection of palatal mucoperiosteum showing the greater palatine nerve and needle near location of nerve, but not in greater palatine block location. *Arrow* shows location of greater palatine foramen. 5. Greater palatine foramen; 6. mucoperiosteum; 7. greater palatine nerve; 21. incisive foramen. (From McMinn RMH, Hutchings RT, Logan BM. *Color Atlas of Head and Neck Anatomy*, 2nd ed. St. Louis, Mosby, 1994.)

Because the overlying palatal tissues are very dense and adhere firmly to the underlying palatal bone, the use of pressure anesthesia created by applying an applicator stick to the site before and during the injection to blanch the tissues will reduce patient discomfort. This pressure anesthesia of the tissues produces a dull ache that blocks pain impulses that arise from needle penetration. The very slow deposition of the anesthetic solution will also reduce patient discomfort.

Target Area and Injection Site for Greater Palatine Block

The target area for the greater palatine block is the greater palatine nerve as it enters the greater palatine foramen from its location between the mucoperiosteum and bone of the hard palate (Figures 9–19 and 9–20). The greater palatine foramen is located at the junction of the maxillary alveolar process and posterior hard palate, at the apex of the maxillary second (in children) or third molar, about 10 mm medial and directly above the lingual gingival margin.

The site of injection is the palatal tissues at the depression created by the greater palatine foramen (Figure 9–21). This depression can be palpated about midway between the median palatine raphe and lingual gingival margin of the molar tooth.

The patient is supine, with the mouth open wide, the neck extended, and the head turned to the left or right, depending on injection side. The needle for the greater palatine block is inserted into the previously blanched palatal tissues at a right angle or 90-degree angle to the palate (Figure 9–22). The needle is advanced during the greater palatine block, applying enough pressure to bow the needle slightly, until the palatine bone is contacted. The depth of penetration of the

FIGURE 9–21 ■ The injection site for the greater palatine block is probed at the depression caused by the greater palatine foramen. The palatal tissues around the greater palatine foramen are blanched to cause pressure anesthesia.

FIGURE 9–22 ■ Needle penetration of the palatal tissues for the greater palatine block is demonstrated at the depression created by the greater palatine foramen. The needle may bow slightly, and the tissue blanching is maintained during the injection. Injection site is highlighted.

needle into the palatal tissue will usually be less than 5 mm. There is no need to enter the greater palatine canal. Although this is not potentially hazardous, it is not necessary for adequate anesthesia.

Symptoms and Possible Complications of Greater Palatine Block

Symptoms of the greater palatine block are numbness in the posterior portion of the palate and absence of discomfort during dental procedures. Some patients may become uncomfortable and may gag if the soft palate becomes inadvertently and harmlessly anesthetized, which is a distinct possibility given the proximity of the lesser palatine nerve.

NASOPALATINE BLOCK

The **nasopalatine block** (nay-zo-**pal**-ah-tine) or **NP block** is useful for anesthesia of the bilateral anterior portion of the hard palate from the mesial of the right maxillary first premolar to the mesial of the left maxillary first premolar. Both the right and left nasopalatine nerves are anesthetized by this block. The nasopalatine block is used when palatal soft tissue anesthesia is required for two or more maxillary anterior teeth, such as with periodontal treatment.

If restorative procedures or extraction are to be performed on the anterior maxillary teeth, additional anesthesia may be indicated, such as the MSA and ASA block or the IO block, since the nasopalatine block does not provide pulpal anesthesia of these teeth.

FIGURE 9–23 ■ Target area for the nasopalatine block is the right and left nasopalatine nerves located at the incisive foramen on the anterior hard palate of the maxilla, lingual to the maxillary central incisors. Area anesthetized is highlighted.

FIGURE 9–24 ■ Saggital section of nerves of the right side of the nasal septum showing the nerves and other structures in the area. 28. Olfactory nerve; 29. nasopalatine nerve; 30. incisive canal; 31. anterior ethmoidal nerve. (From McMinn RMH, Hutchings RT, Logan BM. *Color Atlas of Head and Neck Anatomy*, 2nd ed. St. Louis, Mosby, 1994.)

Because the dense overlying palatal tissues adhere firmly to the underlying maxillary bone, the use of pressure anesthesia created by applying an applicator stick to blanch the tissues will reduce patient discomfort. This pressure anesthesia to the tissues produces a dull ache to block pain impulses that arise from needle penetration. Slow deposition of the anesthetic solution will also help reduce patient discomfort.

In addition, the labial soft tissues between the maxillary central incisors may be anesthetized prior to the palatal injection. This initial injection technique allows some anesthesia of the nasopalatine nerve in the area of the palatal injection before needle insertion in the area.

Some dental professionals follow this initial injection for the nasopalatine block by directing the needle from the labial aspect through the

FIGURE 9–25 ■ The injection site for the nasopalatine block is probed at the palatal tissues lateral to the incisive papilla on the anterior portion of the palate. The palatal tissues lateral to the incisive papilla are blanched to cause pressure anesthesia.

FIGURE 9–26 ■ Needle penetration of the palatal tissues for the nasopalatine block is demonstrated lateral to the incisive papilla. Blanching of the palatal tissues is continued during the injection. Injection site is highlighted.

interdental gingiva or papilla between the maxillary central incisors toward the incisive papilla to anesthetize the nasopalatine nerve. This may be followed by injection into the palatal area of the nerve if needed. This text discusses only a single-needle injection on the palate.

Target Area and Injection Site for Nasopalatine Block

The target area for the nasopalatine block is both the right and left nasopalatine nerves as they enter the incisive foramen from the mucosa of the anterior hard palate, beneath the incisive papilla (Figures 9–23 and 9–24; see also Figure 9–9).

The injection site is the palatal tissues lateral to the incisive papilla, which is located at the midline, about 10 mm lingual to the maxillary central incisor teeth (Figure 9–25). The patient is supine, with the mouth open wide, the neck extended, and the head turned to the left or right, whichever helps with visibility. The needle is inserted for the nasopalatine block into the previously blanched palatal tissues at a 45-degree angle to the palate (Figure 9–26). The initial depth of penetration of the needle into the palatal tissues will be 6–10 mm. The needle is advanced into the tissues until the maxillary bone is contacted. The needle is withdrawn 1 mm from the palatal tissue until the needle tip is directly over the opening of the incisive foramen before depositing the anesthetic solution.

Symptoms and Possible Complications of Nasopalatine Block

Symptoms of the nasopalatine block include numbness in the anterior portion of the palate and absence of discomfort during dental procedures. Complications such as hematoma are extremely rare.

MANDIBULAR NERVE ANESTHESIA

The mandibular nerve and its branches can be anesthetized in a number of ways depending on the tissues requiring anesthesia (Figure 9–1 and Chart 9–2). Infiltration anesthesia of the mandible is not as successful as that of the maxilla since overall the mandible is more dense than the maxilla over similar teeth, especially in the area of the posterior teeth (see Chapter 3). For this reason, nerve blocks are preferred to local infiltrations in most parts of the mandible.

There is also substantial variation in the anatomy of local anesthetic landmarks of the mandibular bone and nerves compared with similar structures in the maxilla, complicating mandibular anesthesia. This text covers some of the most common mandibular variations.

Pulpal anesthesia is achieved through anesthesia of each nerve's dental branches as they extend into the pulp tissue by way of each tooth's apical

CHART 9–2

SUMMARY OF MANDIBULAR LOCAL ANESTHESIA OF THE TEETH AND ASSOCIATED TISSUES

Mandibular Tooth and Tissues	IA Block	Buccal Block	Mental Block	Incisive Block
Central Incisor				
Pulpal	X			X
Facial	X		X	X
Lingual	X			
Lateral Incisor				
Pulpal	X			X
Facial	X		X	X
Lingual	X			
Canine				
Pulpal	X			X
Facial	X		X	X
Lingual	X			
First Premolar				
Pulpal	X			X
Facial	X		X	X
Lingual				
Second Premolar				
Pulpal	X			X
Facial	X		X	X
Lingual	X			
First Molar				
Lingual/pulpal	X			
Buccal		X		
Second Molar				
Lingual/pulpal	X			
Buccal		X		
Third Molar				
Lingual/pulpal	X			
Buccal		X		

The anesthesia for anatomical variants is not included. IA = inferior alveolar.

foramen. The hard and soft tissues of the periodontium are anesthetized by way of each nerve's interdental and interradicular branches.

The inferior alveolar block is used for anesthesia of the mandibular teeth and their associated lingual tissues to the midline, as well as the facial tissues anterior to the mandibular first molar. The buccal block is useful for anesthesia of the tissues buccal to the mandibular molars. The mental block is used for anesthesia of the facial tissues anterior to the mental foramen (usually the mandibular premolars and anterior teeth). The incisive block is used for anesthesia of the teeth and associated facial tissues anterior to the mental foramen (usually the mandibular premolars and anterior teeth). The Gow-Gates mandibular nerve block anesthetizes most of the mandibular nerve and is useful for quadrant dentistry.

INFERIOR ALVEOLAR BLOCK

The **inferior alveolar block** (al-ve-o-lar) or **IA block** or also mandibular block is the most commonly used injection in dentistry. It is used when dental procedures are performed on the mandibular teeth and pulpal anesthesia is needed, such as in the case of restorative procedures and extraction. This block also gives anesthesia of the lingual periodontium of all the mandibular teeth, as well as anesthesia of the facial periodontium of the mandibular anterior and premolar teeth, both of which are needed during periodontal treatment.

Additional use of the buccal nerve block may be considered if anesthesia of the buccal periodontium of the mandibular molars is also needed, such as with the periodontal treatment of these teeth.

Sometimes there is overlap of the left and right incisive nerves. The incisive nerve is a branch of the mandibular nerve that serves the pulp tissue of the mandibular anterior teeth.

If this is the case, a bilateral IA block can be used, but it is not recommended. More often, the use of an incisive block or local infiltration at the apices of the mandibular teeth that fail to achieve initial pulpal anesthesia may be indicated.

Local infiltrations on the facial surface of the anterior mandible are more successful than more posterior injections but less successful than injections over the maxilla in similar locations. Again, these differences in success rates are due to differences in the density of the facial bones.

Bilateral inferior alveolar injections are usually avoided unless absolutely needed. Bilateral mandibular injections produce complete anesthesia of the body of the tongue and floor of the mouth, which can cause difficulty with swallowing and speech, especially in patients with full or partial removable mandibular dentures, until the effects of the anesthetic drug wear off.

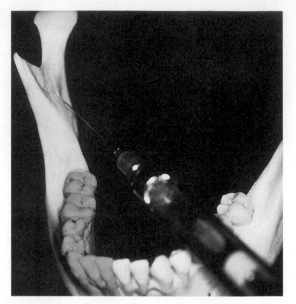

FIGURE 9–27 ■ Area anesthetized by the inferior alveolar block is highlighted.

Comprehensive dental treatment planning can usually prevent the need for bilateral inferior alveolar injections.

Even though the IA block is the most commonly used dental injection, it is not always initially successful. This may mean that the patient must be reinjected to achieve the necessary anesthesia of the tissues. This lack of consistent success is due in part to anatomical variation in the height of the mandibular foramen on the medial side of the ramus and the great depth of soft tissue penetration required to achieve pulpal anesthesia. Other techniques to achieve mandibular anesthesia, such as the Gow-Gates mandibular nerve block, may also be employed.

Target Area and Injection Site for IA Block

The target area for the IA block is slightly superior to the entry point of the inferior alveolar nerve into the mandibular foramen, overhung anteriorly by the lingula (Figures 9–27 and 9–28). The solution must be accurately deposited within 1 mm of the target area to achieve anesthesia. The adjacent anteriorly placed lingual nerve will also be anesthetized as the anesthetic solution diffuses.

The injection site for the IA block is the mandibular tissues on the medial border of the mandibular ramus at the correct height and

FIGURE 9–29 ■ Target area for the IA block is the inferior alveolar nerve located at the mandibular foramen on the medial surface of the mandibular ramus, inferior to the lingula.

anteroposterior direction for the injection (Figures 9–29, 9–30, and 9–31). To locate the injection site, use mainly hard tissues as landmarks, such as the coronoid notch and the occlusal plane of the mandibular molars, to reduce errors caused by

FIGURE 9–28 ■ Deep dissection of the face and right infratemporal fossa after removal of the lateral ptery-goid muscle, zygomatic arch, and portion of mandible to show the nerves in the area. 4. Maxillary nerve; 5. posterior superior alveolar nerve; 6. posterior superior alveolar artery; 9. buccal nerve; 10. medial ptery-goid; 11. lingual nerve; 12. inferior alveolar nerve; 13. inferior alveolar artery; 14. nerve to mylohyoid; 16. maxillary artery; 18. articular disc and head of condyle; 19. capsule; 20. nerve to medial pterygoid; 21. lateral pterygoid plate; 22. chorda tympani; 23. middle meningeal artery; 24. accessory meningeal artery; 25. mandibular nerve; 26. nerve to lateral pterygoid. (From McMinn RMH, Hutchings RT, Logan BM. *Color Atlas of Head and Neck Anatomy*, 2nd ed. St. Louis, Mosby, 1994.)

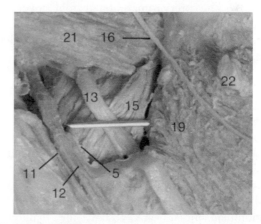

FIGURE 9–30 ■ Dissection of the right infratemporal fossa showing the needle adjacent to the IA nerve. 5. Lingula; 11. inferior alveolar artery; 12. inferior alveolar nerve; 13. lingual nerve; 15. medial pterygoid; 16. buccal nerve; 19. buccinator; 21. lateral pterygoid; 22. parotid duct. (From McMinn RMH, Hutchings RT, Logan BM. *Color Atlas of Head and Neck Anatomy*, 2nd ed. St. Louis, Mosby, 1994.)

FIGURE 9–31 ■ The injection site for the IA block is probed at the depth of the pterygomandibular space on the medial surface of the ramus.

patient soft tissue variance. The patient is supine, with the mouth open wide.

The correct height of the injection for the IA block is determined by palpating the coronoid notch, the greatest depression on the anterior border of the ramus. To determine this level of height, it helps to visualize an imaginary horizontal line that extends posteriorly from the coronoid notch to the pterygomandibular fold as it turns upward toward the palate (Figure 9–32A and B). The pterygomandibular fold covers the deeper pterygomandibular raphe between the buccinator and superior pharyngeal constrictor muscles. This fold is accentuated as the patient opens the mouth wider.

This imaginary horizontal line showing the height of inferior alveolar nerve injection is also parallel to and 6–10 mm above the occlusal plane of the mandibular molar teeth in the majority of adults. In children and small adults, this imaginary horizontal line for the height of the injection should be at the occlusal plane of the mandibular molars. In edentulous patients and when the mandibular molars are absent, the mandibular foramen may appear to be higher than when the dentition is present because the occlusal plane of molars is not present as a guide.

The correct anteroposterior direction of the IA block injection is achieved at the same time as the determination of the correct height of the injection. To determine this direction, it helps to visual-

ize an imaginary vertical line, two thirds to three fourths of the distance between the coronoid notch and the posterior border of the ramus (Figure 9–32 A and B). This area will be at the deepest or most posterior portion of the pterygomandibular space, lateral to the pterygomandibular fold and the sphenomandibular ligament (see Chapter 11 for review). The syringe barrel is usually over the contralateral mandibular second premolar (or at the contralateral labial commissure).

Thus the injection site on the ramus for the IA block is the mandibular tissues at the intersection of the imaginary horizontal line for the height of injection with the imaginary vertical line for the anteroposterior direction of the injection (see Figure 9–32A and B). The needle is inserted into the tissues of the pterygomandibular space until the mandible is contacted (Figures 9–33 and 9–34). The needle is then withdrawn 1 mm from the tissues before injecting the anesthetic solution. The average depth of penetration by the needle into the soft tissues is 20–25 mm. After the injection, have the patient sit upright.

It is not necessary to deposit small amounts of the anesthetic solution as the needle enters the tissue for the IA block to anesthetize the adjacent anteriorly placed lingual nerve since anesthesia of the lingual nerve will occur through diffusion of the anesthetic solution placed near the inferior alveolar nerve. These small amounts injected early will not reduce tissue discomfort for the patient.

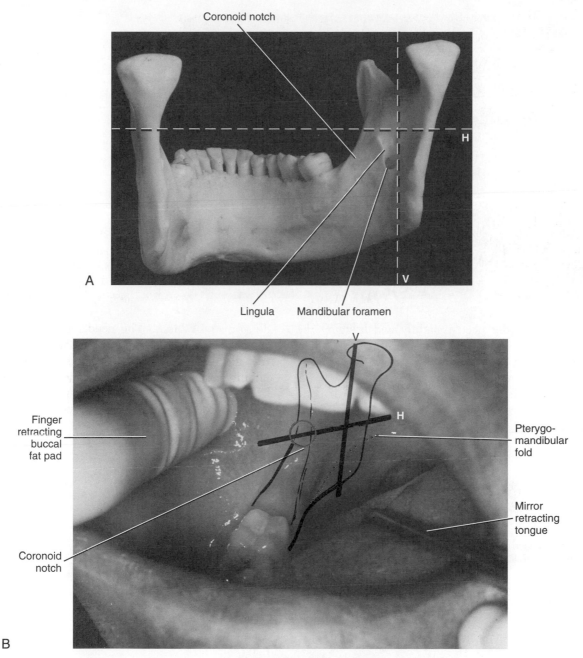

FIGURE 9–32 ■ Imaginary horizontal line showing the correct height and imaginary vertical line showing the correct anteroposterior direction of the injection for the IA block. The intersection of these two lines is the correct injection site for this block. A: Posteromedial surface of the mandible. B: Oral view of the pterygomandibular space.

Trouble-shooting the IA Block

If bone is contacted too soon when trying to administer an IA block, the needle tip is located too far anterior on the ramus. Correction is made by withdrawing the needle slightly and bringing the syringe barrel more closely over the mandibular anterior teeth. This correction moves the needle tip more posteriorly when it is reinserted.

If bone is not contacted when trying to administer an IA block, the needle tip is located too far posterior on the ramus. Correction is made by

FIGURE 9–33 ■ Needle penetration of the mandibular tissues for the IA block is demonstrated at the depth of the pterygomandibular space. Injection site is highlighted.

withdrawing the needle slightly and bringing the syringe barrel more closely over the mandibular molars. This correction moves the needle tip more anteriorly when it is reinserted.

Do not deposit the anesthetic solution if bone is not contacted upon initial insertion of the nee-

dle for an IA block. The needle tip may be too posterior and thus resting within the parotid salivary gland near the facial nerve, resulting in complications (discussed later; Figures 9–34 and 9–35). If the insertion and deposition are too shallow and bone is not contacted, the medially located

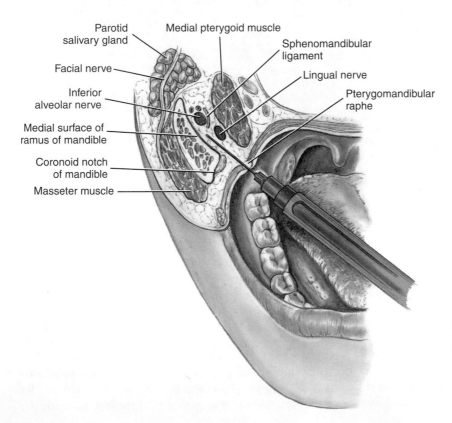

FIGURE 9–34 ■ Correct needle penetration into the pterygomandibular space during an IA block. If the needle is inserted too far posterior, it may enter the parotid salivary gland containing the facial nerve, causing a complication such as transient facial paralysis.

FIGURE 9–35 ■ Dissection of the right infratemporal fossa on horizontal section showing the needle adjacent to the IA nerve. 3. Coronoid notch (external oblique ridge); 4. internal oblique ridge; 5. lingula; 6. mandibular formen; 7. parotid gland; 8. styloid process; 9. maxillary artery; 10. inferior alveolar vein; 11. in-ferior alveolar artery; 12. inferior alveolar nerve; 13. lingual nerve; 14. sphenomandibular ligament; 15. medial pterygoid; 16. buccal nerve; 17. temporalis insertion; 18. pterygomandibular raphe; 19. buccinator, 20. masseter. (From McMinn RMH, Hutchings RT, Logan BM. *Color Atlas of Head and Neck Anatomy*, 2nd ed. St. Louis, Mosby, 1994.)

sphenomandibular ligament can become a physical barrier that stops the important diffusion of the anesthetic solution to the mandibular foramen and inferior alveolar nerve.

If there is failure of anesthesia, there may be accessory innervation of the mandibular teeth. Current thinking supports the mylohyoid nerve as the nerve that may be involved in this accessory mandibular innervation. To correct this problem, anesthesia of the mylohyoid nerve on the lingual border of the mandible is indicated. This additional anesthetic technique is discussed in most current local anesthesia textbooks.

Whenever a bifid inferior alveolar nerve is detected by noting a doubled mandibular canal on a radiograph (see Chapters 3 and 8 for more information), incomplete anesthesia of the mandible may

follow an IA block. In many such cases, a second mandibular foramen, more inferiorly placed, exists. To correct this, deposit more anesthetic solution inferior to the normal anatomical landmarks.

Symptoms and Possible Complications of IA Block

Symptoms of the IA block include harmless numbness or tingling of the lower lip since the mental nerve, a branch of the inferior alveolar nerve, is anesthetized. This is a good indication that the inferior alveolar nerve is anesthetized but is not a reliable indicator of the depth of anesthesia, especially concerning pulpal anesthesia.

Another symptom is harmless numbness or tingling of the body of the tongue and floor of the mouth, which indicates that the lingual nerve, a branch of the mandibular nerve, is anesthetized. It is important to note that this anesthesia of the tongue may occur without anesthesia of the inferior alveolar nerve. Possibly the needle was not advanced deeply enough into the tissues to anesthetize the deeper inferior alveolar nerve. The most reliable indicator of a successful IA nerve block is the absence of discomfort during dental procedures.

Another symptom that sometimes can occur is 'lingual shock' as the needle passes by the lingual nerve. The patient may make an involuntary movement, varying from a slight opening of the eyes to jumping in the chair. This symptom is only momentary, and anesthesia will quickly occur.

One of the complications with an IA block is transient facial paralysis if the facial nerve is mistakenly anesthetized. This can occur because of an incorrect administration of anesthetic into the deeper parotid salivary gland (see Figures 9–34 and 9–35). Symptoms of this paralysis include the inability to close the eyelid and the drooping of the lips on the affected side (see Chapter 4 for more information and Figure 4–6). Other complications such as hematoma can occur (see Chapter 6 for more information and Figure 6–16). Muscle soreness or limited movement of the mandible is rarely seen with this injection. Patient-inflicted trauma can occur, such as lip biting and resulting swelling. The use of stickers with child patients reminds them; reinforce with parents and remind even adult patients of this possibility.

FIGURE 9–36 ■ Target area for the buccal block is the buccal nerve located on the anterior border of the mandibular ramus. Area anesthetized is highlighted.

BUCCAL BLOCK

The buccal block or long buccal block is useful for anesthesia of the buccal periodontium of the mandibular molars, including the gingiva, periodontal ligament, and alveolar bone. This type of anesthesia is needed during dental procedures such as certain restorative procedures or periodontal treatment of these teeth. Some clinicians skip this but should do it after the IA is administered. Many times this block is administered when it is not needed, such as in small occlusal fillings that do not involve the use of a rubber dam. This is a very successful dental injection since the buccal nerve is readily located on the surface of the tissue and not within bone.

Target Area and Injection Site for Buccal Block

The target area for the buccal block is the buccal nerve (or long buccal nerve) as it passes over the

FIGURE 9–37 ■ The injection site for the buccal block is probed in the buccal tissues that are distal and buccal to the most distal molar tooth in the arch.

FIGURE 9–38 ■ Needle penetration of the buccal tissues for the buccal block is demonstrated, distal and buccal to the most distal molar tooth in the arch. Injection site is highlighted.

anterior border of the ramus and through the buccinator muscle before it enters the cheek region (Figure 9–36). Thus the injection site is the buccal tissues distal and buccal to the most distal molar tooth in the arch, on the anterior border of the ramus (Figure 9–37). The patient is supine, with the mouth open wide. Pull the buccal soft tissue laterally until it is taut.

The needle is advanced until it contacts the mandible (Figure 9–38). The usual depth of penetration of the needle into the buccal tissues is only 1–2 mm. If the overlying buccal tissue balloons, deposition of the solution should be stopped. If the solution runs out of the puncture site, the deposition should be stopped and the needle advanced deeper into the tissue before the injection is continued.

Symptoms and Possible Complications of Buccal Block

The patient rarely feels any symptoms of the buccal nerve block because of the location and small size of the anesthetized area. There is usually only absence of discomfort with dental procedures. Sometimes patient-inflicted trauma may occur,

FIGURE 9–39 ■ Target area for the mental block is the mental nerve located at the mental foramen on the surface of the mandible, usually between the apices of the mandibular first and second premolars. Area anesthetized is highlighted.

such as cheek bites. The use of stickers with child patients reminds them; reinforce with parents and remind even adult patients of this possibility. The complication of a hematoma rarely occurs.

MENTAL BLOCK

The **mental block** (**ment**-il) is used to anesthetize the facial periodontium of the mandibular premolars and anterior teeth on one side, including the gingiva, periodontal ligament, and other alveolar tissues. This is useful before dental procedures such as periodontal treatment of these teeth. It is a very successful injection because of the ease of access to the nerve.

If restorative procedures are also to be performed on these mandibular premolar or anterior teeth, local infiltrations at the facial surface of apices of the involved teeth may be additionally performed, or administration of an incisive block may be considered instead (discussed later in this chapter).

Target Area and Injection Site for Mental Block

The target area for the mental block is the mental nerve before it enters the mental foramen to merge with the incisive nerve and form the inferior alveolar nerve (Figures 9–39 and 9–40).

FIGURE 9–40 ■ Dissection showing the needle tip at the opening of the mental foramen. 9. Mental foramen; 10. depressor muscle of angle of mouth; 11. depressor muscle of lower lip; 12. mental nerve and vessels. (From McMinn RMH, Hutchings RT, Logan BM. *Color Atlas of Head and Neck Anatomy*, 2nd ed. St. Louis, Mosby, 1994.)

The mental foramen is usually located on the surface of the mandible between the apices of the first and second mandibular premolars, yet it may be anterior or posterior to this site. The mental foramen in adults faces posterosuperiorly. The mental foramen can be located on a radiograph before performing the injection to allow for a better determination of its position.

To locate the mental foramen for the mental block, palpate intraorally the depth of the mucobuccal fold between the apices of the mandibular first

FIGURE 9–41 ■ The injection site for the mental block is probed at the depression caused by the mental foramen, usually located in the depth of the mucobuccal fold between the apices of the mandibular first and second premolars. This is the same injection site as for the incisive block.

FIGURE 9–42 ■ Needle penetration of the mucobuccal fold tissues for the mental block is demonstrated at the depression created by the mental foramen. Injection site is highlighted.

and second premolars or at a site indicated by a radiograph until a depression is felt, surrounded by smoother bone (Figure 9–41). The patient will comment that pressure in this area produces soreness as the mental nerve is compressed against the mandible near the foramen.

The insertion site for a mental block is the mucobuccal fold tissues directly over or slightly anterior to the depression created by the mental foramen (Figure 9–42). The patient is supine, with the mouth open wide. Pull the buccal soft tissue laterally until it is taut. The needle is advanced until the level of the foramen is reached, avoiding contact with the mandible. The depth of penetration into the tissues will be 5–6 mm. There is no need to enter the mental foramen to achieve facial anesthesia.

Symptoms and Possible Complications of Mental Block

The symptoms of a mental block are harmless tingling or numbness of the lower lip and absence of discomfort during dental procedures. The complication of a hematoma rarely occurs.

INCISIVE BLOCK

The **incisive block** (in-**sy**-ziv) anesthetizes the pulp tissue and facial tissues of the mandibular teeth anterior to the mental foramen (usually the mandibular premolars and anterior teeth). This block is useful when restorative and periodontal treatment procedures are to be done on these teeth. If extraction procedures are to be performed, an inferior alveolar block would be administered instead since the incisive block does not provide lingual anesthesia. This block has a high success rate since the incisive nerve is readily accessible.

FIGURE 9–43 ■ Target area for the incisive nerve block is the mental nerve located at the mental foramen on the surface of the mandible, usually between the apices of the mandibular first and second premolars. Area anesthetized is highlighted.

FIGURE 9–44 ■ Needle penetration of the mucobuccal fold tissues for the incisive block is demonstrated at the depression created by the mental foramen. Pressure near the mental foramen is maintained. Injection site is highlighted.

Target Area and Injection Site for Incisive Block

The target area for the incisive block is the mental foramen, the opening of the mandibular canal where the incisive nerve is located. The mental foramen is also where the mental nerve enters to join with the incisive nerve to form the inferior alveolar nerve (Figure 9–43).

The mental foramen is usually located on the surface of the mandible between the apices of the first and second mandibular premolars, yet it may be anterior or posterior to this site. The mental foramen in adults faces posteriorly. The mental foramen can be located on a radiograph before performing the injection to allow for a better determination of its position.

The injection site for an incisive block is the same as that for a mental nerve block: directly over or slightly anterior to the depression created by the mental foramen, in the depth of the mucobuccal fold between the apices of the first and second mandibular premolars (Figure 9–44). The patient is supine, with the mouth open wide. Pull the buccal soft tissue laterally until it is taut. More anesthetic solution is deposited within the tissue for the incisive block than for the mental block, and pressure is applied during the injection. This pressure forces more anesthetic solution into the mental foramen, thus anesthetizing first the shallow mental nerve and then the deeper incisive nerve. It is important to note that it is not necessary to have the needle enter the mental foramen to a successful incisive block.

While injecting these increased amounts of anesthetic solution during an incisive block, the facial tissue in the area may balloon slightly without complications. Anesthesia of the tissues innervated by the mental nerve will precede that of the deeper incisive nerve's tissues. If an inadequate amount of anesthetic solution is initially placed in the mental foramen, with subsequent lack of pulpal anesthesia, correction can be made by injecting more solution into the proper region and again applying pressure to the site.

Symptoms and Possible Complications of Incisive Block

The symptoms of an incisive block are the same as the symptoms of a mental block, except that there is pulpal anesthesia of the involved teeth. There also is an absence of discomfort during dental procedures. As with a mental block, a hematoma rarely occurs.

GOW-GATES MANDIBULAR NERVE BLOCK

The nerves anesthetized with a **Gow-Gates mandibular nerve block** are the inferior alveolar,

FIGURE 9–45 ■ Area anesthetized by a Gow-Gates mandibular nerve block is highlighted and includes almost the entire mandibular nerve.

mental, incisive, lingual, mylohyoid, auriculotemporal, and buccal (long) nerves in about 75 percent of patients (Figure 9–45). It is a true mandibular block since it anesthetizes almost the entire V_3.

A Gow-Gates technique is indicated for use in quadrant dentistry where the buccal soft tissue anesthesia from most distal molar to midline and lingual soft tissue is needed, and in some cases in which a conventional IA block is unsuccessful. Thus the success rate is higher than that of an IA block—greater than 95 percent—and in many cases it is the only injection necessary for mandibular anesthesia, since the buccal nerve block is not necessary and there is an absence of problems with accessory innervation to mandibular

FIGURE 9–46 ■ Target area for the Gow-Gates mandibular nerve block is located at the anteromedial border of the mandibular condyle neck, just inferior to the insertion of the lateral pterygoid muscle.

FIGURE 9–47 ■ The extraoral line that is followed for the Gow-Gates mandibular nerve block. The line extends from the intertragic notch of the ear to the same side labial commissure.

teeth as there is with the IA block. Its lower positive aspiration rate is also an advantage; it is 2 percent versus 10–15 percent with the IA block.

Target Area and Injection Site for Gow-Gates Mandibular Nerve Block

The target area for the Gow-Gates technique is the anteromedial border of the mandibular condylar neck, just inferior to the insertion of the lateral pterygoid muscle (Figure 9–46). The injection site is located intraorally on the oral mucosa on the mesial of the mandibular ramus, just distal to the height of the mesiolingual cusp of the maxillary second molar, following a line extraorally from the intertragic notch of the ear to the same side labial commissure (Figure 9–47).

The extraoral landmarks of the intertragic notch and labial commissure are first located, while the patient has the neck extended and the

FIGURE 9–48 ■ The injection site for the Gow-Gates mandibular nerve block is probed at the soft tissues just distal to the height of the mesiolingual cusp of the second molar, following a line extraorally from the intertragic notch to the labial commissure of the same side.

FIGURE 9–49 ■ Using the needle to assess the vertical location for the Gow-Gates mandibular nerve block by placing the needle just inferior to the mesiolingual cusp of the maxillary second molar. Note that the barrel of the needle is over the contralateral canine-to-premolar region.

mouth opened comfortably wide for the injection; your thumb is on the condyle (Figure 9–48). The condyle can assume a more frontal position with the mouth open, and the injection site is closer to the mandibular nerve trunk. With a more closed mouth, the condyle will move out of the injection site and the soft tissue will become thicker.

Initially the needle is placed just inferior to the mesiolingual cusp of the maxillary second molar to assess the approximate vertical location for the injection site. The needle is then placed distal to the maxillary second molar, maintaining the established height (Figure 9–49). The barrel of the needle is maintained over the contralateral canine-to-premolar region, such that the angulation of the syringe parallels a line connecting the same-side labial commissure and the intertragic notch. The needle is inserted parallel to the determined line until bony contact is made with the neck of the condyle (Figure 9–50). The average depth of penetration is around 25 mm, although variation can be considerable; it is similar to

FIGURE 9–50 ■ Needle penetration for the Gow-Gates mandibular nerve block is demonstrated at the soft tissues just distal to the maxillary second molar, maintaining the established height. The injection site is highlighted.

that of the IA block. Do not perform the injection if there is no bony contact. This injection is most often missed if attempted too low.

The height of insertion above the mandibular occlusal plane is higher than that of an IA block—around 10–25 mm, depending on the patient's size. When a maxillary third molar is present, the site of injection will be just distal to that tooth. After injection, have the patient sit upright and keep the mouth open for 2 minutes.

Symptoms and Possible Complications of Gow-Gates Mandibular Nerve Block

The mandibular teeth to midline, the buccal mucoperiosteum and mucous membranes, and lingual soft tissues and periosteum will be anesthetized. Inadvertently, the anterior two thirds of the tongue, floor of mouth, and body of the mandible and inferior ramus, as well as the skin over the zygoma and the posterior cheek and temporal regions, are anesthetized. Two of the disadvantages of the Gow-Gates technique are the anesthesia of the lower lip, as well as the temporal area, and the longer time necessary for the anesthetic to take effect. The increased time is due to the larger size of the nerve trunk being anesthetized and the distance of the trunk from the site of deposition, which is 5–10 mm. The injection also lasts longer than the IA block because the area of the injection is less vascular, and a larger volume of anesthetic may be needed. The injection is contraindicated in patients with limited ability to open the mouth; however, trismus is rarely involved.

IDENTIFICATION EXERCISES

Identify the structures on the following diagrams by filling in the blanks with the correct anatomical term. You can check your answers by looking back at the figure indicated in parentheses for each identification diagram.

1. (Figure 9–7)

2. (Figure 9–34)

REVIEW QUESTIONS

1. A hematoma can result from an incorrectly administered PSA block because the needle was overinserted and penetrated the
   A. Parotid salivary gland
   B. Pterygoid plexus of veins
   C. Floor of the nose
   D. Facial or cranial nerve VII

2. Which of the following local anesthetic blocks has the same target area as the incisive block?
   A. Nasopalatine block
   B. Greater palatine block
   C. Inferior alveolar block
   D. Buccal block
   E. Mental block

3. Which of the following nerves is not anesthetized during an inferior alveolar block?
   A. Buccal nerve
   B. Lingual nerve
   C. Mental nerve
   D. Incisive nerve

4. Which of the following anesthetic blocks uses pressure anesthesia of the tissue with an applicator stick to reduce patient discomfort?
   A. PSA block
   B. IO block
   C. Greater palatine block
   D. Inferior alveolar block
   E. Buccal block

5. Which of the following tissues are anesthetized during an IO block?
   A. Bilateral anterior hard palate
   B. Buccal periodontium of maxillary molars
   C. Upper lip, side of nose, and lower eyelid
   D. Lingual periodontium of maxillary anteriors
   E. Side of face, upper eyelid, and bridge of nose

6. If the mesiobuccal root of the maxillary first molar is not anesthetized by a PSA block, the dental professional should
   A. Reinject at the same site as for the PSA block
   B. Perform a buccal block injection
   C. Administer an MSA block injection
   D. Perform a nasopalatine block injection

7. Which of the following is an important landmark to palpate before performing an inferior alveolar block?
   A. Coronoid notch
   B. Tongue
   C. Buccal fat pad
   D. Mental foramen

8. The injection site for the greater palatine block is located on the palate near the
   A. Maxillary first premolar
   B. Maxillary second or third molar
   C. Incisive papilla
   D. Midline portion

9. If an extraction of a maxillary lateral incisor is scheduled, which of the following anesthetic blocks should be administered besides the IO block?
   A. PSA block
   B. MSA block
   C. Nasopalatine block
   D. Greater palatine block

10. Transient facial paralysis can occur with an incorrectly administered
    A. PSA block
    B. MSA block
    C. Nasopalatine block
    D. Inferior alveolar block
    E. Mental block

11. Which block anesthetizes the largest intraoral area?
    A. Long buccal
    B. Inferior alveolar
    C. Mental
    D. Incisive

12. Which of these situations has occurred if bone is contacted too soon in an IA block?
    A. Needle tip is located too far anterior on the ramus
    B. Needle tip is located too far posterior on the maxillary tuberosity
    C. Syringe barrel is mainly over the maxillary posterior teeth
    D. Syringe barrel is mainly over the mandibular posterior teeth

13. In which of the following locations is the outcome most successful when using local infiltrations of local anesthetic?
    A. Facial surface of anterior maxilla
    B. Facial surface of posterior maxilla
    C. Facial surface of anterior mandible
    D. Facial surface of posterior mandible

14. If working within the mandibular anterior sextant, which block is most successful and comfortable for the patient?
    A. Unilateral posterior superior alveolar block
    B. Bilateral lingual block
    C. Bilateral inferior alveolar block
    D. Bilateral incisive block

15. Which depth of penetration is used with a buccal (long) block?
    A. 1–2 mm
    B. 6–10 mm
    C. 10–20 mm
    D. 20–25 mm

REVIEW ACTIVITIES

1. Using a long cotton swab, point out all the landmarks on a skull for each injection.

2. Make a list for each injection, including the teeth and associated structures that are anesthetized with each one.

3. Using a sheathed needle, place it in the correct position in a peer's mouth for each injection.

Lymphatics

CHAPTER OUTLINE

This chapter discusses the following topics:

LEARNING OBJECTIVES

After studying this chapter, the reader should be able to:

1. Define and pronounce all the key words and anatomical terms in this chapter.
2. List and discuss the lymphatic system and its components.
3. Locate and identify all the major groups of lymph nodes of the head and neck on a diagram and extraorally on a patient.
4. Locate and identify all the tonsillar tissues of the head and neck on a diagram and intraorally on a patient.
5. Identify the patterns of lymph drainage for each head and neck tissue or region.
6. Describe and discuss lymphadenopathy of lymphoid tissue.
7. Discuss the spread of cancer in the head and neck region and its relationship to lymph nodes.
8. Correctly complete the identification exercises and review questions and activities for this chapter.
9. Integrate the knowledge about head and neck lymphatics into the clinical practice of patient examination and any related lymphatic diseases of the region.

KEY WORDS

Afferent vessel (af-er-ent) Type of lymphatic vessel in which lymph flows into the lymph node.

Efferent vessel (ef-er-ent) Type of lymphatic vessel in which lymph flows out of the lymph node in the area of the node's hilus.

Hilus (hi-lus) Depression on one side of a lymph node where lymph flows out by way of an efferent lymphatic vessel.

Lymph (limf) Tissue fluid that drains from the surrounding region and into the lymphatic vessels.

Lymphadenopathy (lim-fad-in-**op**-ah-thee) Process in which there is an increase in the size and a change in the consistency of lymphoid tissue.

Lymphatic ducts (lim-**fat-ik**-dukts) Larger lymphatic vessels that drain smaller vessels and then empty into the venous system.

Lymphatic vessels (lim-**fat**-ik **ves**-els) System of channels that drains tissue fluid from the surrounding regions.

Lymph nodes (limf nodes) Organized, bean shaped lymphoid tissue that filters the lymph by way of lymphocytes to fight disease and is grouped into clusters along the connecting lymphatic vessels.

Metastasis (meh-**tas**-tah-sis) Spread of cancer from the original or primary site to another or secondary site.

Primary node Lymph node that drains lymph from a particular region.

Secondary node Lymph node that drains lymph from a primary node.

Tonsillar tissue (ton-sil-lar) Masses of lymphoid tissues located in the oral cavity and pharynx to protect the body against disease processes.

LYMPHATIC SYSTEM

The **lymphatics** (lim-**fat**-iks) are part of the immune system and they help fight disease processes, as well as serve other functions in the body. The lymphatic system consists of a network of lymphatic vessels linking lymph nodes throughout most of the body. Tonsillar tissue located in the oral cavity and pharynx is also part of the lymphatic system. Although not part of the lymphatic system, the thymus gland also works as part of the immune system and is discussed in Chapter 7.

LYMPHATIC VESSELS

The **lymphatic vessels** (lim-**fat**-ik **ves**-els) are a system of channels that mainly parallel the venous blood vessels in location yet are more numerous (Figure 10–1). Tissue fluid drains from the surrounding region into the lymphatic vessels as **lymph** (limf). Not only do the lymphatic vessels drain their region, but they also communicate with each other. Lymphatic vessels are larger and thicker than the blood system's capillaries. Unlike capillaries, lymphatic vessels have valves similar to many veins. These valves ensure a one-way flow of lymph through the lymphatic vessel. Lymphatic vessels are even found within the tooth's pulp tissue.

LYMPH NODES

The **lymph nodes** (limf nodes) are bean-shaped bodies grouped in clusters along the connecting lymphatic vessels (Figure 10–2). Along the lymphatic vessels, the lymph nodes are positioned to filter toxic products from the lymph to prevent their entry into the blood system. The lymph nodes are composed of organized lymphoid tissue and contain lymphocytes, white blood cells of the immune system that actively remove the toxic products. The removal of the toxic products helps fight disease processes in the body.

In healthy patients, lymph nodes are usually small, soft, and free or mobile in the surrounding tissue. The lymph nodes can be superficial in position with the superficial veins or deep in the tissue with the deep blood vessels. Normally lymph nodes cannot be visualized or palpated during an extraoral examination of a healthy patient.

Drainage Patterns of Lymph Nodes

The lymph flows into the lymph node by way of **afferent vessels** (**af**-er-ent). On one side of the node is a depression or **hilus** (**hi**-lus), where the lymph flows out of the node by way of a single **efferent vessel** (**ef**-er-ent).

Lymph nodes can be classified as either a primary or secondary node. Lymph from a particular tissue region drains into a **primary node** or regional node. The primary node may also be called a master node. Primary nodes, in turn, drain into a **secondary node** or central node.

TONSILLAR TISSUE

Tonsillar tissue (**ton**-sil-lar) consists of masses of lymphoid tissue located in the oral cavity and pharynx. Tonsils, like lymph nodes, contain lymphocytes that remove toxic products. Tonsillar tissue is located near airway and food passages to protect the body against disease processes from toxic products.

LYMPHATIC DUCTS

Smaller lymphatic vessels containing lymph converge into larger **lymphatic ducts** (lim-**fat**-ik dukts) (see Figure 10–1), which empty into the venous system of the blood in the chest area. The drainage pattern of the lymphatic vessels into the lymphatic ducts depends on which side of the body is involved.

The lymphatics of the right side of the head and neck converge by way of the right **jugular trunk** (**jug**-you-lar trungk), joining lymphatics from the right arm and thorax to form the right **lymphatic duct,** which drains into the venous system at the junction of the right subclavian and right internal jugular veins.

The lymphatic vessels of the left side of the head and neck converge into the left **jugular**

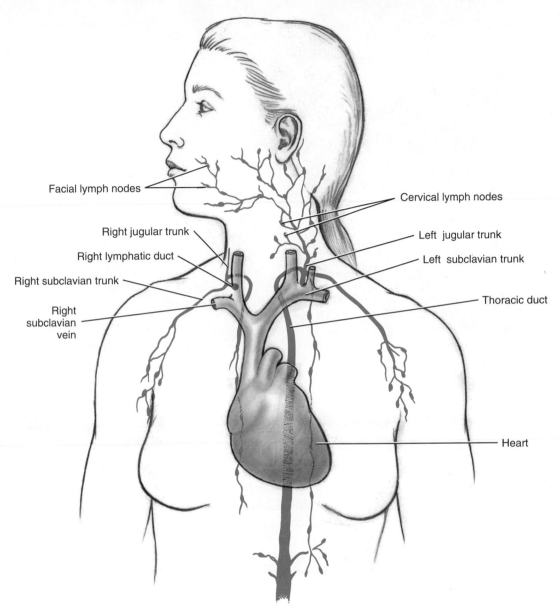

FIGURE 10–1 ■ Lymphatic vessels and lymphatic ducts of the right and left sides of the upper body.

trunk (**jug**-you-lar trungk), actually a short vessel, and then into the **thoracic duct** (tho-**ras**-ik), which joins the venous system at the junction of the left subclavian and left internal jugular veins. Lymphatics from the left arm and thorax also join the thoracic duct. The thoracic duct is much larger than the right lymphatic duct because it drains the lymph from the entire lower half of the body (both right and left sides).

▓ LYMPH NODES OF THE HEAD AND NECK

A dental professional needs to examine carefully for any palpable lymph nodes of the head and neck during an extraoral examination and record whether any are present. The lymph nodes that are palpable may pinpoint where a disease process, such as cancer or infection, is active. The

Afferent lymphatic vessel

Valve

Hilus

Efferent lymphatic vessel

Valve

Blood vessels

FIGURE 10–2 ■ Lymph node and components.

Table 10–1 LYMPH NODE DRAINAGE PATTERN FOR TISSUES OF THE ORAL CAVITY

Tissues	Primary Nodes	Secondary Nodes
Buccal mucosal tissues	Buccal and mandibular	Submandibular
Anterior hard palate	Submandibular and retropharyngeal	Superior deep cervical
Posterior hard palate	Superior deep cervical and retropharyngeal	Inferior deep cervical
Soft palate	Superior deep cervical and retropharyngeal	Inferior deep cervical
Maxillary anterior teeth and associated tissues	Submandibular	Superior deep cervical
Maxillary first and second molars and premolars and associated tissues	Submandibular	Superior deep cervical
Maxillary third molars and associated tissues	Superior deep cervical	Inferior deep cervical
Mandibular incisors and associated tissues	Submental	Submandibular and deep cervical
Mandibular canines, premolars, and molars and associated tissues	Submandibular	Superior deep cervical
Floor of mouth	Submental	Submandibular and deep cervical
Tongue apex	Submental	Submandibular and deep cervical
Tongue body	Submandibular	Superior deep cervical
Tongue base	Superior deep cervical	Inferior deep cervical
Palatine tonsils and lingual tonsil	Superior deep cervical	Inferior deep cervical

role of nodes with cancer is discussed later in this chapter. The examination also may help determine whether the disease process has become widespread and involves a larger region and thus more secondary lymph nodes and related tissues.

This documentation and history concerning palpable lymph nodes will assist in the diagnosis, treatment, and outcome of any disease process that may be present in the patient. It is therefore important that a dental professional understand the relationship between node location and node drainage patterns in the tissues of the oral cavity (Table 10–1), face and scalp (Table 10–2), and neck (Table 10–3).

The dental professional also needs to keep in mind that these lymph nodes drain not only intraoral dental structures, such as the teeth, but also the eyes, ears, nasal cavity, and deeper areas of the throat. Many times a patient needs a referral to a physician when lymph nodes are palpable due to a disease process in these other regions.

LYMPH NODES OF THE HEAD

The lymph nodes of the head are in either a superficial or deep position relative to the surrounding tissues. All the nodes of the head drain either the right or left tissues in the area, depending on their location.

Superficial Lymph Nodes of the Head

There are five groups of superficial lymph nodes in the head: the occipital, retroauricular, anterior auricular, superficial parotid, and facial nodes (Figure 10–3).

OCCIPITAL LYMPH NODES

The **occipital lymph nodes** (ok-**sip**-it-al) (1–3 in number) are located bilaterally on the posterior base of the head in the occipital region and drain this portion of the scalp. Having the patient lean the head forward allows for effective bilateral palpation for these nodes (Figure 10–4). The

Table 10–2 LYMPH NODE DRAINAGE PATTERNS FOR TISSUES OF THE SCALP AND FACE

Tissues	Primary Nodes	Secondary Nodes
Scalp	Occipital, retroauricular, anterior auricular, superficial parotid, and accessory	Superior deep cervical, inferior deep cervical, and supraclavicular
Lacrimal gland	Superficial parotid	Superior deep cervical
External ear	Retroauricular, anterior auricular, and superficial parotid	Superior deep cervical
Middle ear	Deep parotid	Superior deep cervical
Pharyngeal tonsil and tubal tonsil	Superior deep cervical	Inferior deep cervical
Paranasal sinuses	Retropharyngeal	Superior deep cervical
Infraorbital region and nasal cavity	Malar, nasolabial, retropharyngeal, and superior deep cervical	Submandibular and deep cervical
Cheek	Buccal, malar, mandibular, and submandibular	Superior deep cervical
Parotid gland	Deep parotid	Superior deep cervical
Upper lip	Submandibular	Superior deep cervical
Lower lip	Submental	Submandibular and deep cervical
Chin	Submental	Submandibular and deep cervical
Sublingual gland	Submandibular	Superior deep cervical
Submandibular gland	Submandibular	Superior deep cervical

Table 10–3   LYMPH NODE DRAINAGE PATTERNS FOR TISSUES OF THE NECK

Tissues	Primary Nodes	Secondary Nodes
Superficial anterior cervical triangle	Anterior jugular	Inferior deep cervical
Superficial lateral and posterior cervical triangles	External jugular and accessory	Deep cervical and supraclavicular
Deep posterior cervical triangle	Inferior deep cervical	
Pharynx	Retropharyngeal	Superior deep cervical
Thyroid gland	Superior deep cervical	Inferior deep cervical
Larynx	Laryngeal	Inferior deep cervical
Esophagus	Superior deep cervical	Inferior deep cervical
Trachea	Superior deep cervical	Inferior deep cervical

occipital nodes empty into the inferior deep cervical nodes of the neck.

RETROAURICULAR, AURICULAR, AND SUPERFICIAL PAROTID LYMPH NODES

The nodes known as **retroauricular lymph nodes** (ret-ro-aw-**rik**-you-lar) or mastoid or posterior auricular lymph nodes (1–3 in number) are located posterior to each ear, where the sternocleidomastoid muscle inserts on the mastoid process. The **anterior auricular lymph nodes** (aw-**rik**-you-lar) (1–3 in number) are located anterior to each ear.

The **superficial parotid lymph nodes** (pah-**rot**-id) or paraparotid lymph nodes (up to 10 in

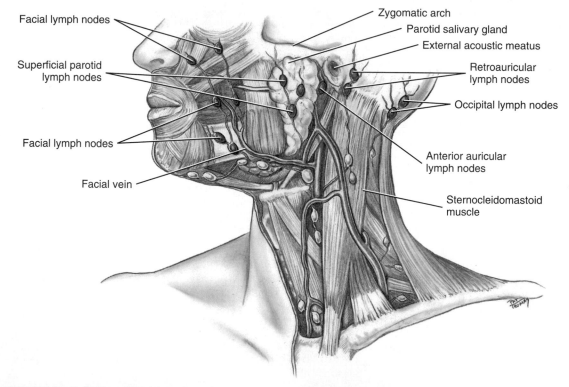

FIGURE 10–3 ■ Superficial lymph nodes of the head and associated structures.

FIGURE 10–4 ■ Palpating the occipital lymph nodes by having the patient's head forward.

number along with the deep parotid group) are just superficial to each parotid salivary gland. Some anatomists group the anterior auricular and superficial parotid lymph nodes together.

The retroauricular, anterior auricular, and superficial parotid nodes drain the external ear, lacrimal gland, and adjacent regions of the scalp and face. All of these nodes empty into the superior deep cervical lymph nodes. During an extraoral examination, standing near the patient bilaterally palpate the auricular nodes (Figure 10–5). Gentle pressure on the face and scalp around each ear will lead to effective palpation for these nodes.

FACIAL LYMPH NODES

The final group of superficial nodes of the head is the **facial lymph nodes** (up to 12 in number), which are positioned along the length of the facial vein. These nodes are typically small and variable in number. The facial nodes are further categorized into four subgroups: malar, nasolabial, buccal, and mandibular nodes.

Nodes in the infraorbital region are the **malar lymph nodes** (**may**-lar) or infraorbital lymph nodes. Nodes near the nose are the **nasolabial lymph nodes** (nay-zo-**lay**-be-al). Nodes at the labial commissure and just superficial to the

FIGURE 10–5 ■ Palpation of auricular lymph nodes using gentle pressure on the face and scalp around each ear.

buccinator muscle are the **buccal lymph nodes.** Nodes over the surface of the mandible, anterior to the masseter muscle, are the **mandibular lymph nodes** (man-**dib**-you-lar).

Each facial node group drains the skin and mucous membranes where the nodes are located. The facial nodes also drain from one to the other, superior to inferior, and then finally drain into the submandibular nodes. To palpate effectively for the facial nodes, apply gentle pressure on each side of the face, moving from the infraorbital region to the labial commissure and then to the surface of the mandible (Figure 10–6A, B, and C).

Deep Lymph Nodes of the Head

There are deep lymph nodes in the head region that can never be palpated during an extraoral examination due to their depth in the tissues. The deep nodes of the face include the deep parotid and retropharyngeal nodes (Figure 10–7).

DEEP PAROTID LYMPH NODES

The **deep parotid lymph nodes** (pah-**rot**-id) (up to 10 in number along with the superficial parotid nodes) are located deep in the parotid salivary gland and drain the middle ear, auditory tube, and parotid salivary gland.

RETROPHARYNGEAL LYMPH NODES

Also located near the deep parotid nodes and at the level of the atlas, the first cervical vertebra, are the **retropharyngeal lymph nodes** (ret-ro-far-**rin**-je-al) (up to 3 in number), which drain the pharynx, palate, paranasal sinuses, and nasal cavity. All of these deep nodes of the head drain into the superior deep cervical lymph nodes of the neck.

CERVICAL LYMPH NODES

Lymph nodes of the neck or cervical lymph nodes can be in either a superficial or deep position in the tissues. All the cervical lymph nodes drain either the right or left portions of the tissues in which they are located, except the midline submental nodes, which drain the tissues in the region bilaterally.

Many clinicians record all the cervical lymph nodes (except those directly inferior to the chin) in relationship to the sternocleidomastoid muscle. Thus, the cervical nodes are placed in three overlapping categories: superior or inferior, anterior

FIGURE 10–6 ■ Palpation of the facial nodes from the molar to the nasolabial to the buccal and then to the mandibular nodes.

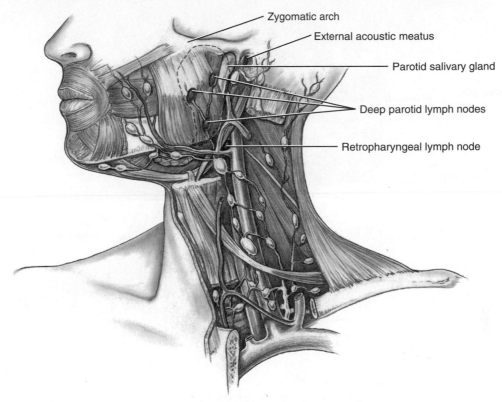

Zygomatic arch

External acoustic meatus

Parotid salivary gland

Deep parotid lymph nodes

Retropharyngeal lymph node

FIGURE 10–7 ■ Deep lymph nodes of the head and associated structures.

or posterior, superficial or deep. This text is more specific but recognizes this other method as workable.

Superficial Cervical Lymph Nodes

There are four groups of superficial cervical lymph nodes: the submental, submandibular, external jugular, and anterior jugular nodes (Figure 10–8).

SUBMENTAL LYMPH NODES

The **submental lymph nodes** (sub-**men**-tal) (2–3 in number) are located inferior to the chin in the submental fascial space. The submental nodes are also just superficial to the mylohyoid muscle, near the midline between the mandible's symphysis and hyoid bone. The submental nodes drain both sides of the chin and the lower lip, floor of the mouth, apex of the tongue, and mandibular incisors and associated tissues. The submental nodes then empty into the submandibular nodes or directly into the deep cervical nodes.

SUBMANDIBULAR LYMPH NODES

Submandibular lymph nodes (sub-man-**dib**-you-lar) (3–6 in number) are located at the inferior border of the ramus of the mandible, just superficial to the submandibular salivary gland, and within the submandibular fascial space. The submandibular nodes drain the cheeks, upper lip, body of the tongue, anterior portion of the hard palate, and teeth and associated tissues, except the mandibular incisors and maxillary third molars.

These nodes may be secondary nodes for the submental nodes and facial regions. Lymphatics from both the sublingual and submandibular salivary glands also drain into the submandibular nodes. The submandibular nodes then empty into the superior deep cervical nodes.

For the submental and submandibular nodes directly inferior to the chin, having the patient lower the chin will allow more effective palpation (Figures 10–9 and 10–10). Pushing the tissue in the area over the bony edge of the mandible where it is being grasped and rolled allows any

FIGURE 10–8 ■ Superficial cervical lymph nodes and associated structures.

palpable nodes to be located. The opposite side is examined in the same way. Some dental professionals recommend that the patient put the chin up with the mouth slightly open and the tip of the tongue on the hard palate to allow palpation of the nodes directly inferior to the chin.

FIGURE 10–9 ■ Palpating the submental lymph nodes.

EXTERNAL JUGULAR LYMPH NODES

The **external jugular lymph nodes** (jug-you-lar) or superficial lateral cervical lymph nodes are located on each side of the neck along the external jugular vein, superficial to the sternocleidomastoid muscle. The external jugular nodes may be secondary nodes for the occipital, retroauricular, anterior auricular, and superficial parotid nodes. These nodes may then empty into the superior or inferior deep cervical nodes.

ANTERIOR JUGULAR LYMPH NODES

The **anterior jugular lymph nodes** (jug-you-lar) or superficial anterior cervical lymph nodes are located on each side of the neck along the length of the anterior jugular vein, anterior to the sternocleidomastoid muscle, to drain the infrahyoid region of the neck. The anterior jugular nodes then empty into the inferior deep cervical nodes.

To palpate effectively for the external and anterior jugular nodes in the mid portion of the neck, having the patient turn the head to the side

FIGURE 10–10 ■ Palpating the submandibular lymph nodes inferior to the chin by having the patient's chin lowered.

FIGURE 10–11 ■ Palpating the external and anterior jugular lymph nodes using a prominent sternocleidomastoid muscle, starting at the ear and continuing down the length of the muscle.

makes the important landmark of the sternocleidomastoid muscle more prominent (Figure 10–11A and B). Palpation of these nodes should start below the ear and continue the whole length of the muscle's surface to the clavicles.

Deep Cervical Lymph Nodes

The **deep cervical lymph nodes** (**ser**-vi-kal) (15–30 in number) are located along the length of the internal jugular vein on each side of the neck, deep to the sternocleidomastoid muscle (Figure 10–12). The deep cervical nodes extend from the base of the skull to the root of the neck, adjacent to the pharynx, esophagus, and trachea.

Unlike the deep nodes of the head, the deep cervical lymph nodes of the neck can be palpated. Again, having the patient turn the head to the side makes the important landmark of the sternocleidomastoid muscle more prominent and increases accessibility for effective palpation of these nodes (Figure 10–13). Palpation of the deep cervical nodes is performed on the underside of the anterior and posterior aspects of the muscle in contrast to the superficial cervical nodes that are on the muscle's surface. Palpation should start below the ear and continue down the length of the muscle to the clavicles.

For those lymph nodes in the most inferior portion of the neck in the area of the clavicles, having the patient raise the shoulders up and forward allows for effective palpation during an extraoral examination (Figure 10–14).

The deep cervical lymph nodes are divided into two groups, the superior and inferior deep cervical nodes. This division is based on whether the nodes are superior or inferior to the point where the omohyoid muscle crosses the internal jugular vein.

SUPERIOR DEEP CERVICAL LYMPH NODES
The superior deep cervical lymph nodes are located deep beneath the sternocleidomastoid muscle, superior to where the omohyoid muscle

Digastric muscle

Jugulodigastric lymph node

Hyoid bone

Superior deep cevical lymph nodes

Internal jugular vein

Jugulo-omohyoid lymph node

Inferior deep cervical lymph nodes

Sternocleidomastoid muscle (cut)

Accessory lymph nodes

Accessory nerve

Omohyoid muscle

Supraclavicular lymph node

Clavicle (cut)

Thoracic duct

FIGURE 10–12 ■ Deep cervical lymph nodes and associated structures.

FIGURE 10–13 ■ Palpating the deep cervical lymph nodes by having the patient's head turned.

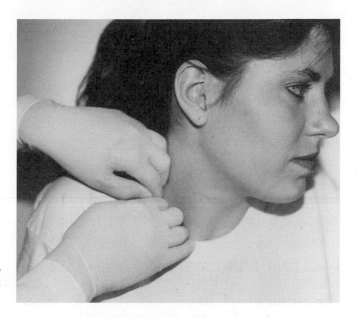

FIGURE 10–14 ■ Palpating the most inferior deep cervical lymph nodes by having the patient's shoulders raised up and forward.

crosses the internal jugular vein. The superior deep cervical nodes are primary nodes for and drain the posterior nasal cavity, posterior portion of the hard palate, soft palate, base of the tongue, maxillary third molars and associated tissues, esophagus, trachea, and thyroid gland.

The superior deep cervical nodes may be secondary nodes for all other nodes of the head and neck, except the occipital nodes and inferior deep cervical nodes. The superior deep cervical nodes empty into the inferior deep cervical nodes or directly into the jugular trunk.

One node of the superior deep cervical nodes, the **jugulodigastric lymph node** (jug-you-lo-di-**gas**-tric) or tonsillar node, easily becomes palpable when the palatine tonsils or pharynx is inflamed. The jugulodigastric node is located below the posterior belly of the digastric muscle.

INFERIOR DEEP CERVICAL LYMPH NODES

The inferior deep cervical lymph nodes are a continuation of the superior deep cervical group. The inferior deep cervical nodes are located deep to the sternocleidomastoid muscle, inferior to where the omohyoid muscle crosses the internal jugular vein, extending into the supraclavicular fossa, superior to each clavicle. The inferior deep cervical nodes are primary nodes for and drain the posterior portion of the scalp and neck, the superficial pectoral region, and a portion of the arm.

A sometimes prominent node of the inferior deep cervical nodes, the **jugulo-omohyoid lymph node** (jug-you-lo-o-mo-**hi**-oid), is located at the actual crossing of the omohyoid muscle and internal jugular vein. The jugulo-omohyoid node drains the tongue and submental region.

The inferior deep cervical nodes may be secondary nodes for the occipital and superior deep cervical nodes. Their efferent vessels form the jugular trunk, which is one of the tributaries of the right lymphatic duct (on the right side) and the thoracic duct (on the left). The inferior deep cervical nodes also communicate with the axillary lymph nodes that drain the breast region. These axillary nodes in the area of the armpit may be involved when the patient has breast cancer (adenocarcinoma), which is discussed later in this chapter.

Accessory and Supraclavicular Lymph Nodes

In addition to the deep cervical lymph nodes, there are also the accessory and supraclavicular node groups in the most inferior portion of the neck. The **accessory lymph nodes** (ak-**ses**-o-ree) (2–6 in number) are located along the accessory nerve (cranial nerve XI) and drain the scalp and neck regions and then drain into the supraclavicular nodes. The **supraclavicular lymph nodes** (soo-prah-klah-**vik**-you-ler) or transverse cervical nodes (1–10 in number) are located along the clavicle and drain the lateral cervical triangles. The supraclavicular nodes may empty into one of the jugular trunks or directly into the right lymphatic duct or thoracic duct.

TONSILS

The **tonsils** (**ton**-sils) are masses of lymphoid tissue located in the oral cavity and pharynx. Unlike lymph nodes, tonsils are not located along lymphatic vessels. All the tonsillar tissue drains into the superior deep cervical lymph nodes, particularly the jugulodigastric lymph node (see Tables 10–1 and 10–2).

PALATINE AND LINGUAL TONSILS

The **palatine tonsils** (**pal**-ah-tine) are two rounded masses of variable size located in the oral cavity between the anterior and posterior faucial pillars (Figure 10–15). The **lingual tonsil** is an indistinct layer of lymphoid tissue located intraorally on the base of the dorsal surface of the tongue (Figure 10–16).

PHARYNGEAL AND TUBAL TONSILS

The **pharyngeal tonsil** (fah-**rin**-je-il) is located on the posterior wall of the nasopharynx (Figure 10–17). This tonsil is also called the **adenoids** (**ad**-in-oidz) and is normally enlarged in children. The **tubal tonsil** (**tube**-al) is also located in the nasopharynx, posterior to the openings of the eustachian or auditory tube (Figure 10–17).

LYMPHADENOPATHY

When a patient has a disease process active in a region, such as cancer or infection, the region's lymph nodes respond. The resultant increase in size and change in consistency of the lymphoid tissue is termed *lymphadenopathy* (lim-fad-in-**op**-ah-thee) (Figure 10–18). Lymphadenopathy results from an increase in both the size of each individual lymphocyte and the overall cell count in the lymphoid tissue. With more and larger lymphocytes, the lymphoid tissue is better able to fight the disease process.

The lymph nodes can also be involved in the spread of infection, such as dental infection from the teeth, which is covered in Chapter 12. This spread of infection occurs along the connecting lymphatic vessels of the involved nodes.

This lymphadenopathy may allow the node to be visualized during an extraoral examination. More important, changes in consistency allow the lymph node to be palpated during the extraoral examination along the even firmer backdrop of

FIGURE 10–15 ■ Palatine tonsils in oral cavity.

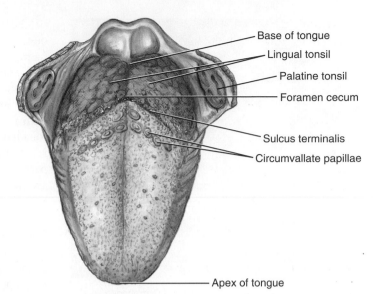

Base of tongue
Lingual tonsil
Palatine tonsil
Foramen cecum

Sulcus terminalis
Circumvallate papillae

Apex of tongue

FIGURE 10–16 ■ Lingual tonsil on the base of the tongue's dorsal surface.

underlying bones and muscles or the examiner's hands.

This change in lymph node consistency can range from firm to bony hard. Lymph nodes can remain mobile or free from the surrounding tissue during a disease. However, they can also become attached or fixed to the surrounding tissues, such as skin, bone, or muscle, as the disease process progresses to involve the regional tissues. When the lymph nodes are involved with lymphadenopathy, the lymph node can also feel tender to the patient when palpated. This tenderness is due to the pressure on the area nerves resulting from the nodes' enlargement.

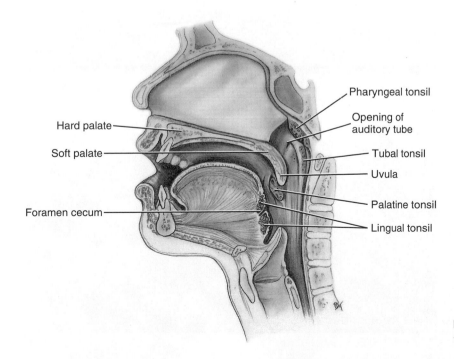

Pharyngeal tonsil
Opening of auditory tube
Tubal tonsil
Uvula
Palatine tonsil
Lingual tonsil

Hard palate
Soft palate
Foramen cecum

FIGURE 10–17 ■ Pharyngeal tonsil and tubal tonsil.

FIGURE 10–18 ■ Excessive unilateral lymphadenopathy of the submandibular lymph nodes causing enlargement and loss of cervical symmetry of the neck.

Again, any palpable lymph nodes found in a patient need to be recorded, and any appropriate physician referrals made by the dental professional. The changes in a lymph node when it is involved with infection are discussed in Chapter 12.

Lymphadenopathy can also occur to the tonsils, causing tissue enlargement. In most cases, this enlargement of the tonsils, with the exception of the tonsils in the pharynx, can be visualized during an intraoral examination of the patient (compare Figures 10–19 and 10–11). The intra-oral tonsils may also be tender when palpated. Lymphadenopathy of the tonsils in both the oral cavity and pharynx may cause airway obstruction with its complications and lead to infection of the tonsillar tissue. A dental professional may need to refer the patient to a physician if lymphadenopathy and infection of intraoral tonsillar tissue are noted.

▓ METASTASIS AND CANCER

Even though the lymph nodes usually assist in fighting the disease process, the lymph nodes can become involved in the spread of certain cancers, called carcinomas, from epithelial tissues in the region they filter. The spread of a cancer from the original or primary site of the tumor to another or secondary site is called *metastasis* (meh-**tas**-tah-sis). Primary nodes are the initial secondary site in which the cancer will metastasize from the tumor.

Many times if the cancer is caught early enough at the primary tumor site or even at the initial secondary site of the primary lymph nodes, surgery to remove the tumor as well as the primary nodes

FIGURE 10–19 ■ Enlarged palatine tonsils undergoing lymphadenopathy (note arrows).

may successfully stop metastasis. If the cancer is not caught early or stopped by the primary nodes, the cancer will spread to secondary nodes, and metastasis will continue to progress. Cancerous cells can slowly travel unchecked in the lymph from node to node if they are not stopped by any of the nodes along the lymphatic vessels.

If the cancer metastasizes past all the nodes, the cancer cells of a carcinoma can enter the blood system by way of the lymphatic ducts. The spread of cancer or metastasis by way of the blood vessels is quicker than by way of the lymph nodes, so the cancer can quickly metastasize to the rest of the body, causing possibly fatal systemic involvement with the cancer. Thus an increase in the number of nodes involved with the cancer before involving the lymphatic duct and associated blood vessels may mean a better outcome for the patient.

When they are involved with cancer, the lymph nodes can become bony hard and possibly fixed to surrounding tissues as the cancer grows and spreads. The cancerous nodes are usually not tender. In comparison, those nodes involved with acute infection are firm, mobile, and tender (see Chapter 12 for more information).

IDENTIFICATION EXERCISES

Identify the structures on the following diagrams by filling in the blanks with the correct anatomical term. You can check your answers by looking back at the figure indicated in parentheses for each identification diagram.

1. (Figure 10–1)

Facial lymph nodes
R jugular trunk
R lymphatic trunk

2. (Figure 10–3)

3. (Figure 10–7)

4. (Figure 10–8)

5. (Figure 10–12)

6. (Figure 10–16)

7. (Figure 10–17)

REVIEW QUESTIONS

1. Which of the following lymph node groups have both superficial and deep nodes within the group?
   A. Facial nodes
   B. Buccal nodes
   C. Parotid nodes
   D. Occipital nodes
   E. Submandibular nodes

2. Which of the following structures leave each individual lymph node at the hilus?
   A. Lymphatic ducts
   B. Tonsillar tissue
   C. Efferent lymphatic vessels
   D. Afferent lymphatic vessels

3. Which of the following lymph nodes are considered part of the facial lymph nodes?
   A. Sublingual, submandibular, zygomatic, and buccal nodes
   B. Infraorbital, nasal, buccal, and submental nodes
   C. Mandibular, lingual, malar, and zygomatic nodes
   D. Malar, buccal, nasolabial, and mandibular nodes
   E. Zygomatic, nasolabial, masseteric, and submental nodes

4. Which of the following components of the lymphatic system have one-way valves?
   A. Arteries
   B. Veins
   C. Vessels
   D. Nodes
   E. Ducts

5. Which of the following nodes drain lymph from a local region before the lymph flows to a more distant region?
   A. Primary
   B. Secondary
   C. Central
   D. Tertiary

6. The buccal lymph nodes are located superficial to the
   A. Sublingual gland
   B. Buccinator muscle
   C. Sternocleidomastoid muscle
   D. Parotid gland
   E. Submandibular gland

7. Which of the following lymph node groups extend from the base of the skull to the root of the neck?
   A. Facial nodes
   B. Deep cervical nodes
   C. Occipital nodes
   D. Jugulodigastric nodes
   E. Anterior jugular nodes

8. The external jugular lymph nodes are located
   A. Anterior to the hyoid bone
   B. Along the external jugular vein
   C. Deep to the sternocleidomastoid muscle
   D. Close to the symphysis of the mandible

9. The thoracic duct empties into the
   A. Aortic arch of the body
   B. Superior vena cava of the body
   C. Junction of the right and left brachiocephalic veins
   D. Junction of the left internal jugular and subclavian veins

10. Which of the following nodes are the primary lymph nodes that drain the skin and mucous membranes of the lower face?
    A. Occipital nodes
    B. Malar nodes
    C. Submandibular nodes
    D. Superficial parotid nodes
    E. Deep parotid nodes

11. Which of the following nodes are secondary lymph nodes for the occipital nodes?
    A. Buccal nodes
    B. Submental nodes
    C. Submandibular nodes
    D. Superior deep cervical nodes
    E. Inferior deep cervical nodes

12. Which of the following pairs of lymph nodes are both considered part of the superficial cervical lymph node group?
    A. External and anterior jugular nodes
    B. Superficial and deep jugular nodes
    C. Medial and lateral jugular nodes
    D. Internal and external jugular nodes

13. Which of the following statements concerning the submental lymph nodes is correct?
    A. Located deep to the mylohyoid muscle
    B. Located between the mandible's symphysis and hyoid bone
    C. Drains the labial commissure and base of tongue
    D. Secondary node for superior deep cervical nodes

14. Which muscle needs to be made more prominent on a patient to achieve effective palpation of the region where the superior deep cervical lymph nodes are located?
    A. Masseter muscle
    B. Trapezius muscle
    C. Sternocleidomastoid muscle
    D. Epicranial muscle

15. The lingual tonsil is located
    A. Posterior to the auditory tube's opening
    B. On the superior posterior wall of the nasopharynx
    C. At the base of the tongue
    D. Between the anterior and posterior faucial pillars

16. Which of the following nodes often become easily palpable when the palatine tonsils are inflamed?
    A. Jugulo-omohyoid node
    B. Jugulodigastric node
    C. Submental nodes
    D. Facial nodes

17. Which of the following are primary nodes for the maxillary third molar if it becomes infected?
    A. Submental nodes
    B. Submandibular nodes
    C. Superior deep cervical nodes
    D. Inferior deep cervical nodes

18. If a patient with breast cancer has involvement with the axillary nodes, which lymph nodes in the neck area primarily communicate with these nodes?
    A. Superior deep cervical nodes
    B. Inferior deep cervical nodes
    C. Submental nodes
    D. Submandibular nodes

19. The palatine tonsils are located at which site intraorally?
    A. Dorsal surface of tongue
    B. Submandibular fossa
    C. Between anterior and posterior faucial pillars
    D. Surrounding the faucial arch

20. Lymph nodes, when involved in the metastasis of cancer, are
    A. Always tender
    B. Usually bony hard
    C. Always mobile
    D. Usually decreased in size

lingual tonsil - base of tongue
palatine tonsil - a+p faucial pillars

REVIEW ACTIVITIES

1. Draw a lymph node and label the various portions including the hilus, lymphatic vessels, and valves, making sure to show the movement of lymph in the node.

2. Create a flow chart of the facial nodes on the left side of the body as they drain and converge into the venous system.

3. Make a list of the superficial cervical lymph nodes and the tissues they drain.

4. Looking in a mirror, palpate the deep cervical lymph nodes, both superior and inferior, or palpate a peer or patient.

5. Looking in a mirror, trace the flow of lymph from an infected mandibular third molar to the venous system, pointing out the lymph nodes along the way.

Fascia and Spaces

LEARNING OBJECTIVES

After studying this chapter, the reader should be able to:

1. Define and pronounce all the key words and anatomical terms in this chapter.
2. Locate and identify the fasciae of the head and neck on a diagram, a skull, and a patient.
3. Locate and identify the major spaces of the head and neck on a diagram, a skull, and a patient.
4. Discuss the communication between the major spaces of the head and neck.
5. Correctly complete the identification exercises and review questions and activities for this chapter.
6. Integrate the knowledge of head and neck fasciae and spaces into the clinical practice of patient examination, administration of local anesthetics, and management of the spread of dental infection.

KEY WORDS

Fascia, fasciae (**fash**-e-ah, **fash**-e-ay) Layers of fibrous connective tissue that underlie the skin and also surround the muscles, bones, vessels, nerves, organs, and other structures of the body.

Fascial spaces (**fash**-e-al) Potential spaces between the layers of fascia in the body.

FASCIA

The *fascia* (plural *fasciae*) (**fash**-e-ah, **fash**-e-ay) consists of layers of fibrous connective tissue. The fascia lies underneath the skin and also surrounds the muscles, bones, vessels, nerves, organs, and other structures of the body. The fasciae of the body can be divided into superficial fascia and deep fascia.

SUPERFICIAL FASCIA

In all areas of the body, the superficial fascia is found just beneath and attached to the skin. The superficial fascia generally separates the skin from the deeper structures of the body, allowing the skin to move independently of these deeper structures. The superficial fascia varies in thickness in different parts of the body. The superficial fascia

FIGURE 11–1 ■ Frontal section (A) of the head highlighting the fasciae of the face. Transverse sections (B) at the oral cavity and neck highlighting the continuous nature of the investing fascia.

is composed of fat, as well as irregularly arranged connective tissue. The vessels and nerves of the skin travel in the superficial fascia.

Superficial Fascia of the Head and Neck

The superficial fascia of the body does not usually enclose muscles, except in the superficial fascia of the head and neck (Figure 11–1A and B). In the face, the superficial fascia encloses the muscles of facial expression. The superficial cervical fascia of the neck contains the platysma muscle, which covers most of the anterior cervical triangle.

DEEP FASCIA

The deep fascia covers the deeper structures of the body, such as the bones, muscles, vessels, and nerves. The deep fascia consists of a dense and inelastic fibrous tissue forming sheaths around these deeper structures.

Deep Fascia of the Face and Jaws

The deep fascia of the face and jaws is divided into fascial layers that are continuous with each other and with the deep cervical fascia (see Figure 11–1). The deep fasciae of the face and jaws include the temporal, masseteric-parotid, and pterygoid fasciae.

The **temporal fascia** (**tem**-poh-ral) covers the temporalis muscle down to the zygomatic arch. The **masseteric-parotid fascia** (mass-et-**tehr**-ik-pah-**rot**-id) is located inferior to the zygomatic arch and over the masseter muscle and also surrounds the parotid salivary gland. The **pterygoid fascia** (**teh**-ri-goid) is located on the medial surface of the medial pterygoid muscle. These fasciae are all continuous with the investing layer of the deep cervical fascia.

Deep Cervical Fascia

The deep cervical fascia (**ser**-vi-kal) is composed of layers that include the investing fascia, carotid sheath, visceral fascia, and vertebral fascia (Figures 11–2 and 11–3). Again, it is important to note that these layers of deep cervical fascia are

FIGURE 11–2 ■ Midsagittal section of the head and neck highlighting the deep cervical fasciae.

continuous with each other and with the deep fascia of the face and jaws.

INVESTING FASCIA

The **investing fascia** (in-**vest**-ing) is the most external layer of deep cervical fascia. The investing fascia surrounds the neck, continuing onto the masseteric-parotid fascia. The investing fascia splits around two glands (submandibular and parotid) and two muscles (sternocleidomastoid and trapezius), enclosing them completely. Branching laminae from the investing fascia also provide the deep fasciae that surround the infrahyoid muscles, from the hyoid bone down to the sternum.

CAROTID SHEATH AND VISCERAL FASCIA

The **carotid sheath** (kah-**rot**-id sheath) is a tube of deep cervical fascia deep to the investing

fascia and sternocleidomastoid muscle, running down each side of the neck from the base of the skull to the thorax. The carotid sheath houses the internal carotid and common carotid arteries and the internal jugular vein, as well as the tenth cranial or vagus nerve. All these structures travel between the braincase and thorax.

Deep to the carotid sheath is the **visceral fascia** (**vis**-er-al) or pretracheal fascia, which is a single, midline tube of deep cervical fascia running down the neck. The visceral fascia surrounds the airway and food way, including the trachea, esophagus, and thyroid gland.

Nearer to the skull, the visceral fascia located posterior and lateral to the pharynx is known as the **buccopharyngeal fascia** (buk-o-fah-**rin**-je-al). This deep cervical fascial layer encloses the entire upper part of the alimentary canal and is continuous with the fascia on the surface of the

FIGURE 11–3 ■ Transverse section of the neck diagramming the deep cervical fasciae.

buccinator muscle, where that muscle and the superior pharyngeal constrictor muscle come together at the pterygomandibular raphe (see Chapter 4 for more information).

VERTEBRAL FASCIA

The deepest layer of the deep cervical fascia, the **vertebral fascia** (**ver**-teh-brahl) or prevertebral fascia, covers the vertebrae, spinal column, and associated muscles. Some clinicians distinguish a branch of the vertebral fascia, called the alar fascia, which is said to run from the base of the skull to connect with the visceral fascia low in the neck.

▥ SPACES

Potential spaces are created between the layers of fascia of the body because of the sheetlike nature of the fasciae. These potential spaces are termed *fascial spaces* (**fash**-e-al) or planes. It is important to remember that these fascial spaces are not actually empty spaces in healthy patients since they contain loose connective tissue. Other spaces are present in the head and neck but not created necessarily by the fascia.

SPACES OF THE HEAD AND NECK

A dental professional must have knowledge of the anatomical aspects of the spaces of the head and neck when examining a patient. These spaces are important because they can be involved in infections arising in dental tissues. These spaces also communicate with each other directly, as well as through their blood and lymph vessels. This communication may allow the spread of dental infection from an initial superficial area to more vital deeper structures. The spread of infection by way of these spaces may result in serious consequences. The role of spaces in the spread of dental infection is discussed further in Chapter 12. The study of these spaces allows the clinician to also form a three-dimensional view of head and neck anatomy.

Table 11–1 MAJOR SPACES OF THE FACE AND JAWS WITH THEIR LOCATIONS, CONTENTS, AND COMMUNICATION PATTERNS

Space	Location	Contents	Communication Patterns
Maxillary vestibular space	Between buccinator muscle and oral mucosa		Maxillary teeth and periodontium
Mandibular vestibular space	Between buccinator muscle and oral mucosa		Mandibular teeth and periodontium, and body of mandible
Canine	Within superficial fascia over canine fossa		Buccal
Buccal	Lateral to buccinator muscle	Buccal fat pad	Canine, pterygomandibular, and body of mandible
Parotid	Within parotid gland	Parotid gland, facial nerve, external carotid artery, and retromandibular vein	
Masticator	Area of mandible and muscles of mastication	Temporal, submasseteric, and infratemporal spaces	All portions communicate with each other and submandibular and parapharyngeal
Temporal	Portion of masticator space between temporal fascia and temporalis muscle	Fat	Infratemporal and submasseteric
Infratemporal	Portion of masticator space between lateral pterygoid plate, maxillary tuberosity, and ramus	Maxillary artery and branches, mandibular nerve and branches, and pterygoid plexus	Temporal, submasseteric, submandibular, and parapharyngeal
Pterygomandibular	Portion of infratemporal space between medial pterygoid muscle and ramus	Inferior alveolar nerve and vessels	Submandibular and parapharyngeal
Submasseteric	Portion of masticator space between masseter muscle and external surface of ramus		Temporal and infratemporal
Body of mandible	Periosteum covering mandible	Mandible and inferior alveolar nerve, artery, and vein	Vestibular space of mandible, buccal, submental, submandibular, and sublingual
Submental	Midline between symphysis and hyoid bone	Submental nodes and anterior jugular vein	Body of mandible, submandibular, and sublingual
Submandibular	Medial to mandible and inferior to mylohyoid muscle	Submandibular nodes and gland and facial artery	Infratemporal, body of mandible, submental, sublingual and parapharyngeal
Sublingual	Medial to mandible and superior to mylohyoid muscle	Sublingual gland and ducts, submandibular duct, lingual nerve and artery, and hypoglossal nerve	Body of mandible, submental, and submandibular

Spaces of the Face and Jaws

The major spaces of the face and jaws include the vestibular spaces of the maxilla and man-

dible; the canine, parotid, buccal, and masticatory spaces; the space of the body of the mandible; and the submental, submandibular, and sublingual spaces (Table 11–1). It is important to remember that these spaces of the face and jaw can communicate with each other and also with the cervical fascial spaces. Unlike the neck, the spaces of the face and jaws are often defined by the arrangement of muscles and bones, in addition to the fasciae. Thus many of the spaces are not fascial spaces.

VESTIBULAR SPACE OF THE MAXILLA

The space of the upper jaw, the **vestibular space of the maxilla** (mak-**sil**-ah), is located medial to the buccinator muscle and inferior to the attachment of this muscle along the alveolar process of the maxilla (Figure 11–4). Its lateral wall is the oral mucosa. This space communicates with the maxillary molar teeth and periodontium and thus can become involved with infections of these tissues.

VESTIBULAR SPACE OF THE MANDIBLE

The **vestibular space of the mandible** (man-di-bl) is located between the buccinator muscle and overlying oral mucosa (see Figure 11–4). This space is bordered by the attachment of the buccinator muscle onto the mandible. This important

space of the lower jaw communicates with the mandibular teeth and periodontium, as well as the space of the body of the mandible.

CANINE SPACE

The **canine space** (**kay**-nine) is located superior to the upper lip and lateral to the apex of the maxillary canine (Figure 11–5). This space is deep to the overlying skin and muscles of facial expression that elevate the upper lip (levator labii superioris and zygomaticus minor). The floor of the space is the canine fossa, which is covered by periosteum. This space is bordered anteriorly by the orbicularis oris muscle and posteriorly by the levator anguli oris muscle. The canine space communicates with the buccal space.

BUCCAL SPACE

The **buccal space** is the fascial space formed between the buccinator muscle (actually the buccopharyngeal fascia) and masseter muscle (see Figure 11–5). Therefore, the buccal space is inferior to the zygomatic arch, superior to the mandible, lateral to the buccinator muscle, and medial and anterior to the masseter muscle.

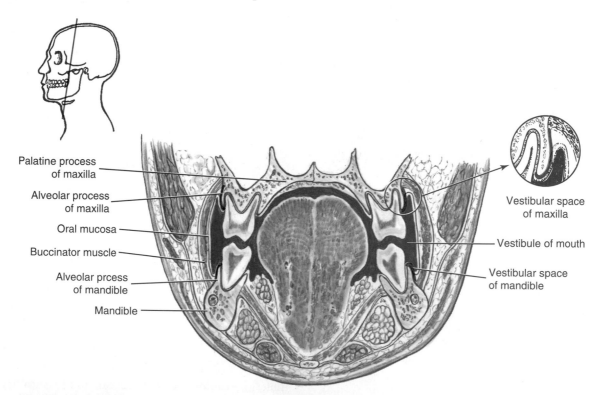

Palatine process of maxilla

Alveolar process of maxilla

Oral mucosa

Buccinator muscle

Alveolar prcess of mandible

Mandible

Vestibular space of maxilla

Vestibule of mouth

Vestibular space of mandible

FIGURE 11–4 ■ Frontal section of the head highlighting the maxillary vestibular space and mandibular vestibular space.

FIGURE 11–5 ■ Frontal view of the head highlighting the canine space and buccal space.

This bilateral space is partially covered by the platysma muscle, as well as by an extension of fascia from the parotid salivary gland capsule. The space contains the buccal fat pad. The buccal space communicates with the canine space, pterygomandibular space, and space of the body of the mandible.

PAROTID SPACE

The **parotid space** (pah-**rot**-id) is a fascial space created inside the investing fascial layer of the deep cervical fascia as it envelops the parotid salivary gland (Figure 11–6). The space contains not only the entire parotid gland but also much of the facial or seventh cranial nerve and a portion of the external carotid artery and retromandibular vein. The fascial boundaries of this space help to keep infections of the parotid gland from spreading to other sites.

MASTICATOR SPACE

The **masticator space** (mass-ti-**kay**-tor) is a general term used to include the entire area of the mandible and muscles of mastication. Thus the masticator space includes the temporal, infratemporal, and submasseteric spaces, as well as the masseter muscle and ramus and body of the mandible. All portions of the masticator space communicate with each other, as well as with the submandibular space and a cervical fascial space, the parapharyngeal space (discussed later in this chapter).

A portion of the masticator space is the **temporal space** (**tem**-poh-ral), which is formed by the temporal fascia covering the temporalis muscle (Figure 11–7). This space is between the fascia and muscle and therefore extends from the superior temporal line down to the zygomatic arch and infratemporal crest. The temporal space contains fat tissue and communicates with the infratemporal and submasseteric spaces.

The **infratemporal space** (in-frah-**tem**-poh-ral) occupies the infratemporal fossa, an area adjacent to the lateral pterygoid plate and maxillary tuberosity (Figures 11–7 and 11–8A). The space is bordered laterally by the medial surface of the mandible and the temporalis muscle. Its roof is formed by the infratemporal surface of the greater wing of the sphenoid bone. Medially, the space is bordered by the lateral pterygoid plate anteriorly and by the pharynx with its visceral layer of deep fascia posteriorly. There is no boundary inferiorly and posteriorly, where the infratemporal space is continuous with the cervical fascial space, the parapharyngeal space (discussed later).

The infratemporal space contains a portion of the maxillary artery as it branches, the mandibular nerve and its branches, and the pterygoid plexus

Facial nerve

Pterygo-
mandibular
vein

External
carotid
artery

Parotid
salivary
gland

Masseter
muscle

Parotid space

Parotid duct

FIGURE 11–6 ■ Transverse section of the head highlighting the parotid space.

of veins. It also houses the medial and lateral pterygoid muscles. This space communicates with the temporal and submasseteric spaces, as well as the submandibular and parapharyngeal spaces.

The **pterygomandibular space** (teh-ri-go-man-**dib**-you-lar) is a portion of the infratemporal space, formed by the lateral pterygoid muscle (roof), medial pterygoid muscle (medial wall), and mandibular ramus (lateral wall) (Figure 11–8A and B).

The pterygomandibular space is important because it contains the inferior alveolar nerve and vessels and is the site for the inferior alveolar nerve anesthetic block (see Chapter 9). This space communicates with the submandibular space and the parapharyngeal space of the neck (discussed later).

Another portion of the masticator space, the **submasseteric space** (sub-mas-et-**tehr**-ik) is located between the masseter muscle and external surface of the vertical ramus (Figure 11–9). This space communicates with the temporal and infratemporal spaces.

SPACE OF THE BODY OF THE MANDIBLE

The **space of the body of the mandible** (**man**-di-bl) is formed by the periosteum, covering the body of the mandible from its symphysis to the anterior borders of the masseter and medial pterygoid muscles (Figure 11–10).

This potential space of the body of the mandible contains the mandible, a portion of the inferior alveolar nerve, artery, and vein, and the dental and alveolar branches of these vessels, as well as the mental and incisive branches. The space of the mandible communicates with the vestibular space of the mandible, as well as the buccal, submental, submandibular, and sublingual spaces.

SUBMENTAL SPACE

The **submental space** (sub-**men**-tal) is located in the midline between the mandibular symphysis

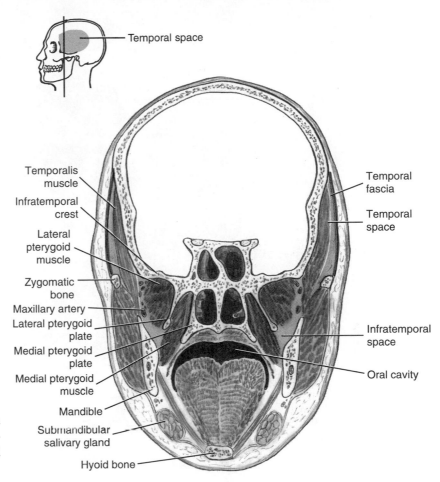

FIGURE 11–7 ■ Frontal section of the head highlighting the temporal space and infratemporal space.

and hyoid bone (Figure 11–11). The floor of this space is the superficial cervical fascia over the suprahyoid muscles. The roof is the mylohyoid muscle, covered by the investing fascia. Forming the lateral boundaries of this space are the diverging anterior bellies of the digastric muscles.

The submental space contains the submental lymph nodes and the origin of the anterior jugular vein. The submental space communicates with the space of the body of the mandible and the submandibular and sublingual spaces.

SUBMANDIBULAR SPACE

The **submandibular space** (sub-man-**dib**-you-lar) is located lateral and posterior to the submental space on each side of the jaws (Figures 11–11 and 11–12). The cross-sectional shape of this bilateral potential space is triangular, with the mylohyoid

line of the mandible being its superior boundary. The mylohyoid muscle forms the medial as well as the superior boundary of the space, and the hyoid bone creates its medial apex.

The submandibular space contains the submandibular lymph nodes, most of the submandibular salivary gland, and portions of the facial artery. This space communicates with the infratemporal, submental, and sublingual spaces and the parapharyngeal space of the neck (discussed later in this chapter).

SUBLINGUAL SPACE

The **sublingual space** (sub-**ling**-gwal) is located deep to the oral mucosa, thus making this tissue its roof (see Figure 11–12). The floor of this space is the mylohyoid muscle. Thus this muscle creates the division between the submandibular and

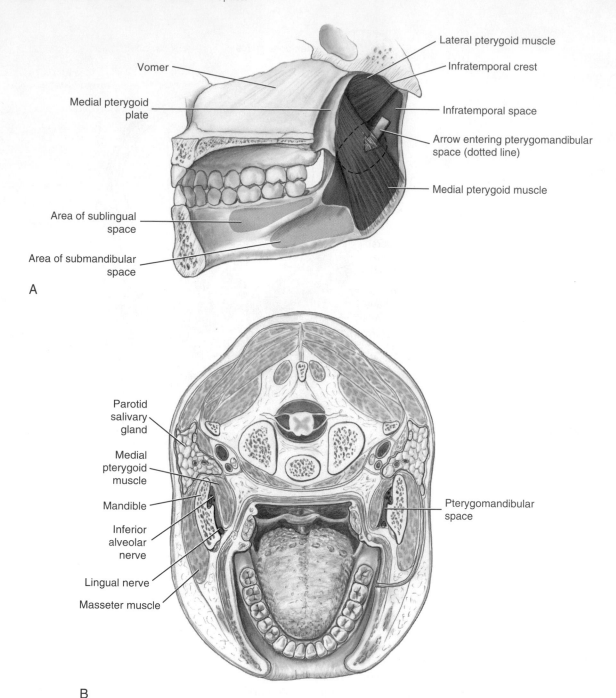

FIGURE 11–8 ■ A: Median section of the skull highlighting the infratemporal space and pterygomandibular space. B: Transverse section of the head highlighting the pterygomandibular space.

sublingual spaces. The tongue and its intrinsic muscles form the medial boundary of the sublingual space, and the mandible forms its lateral wall.

The sublingual space contains the sublingual salivary gland and ducts, the duct of the subman- dibular salivary gland, a portion of the lingual nerve and artery, and the twelfth cranial or hypoglossal nerve. The sublingual space commu- nicates with the submental and submandibular spaces and the space of the body of the mandible.

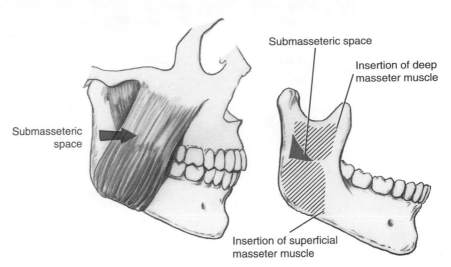

FIGURE 11–9 ■ Lateral views of the face and mandible highlighting the submasseteric space.

Cervical Fascial Spaces

The major cervical fascial spaces (**ser**-vi-kal) include the parapharyngeal, retropharyngeal, and previsceral spaces (Figures 11–13 and 11–14A and B, Table 11–2). These fascial spaces of the neck can communicate with the spaces of the face and jaws, as well as with each other. Most important, these spaces connect the spaces of the head and neck with those of the thorax, allowing dental infections to spread to vital organs, such as the heart and lungs.

PARAPHARYNGEAL SPACE

The **parapharyngeal space** (pare-ah-fah-**rin**-je-al) is a fascial space lateral to the pharynx and medial to the medial pterygoid muscle, paralleling the carotid sheath. The parapharyngeal space in its posterior portion is adjacent to the carotid sheath, which contains the internal and common carotid arteries and the internal jugular vein, as well as the tenth cranial or vagus nerve. It is also adjacent to the ninth, eleventh, and twelfth cranial nerves as they exit the cranial cavity.

FIGURE 11–10 ■ Frontal section of the head highlighting the space of the body of the mandible.

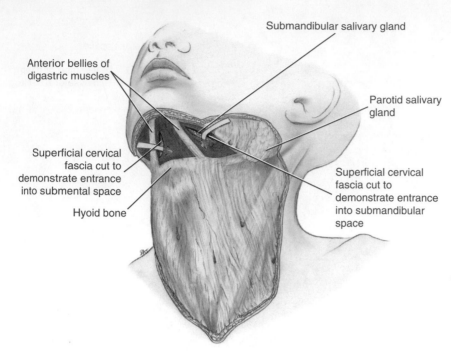

FIGURE 11–11 ■ Anterolateral view of the neck. The skin has been removed, leaving the superficial cervical fascia in place (platysma has been omitted). The location of the submental space at the midline and the two lateral submandibular spaces are indicated.

Anteriorly, the parapharyngeal space extends to the pterygomandibular raphe, where it is continuous with the infratemporal and buccal spaces. The parapharyngeal space anteriorly contains a few lymph nodes. Posteriorly, the space extends around the pharynx, where it is continuous with another cervical fascial space, the retropharyngeal space. Dental infections become dangerous when they reach the parapharyngeal space also because of its connection to the retropharyngeal space (see Chapter 12 for more information).

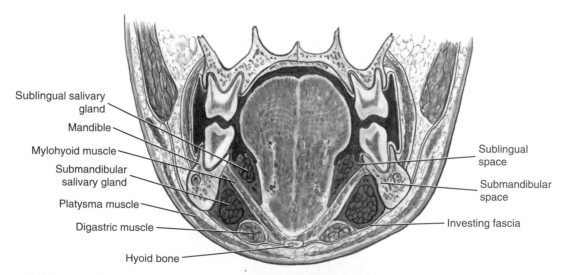

FIGURE 11–12 ■ Frontal section of the head and neck highlighting the submandibular space and sublingual space.

Vertebral muscles

Sternocleidomastoid muscle

Internal jugular vein

Internal carotid artery

Superior pharyngeal constrictor muscle

Pharynx

Medial pterygoid muscle

Mandible

Pterygomandibular raphe

Masseter muscle

Buccinator muscle

Vertebral fascia

Parapharyngeal space

Retropharyngeal space

Buccopharyngeal fascia

Buccal space

FIGURE 11–13 ■ Transverse section of the oral cavity highlighting the retropharyngeal space and parapharyngeal space.

Table 11–2 MAJOR CERVICAL FASCIAL SPACES WITH THEIR LOCATIONS, CONTENTS, AND COMMUNICATION PATTERNS

Fascial Space	Location	Contents	Communication Patterns
Parapharyngeal	Lateral to the visceral fascia around pharynx	Nodes	Masticator, submandibular, retropharyngeal, previsceral, and adjacent to carotid sheath
Retropharyngeal	Between vertebral and visceral fasciae		Parapharyngeal
Previsceral	Between visceral and investing fasciae	Nodes and cervical vessels	Parapharyngeal

FIGURE 11–14 ■ A: Midsagittal section of the head and neck highlighting the retropharyngeal space and previsceral space. B: Transverse section of the neck highlighting the retropharyngeal space and previsceral space.

RETROPHARYNGEAL SPACE

The **retropharyngeal space** (re-troh-fah-**rin**-je-al) is a fascial space located immediately posterior to the pharynx, between the vertebral and visceral fasciae. The retropharyngeal space extends from the base of the skull, where it is posterior to the superior pharyngeal constrictor muscle, down to the thorax.

Because of the rapidity with which dental infections can travel down the retropharyngeal space, it is also known as the danger space (see Chapter 12 for more information). This space communicates with the parapharyngeal spaces.

PREVISCERAL SPACE

The **previsceral space** (pre-**vis**-er-al) is located between the visceral and investing fasciae, anterior to the trachea. The previsceral space communicates with the parapharyngeal spaces.

IDENTIFICATION EXERCISES

Identify the structures on the following diagrams by filling in the blanks with the correct anatomical term. You can check your answers by looking back at the figure indicated in parentheses for each identification diagram.

1. (Figure 11–8B)

Parotid Salivary Gland

Med. Ptery mus

mandible

I A N

lingual N

masseter

2. (Figure 11–12)

3. (Figure 11–13)

REVIEW QUESTIONS

1. Which of the following describes deep fascia?
   A. Dense and inelastic tissue forming sheaths around deep structures
   B. Fatty and elastic fibrous tissue found just beneath the skin
   C. Potential spaces containing loose connective tissue
   D. Fatty and elastic fibrous tissue forming spaces under the skin
   E. Dense and inelastic deep structures of the vascular system

2. Which of the following is covered by the carotid sheath?
   A. Internal and common carotid arteries and tenth cranial nerve
   B. External and common carotid arteries and fifth cranial nerve
   C. External jugular vein and tenth cranial nerve
   D. Internal jugular vein and fifth cranial nerve

3. In which of the following spaces is the pterygoid plexus of veins located?
   A. Parotid space
   B. Temporal space
   C. Infratemporal space
   D. Buccal space
   E. Parapharyngeal space

4. The masticator space includes the submasseteric space and the
   A. Submental space
   B. Submandibular space
   C. Sublingual space
   D. Pterygomandibular space
   E. Retropharyngeal space

5. Which of the following tissues surrounds the space of the body of the mandible?
   A. Fatty tissue
   B. Loose connective tissue
   C. Periosteum
   D. Elastic tissue

6. The submandibular space communicates most directly with the
   A. Temporal space
   B. Parotid space
   C. Buccal space
   D. Sublingual space
   E. Canine space

7. The parapharyngeal space is located between the superior pharyngeal constrictor muscle and the
   A. Lateral pterygoid muscle
   B. Medial pterygoid muscle
   C. Mylohyoid muscle
   D. Masseter muscle
   E. Buccinator muscle

8. Which space is located in the midline between the mandibular symphysis and the hyoid bone?
   A. Retropharyngeal space
   B. Sublingual space
   C. Submandibular space
   D. Submental space
   E. Submasseteric space

9. Which of the following nerves is located in the pterygomandibular space?
   A. Infraorbital nerve
   B. Posterior superior alveolar nerve
   C. Inferior alveolar nerve
   D. Anterior superior alveolar nerve

10. Which of the following areas directly communicates with the retropharyngeal space?
    A. Masticator space
    B. Submandibular space
    C. Previsceral space
    D. Parapharyngeal space

REVIEW ACTIVITIES

1. Using a cotton swab, demonstrate the fascial spaces of the face and jaws.

2. Create a flow chart of an infection of a mandibular third molar and the fascial spaces it may involve with the spread of infection.

3. Draw the pterygomandibular space and label its contents.

Spread of Dental Infection

12

LEARNING OBJECTIVES

After studying this chapter, the reader should be able to:

1. Define and pronounce all the key words and anatomical terms in this chapter.
2. Discuss the spread of infection to the sinuses and by the blood system, lymphatics, and spaces to other areas in the head and neck region.
3. Trace the routes of the spread of dental infection in the head and neck region on a diagram, a skull, and a patient.
4. Discuss the lesions and complications that can occur with the spread of dental infection in the head and neck region.
5. Discuss the prevention of the spread of dental infection during patient care.
6. Correctly complete the review questions for this chapter and the case histories at the end of the textbook in the Appendices.
7. Integrate the knowledge of the spread of dental infection into the ability to prevent and manage the spread of dental infection.

KEY WORDS

Abducens nerve paralysis (ab-**doo**-senz pah-**ral**-i-sis) Loss of function of the sixth cranial nerve.

Abscess (**ab**-ses) Infection with suppuration resulting from the entrapment of pathogens in a contained space.

Bacteremia (bak-ter-**ee**-me-ah) Bacteria traveling within the blood system.

Cavernous sinus thrombosis (**kav**-er-nus **sy**-nus throm-**bo**-sus) Infection of the cavernous venous sinus.

Cellulitis (sel-you-**lie**-tis) Diffuse inflammation of soft tissue.

Embolus, emboli (**em**-bol-us, **em**-bol-eye) Foreign material or thrombus traveling in the blood that can block the vessel.

Fistula, fistulae (**fis**-chool-ah, **fis**-chool-ay) Passageway in the skin, mucosa, or even bone allowing drainage of an abscess at the surface.

Ludwig's angina (**lood**-vigz an-**ji**-nah) Serious infection of the submandibular space, with a risk of spread to the neck and chest.

Lymphadenopathy (lim-fad-in-**op**-ah-thee) Process in which there is an increase in the size and a change in the consistency of lymphoid tissue.

Maxillary sinusitis (sy-nu-**si**-tis) Infection of the maxillary sinus.

Meningitis (men-in-**jite**-is) Inflammation of the meninges of the brain or spinal cord.

Normal flora (**flor**-ah) Resident microorganisms that usually do not cause infections.

(continued)

Opportunistic infections (op-or-tu-**nis**-tik) Normal flora creating an infectious process because the body's defenses are compromised.

Osteomyelitis (os-tee-o-my-il-**ite**-is) Inflammation of bone marrow.

Paresthesia (par-es-**the**-ze-ah) Abnormal sensation from an area, such as burning or prickling.

Pathogens (**path**-ah-jens) Flora that are not normal body residents and can cause an infection.

Perforation (per-fo-**ray**-shun) Abnormal hole in a hollow organ, such as in the wall of a sinus.

Primary node Lymph node that drains lymph from a particular region.

Pustule (**pus**-tule) Small, elevated, circumscribed suppuration-containing lesion of either the skin or the oral mucosa.

Secondary node Lymph node that drains lymph from a primary node.

Stoma (**stow**-mah) Opening, such as that which occurs with a fistula.

Suppuration (sup-u-**ray**-shun) Pus containing pathogenic bacteria, white blood cells, tissue fluid, and debris.

Thrombus, thrombi (**throm**-bus, **throm**-by) Clot that forms on the inner blood vessel wall.

INFECTIOUS PROCESS

A dental professional should understand the **infectious process** that allows a microorganism to create disease. The healthy body usually lives in balance with a number of resident *normal flora* (**flor**-ah). However, certain nonresident microorganisms called *pathogens* (**path**-ah-jens) can invade and initiate an infection process. Pathogens contain certain factors that help further the infection process, such as capsules, spores, and toxins.

DENTAL INFECTIONS

Dental infections or odontogenic infections involving the teeth or associated tissues are caused by oral pathogens that are predominantly anaerobic and usually of more than one species. These infections can be of dental origin or can arise from a nonodontogenic source. Infections of dental origin usually originate from progressive dental caries or extensive periodontal disease. Pathogens can also be introduced deeper into the oral tissues by the trauma caused by dental procedures, such as the contamination of dental surgical sites (e.g., tooth extraction) and needle tracks made during local anesthetic administration. Treatment consists of removal of the source of infection, systemic antibiotics, and area drainage.

Some dental infections are secondary infections incited by an infection from the tissues surrounding the oral cavity, such as the skin, tonsils, ears, or sinuses. These nonodontogenic sources of infections must be diagnosed and treated early. Prompt referral to the patient's physician will prevent further spread and potential complications.

DENTAL INFECTION LESIONS

Dental infections can result in various types of lesions, depending on the location of the infection and thus the type of tissue involved. Dental infections can result in an abscess, cellulitis, or osteomyelitis in the head and neck region.

Abscess

An oral *abscess* (**ab**-ses) occurs when there is localized entrapment of pathogens from a dental infection in a closed tissue space, such as that created by the oral mucosa (Figures 12–1, 12–2, 12–3, and 12–4). The abscess is filled with *suppuration* (sup-u-**ray**-shun). Periapical abscess formation can occur with progressive caries, when pathogens invade the pulp and the infection spreads apically. Pathogens can also become entrapped in deep pockets in cases of severe periodontal disease and cause a periodontal abscess. An erupting third molar can cause a pericoronal abscess (pericoronitis).

Abscess formation may not be detectable radiographically during the early stages. In the later stages of infection, abscess formation can lead to the formation of a passageway or *fistula* (plural, **fistulae**) (**fis**-chool-ah, **fis**-chool-ay) in the skin, oral mucosa, or even bone that allows drainage of the infection and creates suppuration on a surface (Figures 12–2 and 12–3). The infectious process causes the overlying tissue to undergo necrosis,

FIGURE 12–1 ■ Intact periodontal abscess formation noted between the apices of the permanent mandibular first and second molars.

which allows this tract or canal to form in the tissue. The opening of the fistula is called a *stoma* (**stow**-mah). If the dental infection is surrounded by the alveolar bone, it will break down the bone in its thinnest portion (either the facial or lingual cortical plate), following the path of least resistance, and thus will be noted radiographically. The abscess can be either acute or chronic in nature.

The soft tissue over a fistula in the alveolar bone may also have an extraoral or intraoral *pustule*, a small, elevated, circumscribed, suppuration-containing lesion of either the skin or oral mucosa. The position of the pustule is determined largely by the relationship between the fistula and the overlying muscle attachments. Again the infection will follow the path of least resistance (Table 12–1). The muscle attachments to the bones, unlike the other facial soft tissues, serve as barriers to the spread of infection.

FIGURE 12–2 ■ Abscess on the buccal skin surface resulting from the formation of a fistula and stoma caused by periapical involvement of the permanent mandibular second molar. (Courtesy of Dr. Mark Gabrielson.)

FIGURE 12–3 ■ Periodontal abscess of the permanent maxillary central incisor with fistula and stoma formation (probe inserted) in the maxillary vestibule.

FIGURE 12–4 ■ Pericoronitis of the mandibular third molar with abscess formation.

Cellulitis

Cellulitis (sel-you-**lie**-tis) of the face and neck can also occur with dental infections, resulting in the diffuse inflammation of soft tissue spaces (Figure 12–5). The clinical signs and symptoms are pain, tenderness, redness, and diffuse edema of the involved soft tissue space, causing a massive and firm swelling (Table 12–2). There also may be difficulty swallowing (dysphagia) or restricted eye opening (ptosis) if the cellulitis occurs within the pharynx or orbital regions, respectively. Usually the infection remains localized and a facial abscess tends to form; if not initially treated, it may discharge upon the facial surface. Without treatment, cellulitis can possibly spread, due to perforation of the surrounding bone, causing serious complications

Table 12–1 TEETH AND ASSOCIATED PERIODONTIUM MOST COMMONLY INVOLVED IN CLINICAL PRESENTATIONS OF ABSCESSES AND FISTULAE

Clinical Presentation of Lesion	Teeth and Associated Periodontium Most Commonly Involved
Maxillary vestibule	Maxillary central or lateral incisor, all surfaces and root
	Maxillary canine, all surfaces and root (short root inferior to levator anguli oris)
	Maxillary premolars, buccal surfaces and roots
	Maxillary molars, buccal surfaces or buccal roots (short roots inferior to buccinator)
Penetration of nasal floor	Maxillary central incisor, root
Nasolabial skin region	Maxillary canine, all surfaces and root (long root superior to levator anguli oris)
Palate	Maxillary lateral incisor, lingual surface and root
	Maxillary premolars, lingual surfaces and roots
	Maxillary molars, lingual surfaces or palatal roots
Perforation into maxillary sinus	Maxillary molars, buccal surface and buccal roots (long roots)
Buccal skin surface	Maxillary molars, buccal surfaces and buccal roots (long roots superior to buccinator)
	Mandibular first and second molars, buccal surfaces and buccal roots (long roots inferior to buccinator)
Mandibular vestibule	Mandibular incisors, all surfaces and roots (short roots superior to mentalis)
	Mandibular canine and premolars, all surfaces and roots (all roots superior to depressors)
	Mandibular first and second molars, buccal surfaces and roots (short roots superior to buccinator)
Submental skin region	Mandibular incisors, root (long roots inferior to mentalis)
Sublingual region	Mandibular first molar, lingual surface and roots (all roots superior to mylohyoid)
	Mandibular second molar, lingual surface and roots (short roots superior to mylohyoid)
Submandibular skin region	Mandibular second molar, lingual surface and roots (long roots inferior to mylohyoid)
	Mandibular third molars, all surfaces and roots (all roots inferior to myohyoid)

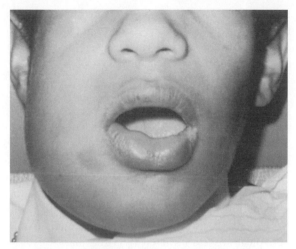

FIGURE 12–5 ■ Cellulitis involving the buccal space resulting from an abscess of the permanent mandibular first molar with swelling noted. (Courtesy of Dr. Mark Gabrielson.)

such as Ludwig's angina (discussed later in this chapter). Cellulitis is treated by administration of antibiotics and removal of the cause of the infection.

Osteomyelitis

Another type of lesion that can be related to dental infections is *osteomyelitis* (os-tee-o-my-il-**ite**-is), an inflammation of the bone marrow. Osteomyelitis can locally involve any bone in the body or can be generalized. This inflammation develops from the invasion of the tissue of a long

FIGURE 12–6 ■ Osteomyelitis of the mandible with swelling noted.

bone by pathogens, usually from a skin or pharyngeal infection. In osteomyelitis involving the jaw bones, the pathogens are most likely to derive from a periapical abscess, from an extension of cellulitis, or from contamination of a surgical site (Figure 12–6). Osteomyelitis most commonly occurs in the mandible; it occurs only rarely in the maxilla because of the mandible's thicker cortical plates and reduced vascularization.

Continuation of osteomyelitis leads to bone resorption and formation of sequestra, pieces of dead bone separated from the sound bone within the area. This bone damage is detected by radiographic evaluation. *Paresthesia* (par-es-**the**-ze-ah), evidenced by burning or prickling, may develop in the mandible if the infection involves the mandibular canal carrying the inferior alveolar nerve. Localized paresthesia of the lower lip may

Table 12–2   SPACE TEETH AND PERIODONTIUM POSSIBLY INVOLVED WITH A CLINICAL PRESENTATION OF CELLULITIS RESULTING FROM THE SPREAD OF DENTAL INFECTION

Clinical Presentation of Lesion	Space Involved	Teeth and Associated Periodontium Most Commonly Involved in Infection
Infraorbital, zygomatic, and buccal regions	Buccal space	Maxillary premolars and maxillary and mandibular molars
Posterior border of mandible	Parotid space	Not generally of odontogenic origin
Submental region	Submental space	Mandibular anterior teeth
Unilateral submandibular region	Submandibular space	Mandibular posterior teeth
Bilateral submandibular region	Submental, sublingual, and submandibular spaces with Ludwig's angina	Spread of mandibular dental infection
Lateral cervical region	Parapharyngeal space	Spread of mandibular dental infection

occur if the infection is distal to the mental foramen where the mental nerve exits. Treatment consists of drainage, surgical removal of any sequestra, and antibiotic administration; in some patients, the additional use of hyperbaric oxygen may be necessary. Today osteomyelitis of the jaw is uncommon since dental care and antibiotics are readily available.

MEDICALLY COMPROMISED PATIENTS

Normal flora usually do not create an infectious process. If, however, the body's natural defenses are compromised, then they can create *opportunistic infections* (**op**-or-tu-**nis**-tik). Medically compromised individuals include those with AIDS, diabetes, or cancer and those undergoing cancer or transplant therapy. Some patients have a higher risk of complications resulting from dental infections because of their medical histories. Patients in this category include those at risk for infective endocarditis.

▓ SPREAD OF DENTAL INFECTIONS

Many infections that start in the teeth and associated oral tissues can have significant consequences if they spread to vital tissues or organs. Usually a localized abscess establishes a fistula in the skin, oral mucosa, or associated bone, allowing natural drainage of the infection and diminishing the risk of spread of the infection. However, fistula formation or even establishment of drainage does not always occur. Occasionally, a dental infection can spread to the paranasal sinuses or can be spread by the blood system, lymphatics, or spaces in the head and neck. It is important review the communication patterns that are possible in these various tissues so as to understand the possible routes of infection that may occur (see Chapters 3, 6, 10, and 11 for more information).

SPREAD TO THE PARANASAL SINUSES

The **paranasal sinuses** of the skull can become infected as a result of the direct spread of infection from the teeth and associated oral tissues, resulting in a *secondary sinusitis* (sy-nu-**si**-tis). A *perforation* (per-fo-**ray**-shun), an abnormal hole in the wall of the sinus, can also be caused by an infection.

Maxillary Sinusitis

Secondary sinusitis of dental origin occurs mainly in the **maxillary sinuses,** since the maxillary posterior teeth and associated tissues are in close proximity to these sinuses (see Chapter 3 for more information). Thus *maxillary sinusitis* (sy-nu-**si**-tis) can result from the spread of infection from a periapical abscess initiated by a maxillary posterior tooth that perforates the sinus floor to involve the sinus mucosa. Also, a contaminated tooth or root fragments can be displaced into the maxillary sinus during an extraction, creating an infection.

However, most infections of the maxillary sinuses are not of dental origin but are caused by an upper respiratory infection, an infection in the nasal region that spreads to the sinuses. An infection in one sinus can travel through the nasal cavity to other sinuses and lead to serious complications for the patient, such as infection of the cranial cavity and brain. Thus it is important that any sinusitis be treated aggressively by the patient's physician to eliminate the initial infection.

The symptoms of sinusitis are headache, usually near the involved sinus, and foul-smelling nasal or pharyngeal discharge, possibly with fever and weakness. The skin over the involved sinus can be tender, hot, and red due to the inflammation in the area. Difficulty in breathing (dyspnea) occurs, as well as pain, when the nasal passages become blocked by the effects of tissue inflammation. Early radiographic evidence of sinusitis is the thickening of the sinus walls, with subsequent radiographic evaluation showing increased opacity and possibly perforation. A panoramic radiographic view of the skull is helpful because bilateral comparisons can be made.

Acute sinusitis usually responds to antibiotic therapy, while drainage is aided by the use of decongestants. Surgery may be needed in cases of chronic maxillary sinusitis to enlarge the ostia of the lateral walls in the nasal cavity so that adequate drainage can diminish the effects of the infection. The surgical approach to the maxillary sinus is through the thin bone of the canine fossa.

SPREAD BY BLOOD SYSTEM

The blood system of the head and neck can allow the spread of infection from the teeth and associated oral tissues because pathogens can travel in the veins and drain the infected oral site into other tissues or organs (see Chapter 6 for more information). The spread of dental infection by way of the blood system can occur because of bacteremia or an infected thrombus.

Bacteremia

Bacteria traveling in the blood can cause transient *bacteremia* (bak-ter-ee-me-ah), which can occur during dental treatment. In an individual with a high risk for infective endocarditis, these bacteria may lodge in the compromised tissues and set up serious infection deep in the heart, which can result in massive and fatal heart damage. Such a patient may need antibiotic premedication to prevent bacteremia from occurring during dental treatment.

Cavernous Sinus Thrombosis

An infected intravascular clot or *thrombus* (plural *thrombi*) (**throm**-bus, **throm**-by) can dislodge from the inner blood vessel wall and travel as an *embolus* (plural *emboli*) (**em**-bol-us, **em**-bol-eye). Emboli can travel in the veins, draining the oral cavity into areas such as the dural **venous sinuses** within the cranial cavity (see Chapter 6 for more information). These dural sinuses are channels by which blood is conveyed from the cerebral veins into the veins of the head and neck, particularly the internal jugular vein. However, because these veins lack functional valves, venous blood can flow both into and out of the cranial cavity.

The cavernous sinus is most likely to be involved in the possible fatal spread of dental infection. An infection of this venous sinus is called *cavernous sinus thrombosis* (**kav**-er-nus **sy**-nus throm-**bo**-sus). The cavernous sinus is located on the side of the body of the sphenoid bone. Each cavernous venous sinus communicates with the one on the opposite side and also with the **pterygoid plexus of veins** and the **superior ophthalmic vein,** which anastomoses with the **facial vein.** These major veins drain teeth through the **posterior superior** and **inferior**

alveolar veins and the lips through the **superior** and **inferior labial veins.**

None of these major veins that communicate with the cavernous sinus have valves to prevent the retrograde flow of blood back into the cavernous sinus. Therefore, dental infections that drain into these major veins may initiate an inflammatory response resulting in an increase in blood stasis, thrombus formation, and increasing extravascular fluid pressure. Increased pressure can reverse the direction of venous blood flow, enabling the transport of the infected thrombus into this venous sinus and thus causing cavernous sinus thrombosis.

Needle-track contamination can also result in a spread of infection to the pterygoid plexus if a posterior superior alveolar anesthetic block is incorrectly administered. Nonodontogenic infections of the area physicians consider the dangerous triangle of the face—the orbital region, nasal region, and paranasal sinuses—also may result in the spread of infection to the cavernous venous sinus.

The signs and symptoms of cavernous sinus thrombosis include fever, drowsiness, and rapid pulse. In addition, there is loss of function of the abducens nerve, since it runs through the cavernous venous sinus, resulting in *abducens nerve paralysis* (ab-**doo**-senz pah-**ral**-i-sis). Because the muscle supplied by the abducens moves the eyeball laterally, inability to perform this movement suggests nerve damage. Additionally, the patient will usually have double vision (diplopia) because of the restricted movement of the one eye, as well as edema of the eyelids and conjunctivae, tearing (lacrimation), or extruded eyeballs (exophthalmus), depending on the course of the infection.

With cavernous sinus thrombosis there may also be damage to the other cranial nerves, such as the **oculomotor nerve** (third) and **trochlear nerve** (fourth), as well as to the **ophthalmic and maxillary divisions of the trigeminal nerve** (fifth) and changes in the tissues they innervate, since all these nerves travel in the cavernous sinus wall. Finally, this infection can be fatal because it may lead to *meningitis* (men-in-**jite**-is), inflammation of the meninges in the brain or spinal cord, which requires immediate hospitalization with intravenous antibiotics and anticoagulants.

SPREAD BY LYMPHATICS

The **lymphatics** of the head and neck can allow the spread of infection from the teeth and associated oral tissues. This occurs because the pathogens can travel in the lymph through the lymphatic vessels that connect the series of nodes from the oral cavity to other tissues or organs (see Chapter 10 for more information). Thus these pathogens can move from a *primary node* near the infected site to a *secondary node* at a distant site.

The route of dental infection traveling through the nodes varies according to the teeth involved. The **submental nodes** drain the mandibular incisors and their associated tissues. Then the submental nodes empty into the submandibular nodes or directly into the deep cervical nodes. The **submandibular nodes** are the primary nodes for all the teeth and associated tissues, except the mandibular incisors and maxillary third molars. The submandibular nodes then empty into the superior deep cervical nodes

The **superior deep cervical nodes** are the primary nodes for the maxillary third molars and their associated tissues, and they empty into either the **inferior deep cervical nodes** or directly into the **jugular trunk** and then into the vascular system. Once the infection is in the vascular system, it can be spread to all tissues and organs, as previously discussed.

Lymphadenopathy

A lymph node involved in infection undergoes *lymphadenopathy* (lim-fad-in-**op**-ah-thee), which results in a size increase and a change in the consistency of the lymph node so it becomes palpably firm. This change in the lymph node allows it to be better able to fight the infectious process. Evaluation of the involved nodes can determine the degree of regional involvement in the infectious process, which is instrumental in diagnosis and management of the infectious process.

SPREAD BY SPACES

The **fascial spaces** of the head and neck can allow the spread of infection from the teeth and associated oral tissues because the pathogens can travel within the fascial planes, from one space near the infected site to another, distant space by means of the spread of the related inflammatory exudate (see Chapter 11 for more information). When involved in infections, the space can undergo cellulitis (see Table 12–2), which can cause a change in the normal proportions of the face (see Chapter 2 for more information).

If the maxillary teeth and associated tissues are infected, the infection can spread into the **maxillary vestibular space, buccal space,** or **canine space.** If the mandibular teeth and associated tissues are infected, the infection can spread into the **mandibular vestibular space, buccal space, submental space, sublingual space, submandibular space,** or the **space of the body of the mandible.** From these spaces, the infection can spread into other spaces of the jaws and neck, possibly causing serious complications such as Ludwig's angina.

Ludwig's Angina

One of the most serious lesions of the jaw region is *Ludwig's angina* (**lood**-vigz an-**ji**-nah), cellulitis of the **submandibular space** (Figure 12–7). It involves the spread of infection from any of the mandibular teeth or associated tissues to one space initially, the submental, the sublingual, or even the submandibular space itself.

FIGURE 12–7 ■ Ludwig's angina showing involvement of the submandibular and submental spaces resulting from an abscess of the permanent mandibular third molar. (Courtesy of Dr. Mark Gabrielson.)

The infection then spreads to the submandibular space bilaterally, with a risk of spreading to the **parapharyngeal space** of the neck. With this complication, there is massive bilateral submandibular regional swelling, which extends down the anterior cervical triangle to the clavicles. Swallowing, speaking, and breathing may be difficult, and high fever and drooling are evident. Respiratory obstruction may rapidly develop because the continued swelling displaces the tongue upward and backward, thus blocking the pharyngeal airway. As the **retropharyngeal space** or danger space becomes involved, edema of the larynx may cause complete respiratory obstruction, asphyxiation, and death. Ludwig's angina is an acute medical emergency requiring immediate hospitalization, and it may necessitate an emergency cricothyrotomy to create a patent airway. With the advent of earlier care of abscessed teeth and routine antibiotic treatment, Ludwig's angina has become an uncommon dental emergency.

■ PREVENTION OF THE SPREAD OF DENTAL INFECTIONS

Early diagnosis and treatment of dental infections must occur in all patients. Particular care must be taken not to contaminate surgical sites, such as those resulting from extraction, implant placement, or periodontal treatment. There must also be strict adherence to aseptic protocol during nonsurgical dental treatment so as to prevent the spread of infection during, for example, restorative and periodontal debridement therapy such as the removal of heavy plaque accumulations. Using an antiseptic rinse prior to treatment and using a rubber dam or an antimicrobial-laced external water supply during treatment when ultrasonics or irrigators are used may be of help in preventing the spread of infection. It is also important not to administer a local anesthetic through an area of dental infection so as to avoid moving the pathogens deeper into the tissues. After treatment, an antiseptic home rinse or antibiotic coverage might be prescribed.

A thorough medical history with periodic updates will allow the dental professional to perform safe treatment of medically compromised patients and avoid serious complications due to dental diseases. These patients may require antibiotic premedication before dental treatment or other changes in the dental treatment plan so as to prevent serious sequelae. A medical consultation is indicated when there is uncertainty as to the risk of opportunistic infection for an individual patient.

Dental infections can have significant medical ramifications, including death. As the healthcare professional most familiar with a patient's oral health, the dental professional must be knowledgeable about the appearances, causes, and symptoms of the lesions of dental infections as well as being expert in the means of their prevention.

REVIEW QUESTIONS

1. Which of the following complications is likely with untreated Ludwig's angina?
   A. Abducens nerve paralysis
   B. Meningitis
   C. Respiratory obstruction
   D. Sinus perforation
   E. Double vision

2. Which of the following cranial nerves may be involved with cavernous sinus thrombosis?
   A. Oculomotor and trochlear nerves
   B. Vagus and glossopharyngeal nerves
   C. Hypoglossal and accessory nerves
   D. Optic and olfactory nerves

3. Which of the following statements correctly describes an oral abscess?
   A. Inflammation of the bone
   B. Inflammation of the meninges
   C. Infection confined in oral mucosal space
   D. Diffuse inflammation of soft tissue

4. Which of the following statements concerning cavernous sinus thrombosis is correct?
   A. Associated major veins have valves
   B. Only dental infections can spread to the sinus
   C. Eye tissues are not affected
   D. Needle-track contamination may be involved

5. If an infection involves the lingual surface of the mandibular third molar, a swelling is most likely to be observed
   A. In the mandibular vestibule
   B. Beneath the tongue
   C. In the submandibular region
   D. In the buccal and submental regions

BIBLIOGRAPHY

American Academy of Periodontology. Parameter on acute diseases. *J Periodontol* 2000;71:863–866.

American Academy of Periodontology. Parameter on occlusal traumatism in patients with chronic periodontitis. *J Periodontol* 2000;71:873–875.

Bath-Balogh M, Fehrenbach MJ. *Illustrated Dental Embryology, Histology, and Anatomy*. WB Saunders, Philadelphia, 1997.

Beck JD, Pankow J, Tyroler HA, Offenbacher S. Dental infections and atherosclerosis. *Am Heart J* 1999;138(5):528–533.

Bridgeman A, Wiesenfeld D, Newland S. Anatomical considerations in the diagnosis and management of acute maxillofacial bacterial infections. *Aust Dent J* 1996;41(4):238–245.

Budenz AW. Local anesthetics and medically complex patients. *J Calif Dent Assoc* 2000; 28(8):611–619.

Cawson RA. *Aids to Oral Pathology and Diagnosis*. Churchill and Livingstone, Edinburgh, London, Melbourne, and New York, 1981.

Clemente CD. *Anatomy*, 3rd edition. Urban and Schwarzenberg, Baltimore, 1987.

Darby ML, Walsh MM. *Dental Hygiene Theory and Practice*. WB Saunders, Philadelphia, 1995.

Djurdjanovic D, Widmalm SE, Williams WJ, Koh CK, Yang KP. Computerized classification of temporomandibular joint sounds. *IEEE Trans Biomed Eng* 2000;47(8):977–984.

Dorland's Medical Dictionary, 28th edition. WB Saunders, Philadelphia, 1994.

DuBrul EL. *Sicher and DuBrul's Oral Anatomy*, 8th edition. Ishiyaku EuroAmerica, St. Louis, 1988.

Evers H, Haegerstam G. *Introduction to Dental Local Anaesthesia*, 2nd edition. BC Decker, Philadelphia, and Mediglobe, Fribourg, 1990.

Friedman MJ, Hochman MN. The AMSA injection: A new concept for local anesthesia of maxillary teeth using a computer-controlled injection system. *Quintessence Int* 1988;29(5):297–303.

Gage TW, Pickett FA. *Dental Drug Reference*. Mosby, St. Louis, 1997.

Gray H. *Gray's Anatomy*, 37th edition. Churchill and Livingstone, Edinburgh, London, Melbourne, and New York, 1989.

Herrera D, Roldan S, Sanz M. The periodontal abscess: A review. *J Clin Periodontol* 2000;27(6):377–386.

Hohl TH, Whitacre RJ, Hooley JR, Williams BL. *Diagnosis and Treatment of Odontogenic infections*. Stoma Press, Seattle, 1983.

Ibsen AC, Phelan JA. *Oral Pathology for the Dental Hygienist*, 2nd edition. WB Saunders, Philadelphia, 2000.

Jibiki M, Shimoda S, Nakagawa Y, Kawasaki K, Asada K, Ishibashi K. Calcifications of the disc of the temporomandibular joint. *J Oral Pathol Med* 1999;28(9):413–419.

Johnson BR, Remeikis NA, Van Cura JE. Diagnosis and treatment of cutaneous facial sinus tracts of dental origin. *J Am Dental Assoc* 1999;130(6):832–836.

Kasle MJ. *An Atlas of Dental Radiographic Anatomy*, 3rd edition. WB Saunders, Philadelphia, 1990.

Leonard PC. *Medical Terminology*. WB Saunders, Philadelphia, 1990.

Li X, Tronstad L, Olsen I. Brain abscesses caused by oral infection. *Endod Dent Traumatol* 1999;15(3):95–101.

Li X, Kolltveit KM, Tronstad L, Olsen I. Systemic diseases caused by oral infection. *Clin Microbiol Rev* 2000;13(4):547–558.

Little JW, Falace DA, Miller CS, Rhodus NL. *Dental Management of the Medically Compromised Patient*, 5th edition. Mosby, St. Louis, 1997.

Malamed SF. *Handbook of Local Anesthesia*, 4th edition. Mosby, St. Louis, 1997.

Malamed SF. Morbidity, mortality and local anesthesia. *Prim Dent Care* 1999;6(1):11–15.

Michalowicz BS, Pihlstrom BL, Hodges JS, Bouchard TJ Jr. No heritability of temporomandibular joint signs and symptoms. *J Dent Res* 2000;79(8):1573–1578.

Miles DA, Van Dis ML, Razmus TF. *Oral and Maxillofacial Radiology: Radiologic/Pathologic Correlations*. WB Saunders, Philadelphia, 1991.

Nakai Y, Milgrom P, Mancl L, Coldwell SE, Domoto PK, Ramsay DS. Effectiveness of local anesthesia in pediatric dental practice. *J Am Dent Assoc* 2000; 131(12):1699–1705.

Niwa H, Satoh Y, Matsuura H. Cardiovascular responses to epinephrine-containing local anesthetics for dental use: A comparison of hemodynamic responses to infiltration anesthesia and ergometer-stress testing. *Oral Surg Oral Med Oral Pathol Oral Radiol Endod* 2000; 90(2):171–181.

Nomina Anatomica, 6th edition. Churchill and Livingstone, Edinburgh, London, Melbourne, and New York, 1989.

Olsen I, Golberg CO, Finegold SM. A primer on anaerobic bacteria and anaerobic infections for the uninitiated. *Infection* 1999;27(3):159–165.

O'Toole M. *Miller-Keane Encyclopedia and Dictionary of Medicine, Nursing and Allied Health*, 5th edition. WB Saunders, Philadelphia, 1992.

Peretz B, Bimstein E. The use of imagery suggestions during administration of local anesthetic in pediatric dental patients. *ASDC J Dent Child* 2000;67(4):231, 263–267.

Perry DA, Beemsterboer PL, Taggart EJ. *Periodontology for the Dental Hygienist*. WB Saunders, Philadelphia, 1996.

Pogrel MA, Thamby S. Permanent nerve involvement resulting from inferior alveolar nerve blocks. *J Am Dent Assoc* 2000;131(7):901–907.

Quinn JH. Inferior alveolar nerve block using the internal oblique ridge. *J Am Dent Assoc* 1998;129(8): 1147–1148.

Rammelsberg P, Jager L, Duc JM. Magnetic resonance imaging–based joint space measurements in temporomandibular joints with disk displacements and in contols. *Oral Surg Oral Med Oral Pathol Oral Radiol Endod* 2000;90(2): 240–248.

Reed GM, Sheppard VF. *Basic Structures of the Head and Neck*. WB Saunders, Philadelphia, 1976.

Regezi JA, Sciubba JJ, Pogrel MA. *Atlas of Oral and Maxillofacial Pathology*. WB Saunders, Philadelphia, 1999.

Roda RS, Blanton PL. The anatomy of local anesthesia. *Tex Dent J* 1998;115(5):15–25.

Rohen JW, Yokochi C. *Color Atlas of Anatomy*. Igaku-Shoin, New York, 1983.

Saso M, Isen D, Nenniger S, Gardner M. Mandibular nerve block. *J Can Dent Assoc* 1997;63(11):805–808.

Scannapieco FA. Role of oral bacteria in respiratory infections. *J Periodontol* 1999;70(7):793–802.

Schumacher G-H. *Anatomie für Stomatologen*. JA Barth, Leipzig, Germany, 1984.

Solomon EP. *Introduction to Human Anatomy and Physiology*. WB Saunders, Philadelphia, 1992.

Toyama M, Kurita K, Koga K, Rivera G. Magnetic resonance arthrography of the temporomandibular joint. *J Oral Maxillofac Surg* 2000;58(9):978–984.

Wilson-Pauwels LW, Akesson EJ, Stewart PA. *Cranial Nerves*. BC Decker, Toronto and Philadelphia, 1988.

ANSWERS TO REVIEW QUESTIONS

CHAPTER 1
1. B
2. B
3. D
4. B
5. B
6. A
7. B
8. C
9. C
10. D

CHAPTER 2
1. C
2. C
3. C
4. B
5. C
6. B
7. A
8. B
9. A
10. D

CHAPTER 3
1. C
2. D
3. A
4. D
5. A
6. D
7. D
8. B
9. C
10. B
11. B
12. A
13. B
14. C
15. C
16. B
17. E
18. D

19. C
20. A
21. C
22. B
23. A
24. C
25. B

CHAPTER 4
1. C
2. D
3. C
4. D
5. D
6. C
7. A
8. E
9. B
10. D
11. A
12. C
13. A
14. C
15. B
16. B
17. B
18. B
19. A
20. B
21. D
22. A
23. A
24. C
25. A

CHAPTER 5
1. C
2. B
3. C
4. C
5. C
6. E

7. A
8. B
9. D
10. C
11. C
12. C
13. A
14. C
15. A

CHAPTER 6
1. A
2. C
3. B
4. A
5. B
6. A
7. C
8. B
9. C
10. A
11. B
12. A
13. B
14. D
15. B

CHAPTER 7
1. A
2. B
3. B
4. B
5. A
6. B
7. D
8. A
9. D
10. C
11. B
12. B
13. D
14. A
15. A

CHAPTER 8
1. C
2. B
3. A
4. C
5. D
6. B
7. D
8. B
9. C
10. B
11. B
12. D
13. B
14. B
15. A
16. B
17. A
18. B
19. C
20. D

CHAPTER 9
1. B
2. E
3. A
4. C
5. C
6. C
7. A
8. B
9. C
10. D
11. B
12. A
13. A
14. D
15. A

CHAPTER 10
1. C
2. C

3. D
4. C
5. A
6. B
7. B
8. B
9. D
10. C
11. E

12. A
13. B
14. C
15. C
16. B
17. C
18. B
19. C
20. B

CHAPTER 11
1. A
2. A
3. C
4. D
5. C
6. D
7. B
8. D

9. C
10. D

CHAPTER 12
1. C
2. A
3. C
4. D
5. C

GLOSSARY
of Key Words and Anatomical Terms

A

Abducens nerve (ab-**doo**-senz) Sixth cranial nerve (VI) that serves an eye muscle.

Abducens nerve paralysis (ab-**doo**-senz pah-**ral**-i-sis) Loss of function of the sixth cranial nerve.

Abscess (**ab**-ses) Infection with suppuration resulting from the entrapment of pathogens in a contained space.

Accessory lymph nodes (ak-**ses**-o-ree) Deep cervical nodes located along the accessory nerve.

Accessory nerve (ak-**ses**-o-ree) Eleventh cranial nerve (XI) that serves the trapezius and sternocleidomastoid muscles, as well as muscles of the soft palate and pharynx.

Action (**ak**-shun) Movement accomplished by a muscle when the muscle fibers contract.

Action potential (po-**ten**-shal) Rapid depolarization of a cell membrane that results in propagation of the nerve impulse along the membrane.

Adenoids (**ad**-in-oidz) Another term for the pharyngeal tonsils.

Afferent nerve (**af**-er-ent) Sensory nerve that carries information from the periphery of the body to the brain or spinal cord.

Afferent nervous system (**af**-er-ent) Or sensory nerve system, a division of the PNS, that carries information from receptors to the brain or spinal cord.

Afferent vessels (**af**-er-ent) Type of lymphatic vessel in which lymph flows into the lymph node.

Ala, alae (**a**-lah, **a**-lay) Winglike cartilaginous structures that laterally bound the nares.

Alveolar mucosa (al-**ve**-o-lar) Mucosa that lines the vestibules of the oral region.

Alveolar process of the mandible (al-**ve**-o-lar) Portion of the mandible that contains the roots of the maxillary teeth.

Alveolar process of the maxilla (al-**ve**-o-lar) Ridge of maxillary bone that houses the roots of the maxillary teeth.

Anastomosis, anastomoses (ah-nas-tah-**moe**-sis, ah-nas-tah-**moe**-sees) Communication of a blood vessel with another by a connecting channel.

Anatomical nomenclature (an-ah-**tom**-ik-al **no**-men-kla-cher) System of names of anatomical structures.

Anatomical position (an-ah-**tom**-ik-al) Position in which the body is erect, arms at the sides, palms and toes directed forward, and eyes looking forward.

Angle of the mandible Angle at the intersection of the posterior and inferior borders of the ramus.

Angular artery (**ang**-u-lar) Arterial branch that is a termination of the facial artery and supplies the tissues along the side of the nose.

Anterior (an-**tere**-ee-or) Front of an area of the body.

Anterior arch Arch of the atlas or first cervical vertebra.

Anterior auricular lymph nodes (aw-**rik**-you-lar) Superficial nodes located anterior to the ear.

Anterior cervical triangle (**ser**-vi-kal) Anterior region of the neck.

Anterior ethmoidal nerve (eth-**moy**-dal) Nerve from the nasal cavity and paranasal sinuses that converges with other orbital branches to form the nasociliary nerve.

Anterior jugular lymph nodes (**jug**-you-lar) Superficial cervical nodes located along the anterior jugular vein.

315

Anterior jugular vein (**jug**-you-lar) Vein that begins below the chin, descends near the midline, and drains into the external jugular vein.

Anterior superior alveolar artery (al-**ve**-o-lar) Arterial branch from the infraorbital artery that gives off dental and alveolar branches that supply the pulp tissue and periodontium of the anterior maxillary teeth.

Anterior superior alveolar (ASA) block (al-**ve**-o-lar) Local anesthetic block that achieves anesthesia of the pulp of the maxillary canine and incisor and their associated facial tissues.

Anterior superior alveolar (ASA) nerve (al-**ve**-o-lar) Nerve that serves the maxillary anterior teeth and tissues and is formed from dental and interdental branches and later joins the infraorbital nerve.

Anterior suprahyoid muscle group (soo-prah-**hi**-oid) Suprahyoid muscles located anterior to the hyoid bone that include the anterior belly of the digastric, mylohyoid, and geniohyoid muscles.

Anterior faucial pillar (**faw**-shawl **pil**-er) Vertical fold anterior to each palatine tonsil created by the palatoglossal muscle.

Antitragus (an-tie-**tra**-gus) Flap of tissue opposite the tragus of the ear.

Aorta (ay-**ort**-ah) Major artery that gives rise to the common carotid and subclavian arteries on the left side of the body and to the brachiocephalic artery on the right side.

Aperture (**ap**-er-cher) Opening or orifice in bone.

Apex (**ay**-peks) Pointed end of a conical structure.

Apex of the nose Tip of the nose.

Apex of the tongue Tip of the tongue.

Arch (arch) Prominent bridgelike bony structure.

Arteriole (ar-**ter**-ee-ole) Smaller artery that branches off an artery and connects with a capillary.

Artery (**art**-er-ee) Type of blood vessel that carries blood away from the heart.

Articular eminence (ar-**tik**-you-ler) Eminence on the temporal bone that articulates with the mandible at the temporomandibular joint.

Articular fossa (ar-**tik**-you-ler) Fossa on the temporal bone that articulates with the mandible at the temporomandibular joint.

Articulating surface of the condyle (ar-**tik**-you-late-ing) Portion of the head of the condyle that articulates with the temporal bone at the temporomandibular joint.

Articulation (ar-tik-you-**lay**-shin) Area where the bones are joined to each other.

Ascending palatine artery (ah-**send**-ing **pal**-ah-tine) Arterial branch from the facial artery that supplies the palatine muscles and tonsils.

Ascending pharyngeal artery (ah-**send**-ing fah-**rin**-je-al) Medial arterial branch from the external carotid artery that supplies the pharyngeal walls, soft palate, and brain tissue.

Atlas (**at**-lis) First cervical vertebra, which articulates with the occipital bone.

Attached gingiva (jin-**ji**-vah) Gingiva that tightly adheres to the bone over the roots of the teeth.

Auricle (**aw**-ri-kl) Oval flap of the external ear.

Auriculotemporal nerve (aw-**rik**-yule-lo-**tem**-poh-ral) Nerve that serves tissues of the ear and scalp and the parotid salivary gland and joins the posterior trunk of the mandibular division of the trigeminal nerve.

Autonomic nervous system (ANS) (awt-o-**nom**-ik) Portion of the peripheral nervous system that operates without conscious control and is divided into the sympathetic and parasympathetic nervous systems.

Axis (**ak**-sis) Second cervical vertebra, which articulates with the first and third cervical vertebrae.

B

Bacteremia (bak-ter-**ee**-me-ah) Bacteria traveling within the blood system.

Base of the tongue The posterior one third or root of the tongue.

Bell's palsy (**pawl**-ze) Type of unilateral facial paralysis involving the facial nerve.

Body of the hyoid bone (**hi**-oid) Anterior midline portion of the hyoid bone.

Body of the mandible Horizontal portion of the mandible.

Body of the maxilla Portion of the maxilla that contains the maxillary sinus.

Body of the sphenoid bone (**sfe**-noid) Middle portion of the bone containing the sphenoid sinuses.

Body of the tongue Anterior two thirds of the tongue.

Bones (bones) Mineralized structures of the body that protect internal soft tissues and serve as the biomechanical basis for movement.

Brachiocephalic artery (bray-kee-oo-sah-**fal**-ik) Artery that branches directly off the aorta on the right side of the body and gives rise to the right common carotid and subclavian arteries.

Brachiocephalic vein (bray-kee-oo-sah-**fal**-ik) Vein that is formed from the merger of the internal jugular and subclavian veins with the right and left brachiocephalic veins, forming the superior vena cava.

Brain Major regions include the cerebrum, the cerebellum, and the brainstem.

Brainstem Includes the medulla, the pons, and the midbrain.

Bridge of the nose Bony structure inferior to the nasion in the nasal region.

Buccal (**buk**-al) Structures closest to the inner cheek.

Buccal artery Arterial branch from the maxillary artery that supplies the buccinator muscle and cheek tissues.

Buccal fascia Space formed between the buccinator and masseter muscles.

Buccal fat pad Dense pad of tissue covered by the buccal mucosa.

Buccal lymph nodes Superficial nodes of the face located at the mouth angle and superficial to the buccinator muscle.

Buccal mucosa Mucosa that lines the inner cheek.

Buccal nerve Nerve that serves the skin of the cheek and buccal tissue of the mandibular molar teeth and joins with the muscular nerve branches to form the anterior trunk of the mandibular division of the trigeminal nerve.

Buccal region (**buk**-al) Region of the head that is composed of the soft tissues of the cheek of the face.

Buccal space Fascial space between buccinator and masseter muscles.

Buccinator muscle (buck-**sin**-nay-tor) Muscle of facial expression that forms a portion of the cheek.

Buccopharyngeal fascia (buk-o-fah-**rin**-je-al) Deep cervical fascia that encloses the entire upper part of the alimentary canal.

C

Canal (kah-**nal**) Opening in bone that is long, narrow, and tubelike.

Canine eminence (**kay**-nine) Facial ridge of bone over the maxillary canine.

Canine fossa (**kay**-nine) Fossa at the roots of the maxillary canine teeth.

Canine space (**kay**-nine) Space located lateral to the apex of the maxillary canine.

Capillary (**kap**-i-lare-ee) Smaller blood vessel that branches off an arteriole to supply blood directly to tissue.

Carotid canal (kah-**rot**-id) Canal in the temporal bone that carries the internal carotid artery.

Carotid pulse (kah-**rot**-id) Reliable pulse palpated from the common carotid artery.

Carotid sheath (kah-**rot**-id sheeth) Deep cervical fascia forming a tube running down the side of the neck.

Carotid sinus (kah-**rot**-id **sy**-nus) Swelling in the artery just before the common carotid artery bifurcates into the internal and external carotid arteries.

Cavernous sinus thrombosis (**kav**-er-nus **sy**-nus throm-**bo**-sus) Infection of the cavernous venous sinus.

Cavernous venous sinus (**kav**-er-nus) Venous sinus located on the side of the sphenoid bone that communicates with the pterygoid plexus and superior ophthalmic vein.

Cellulitis (sel-you-**lie**-tis) Diffuse inflammation of soft tissue.

Central nervous system (CNS) Portion of the nervous system that consists of the spinal cord and brain.

Cerebellum (ser-e-**bel**-um) Second largest portion of the brain; it coordinates muscles and maintains normal muscle tone and posture, as well as coordinating balance.

Cerebrum (ser-**e**-brum) Largest portion of the brain; it coordinates sensory data and motor functions, as well as governing many aspects of intelligence and reasoning, learning and memory.

Cervical muscles (**ser**-vi-kal) Muscles of the neck that include the sternocleidomastoid and trapezius muscles.

Cervical vertebrae (**ser**-vi-kal **ver**-teh-bray) Vertebrae in the vertebral column between the skull and thoracic vertebrae.

Chorda tympani nerve (**kor**-dah **tim**-pan-ee) Branch of the facial nerve that serves the submandibular and sublingual salivary glands and tongue.

Ciliary nerves (**sil**-ee-a-re) Nerves to or from the eyeball, with some ciliary nerves converging with branches from the nose to form the nasociliary nerve.

Circumvallate lingual papillae (serk-um-**val**-ate) Large lingual papillae anterior to the sulcus terminalis.

Common carotid artery (**kom**-in kah-**rot**-id) Artery that travels in the carotid sheath up the neck to branch into the internal and external carotid arteries.

Condyle (**kon**-dyl) Oval bony prominence typically found at articulations.

Condyle of the mandible Projection of bone from the ramus of the mandible that participates in the temporomandibular joint.

Conjunctiva (kon-junk-**ti**-vah) Membrane lining the inside of the eyelids and front of the eyeball.

Contralateral (kon-trah-**lat**-er-il) Structures on the opposite side of the body.

Cornu (**kor**-nu) Small hornlike prominence.

Coronal suture (kor-**oh**-nahl) Suture between the frontal and parietal bones.

Coronoid notch (**kor**-ah-noid) Notch in the anterior border of the ramus.

Coronoid process (**kor**-ah-noid) Anterior superior projection of the ramus of the mandible.

Corrugator supercilii muscle (cor-rew-**gay**-tor soo-per-**sili**-eye) Muscle of facial expression in the eye region that is used when frowning.

Cranial bones (**kray**-nee-al) Skull bones that form the cranium and include the occipital, frontal, parietal, temporal, sphenoid, and ethmoid bones.

Cranial nerves (**kray**-nee-al) Portion of the peripheral nervous system that is connected to the brain and carries information to and from the brain.

Cranium (**kray**-nee-um) Structure that is formed by the cranial skull bones and includes the occipital, frontal, parietal, temporal, sphenoid, and ethmoid bones.

Crest (krest) Roughened border or ridge on the bone surface.

Cribriform plate (**krib**-ri-form) Horizontal plate of the ethmoid bone that is perforated with foramina for the olfactory nerves.

Crista galli (**kris**-tah **gal**-lee) Vertical midline continuation of the perpendicular plate of the ethmoid bone into the cranial cavity.

D

Deep (deep) Structures located inward, away from the body surface.

Deep cervical lymph nodes (**ser**-vi-kal) Nodes located along the internal jugular vein that are divided into two groups, superior and inferior, based on the point where the omohyoid muscle crosses the vein.

Deep parotid lymph nodes (pah-**rot**-id) Nodes located deep to the parotid salivary gland.

Deep temporal arteries (**tem**-poh-ral) Arterial branches from the maxillary artery that supply the temporalis muscle.

Deep temporal nerves (**tem**-poh-ral) Muscular nerve branches that form the anterior trunk of the mandibular division of the trigeminal nerve and innervate the deep surface of the temporalis muscle.

Dens (denz) Odontoid process of the second cervical vertebra.

Depression of the mandible (de-**presh**-in) Lowering of the lower jaw.

Depressor anguli oris muscle (de-**pres**-er **an**-gu-lie **or**-is) Muscle of facial expression in the mouth region that depresses the angle of the mouth.

Depressor labii inferioris muscle (de-**pres**-er **lay**-be-eye in-**fere**-ee-o-ris) Muscle of facial expression in the mouth region that depresses the lower lip.

Diencephalon (di-en-**sef**-a-lon) Portion of the brain that consists of the thalamus and hypothalamus.

Digastric muscle (di-**gas**-trik) Suprahyoid muscle with an anterior and a posterior belly.

Disc of the temporomandibular joint (disk) Fibrous disc located between the temporal bone and condyle of the mandible.

Distal (**dis**-tl) Area that is farther away from the median plane of the body.

Dorsal (**dor**-sal) Back of an area of the body.

Dorsal surface of the tongue Top surface of the tongue.

Duct (dukt) Passageway to carry the secretion from the exocrine gland to the location where it will be used.

E

Efferent nerve (**ef**-er-ent) Motor nerve that carries information away from the brain or spinal cord to the periphery of the body.

Efferent nervous system (**ef**-er-ent) Or motor nerve system, which carries information from the brain or spinal cord to muscles or glands.

Efferent vessel (**ef**-er-ent) Type of lymphatic vessel in which lymph flows out of the lymph node in the area of the node's hilus.

Elevation of the mandible (el-eh-**vay**-shun) Raising of the lower jaw.

Embolus, emboli (**em**-bol-us, **em**-bol-eye) Foreign material, or thrombus, traveling in the blood that can block the vessel.

Eminence (**em**-i-nins) Tubercle or rounded elevation on the bony surface.

Endocrine gland (**en**-dah-krin) Type of gland without a duct, with the secretion being poured directly into the blood, which then carries the secretion to the region being used.

Epicondyle (ep-ee-**kon**-dyl) Small prominence that is located above or upon a condyle.

Epicranial aponeurosis (ep-ee-**kray**-nee-all ap-o-new-**row**-sis) Scalpal tendon from which the frontal belly of the epicranial muscle arises.

Epicranial muscle (ep-ee-**kray**-nee-al) Muscle of facial expression in the scalp region that has a frontal and an occipital belly.

Ethmoid bone (**eth**-moid) Single midline cranial bone of the skull.

Ethmoid sinuses (**eth**-moid **sy**-nus-es) Paired paranasal sinuses located in the ethmoid bone, which are also called ethmoid air cells.

Exocrine gland (**ek**-sah-krin) Type of gland with an associated duct that serves as a passageway for the secretion to be emptied directly into the location where the secretion is to be used.

External (eks-**tern**-il) Outer side of the wall of a hollow structure.

External acoustic meatus (ah-**koos**-tik me-**ate**-us) Canal leading to the tympanic cavity.

External carotid artery (kah-**rot**-id) Artery that arises from the common carotid artery and supplies the extracranial tissues of the head and neck, including the oral cavity.

External jugular lymph nodes (**jug**-you-lar) Superficial cervical nodes located along the external jugular vein.

External jugular vein (**jug**-you-lar)   Vein that forms from the posterior division of the retromandibular vein.

External nasal nerve (**nay**-zil)   Nerve from portions of the nose skin that converges with other branches to form the nasociliary nerve.

External oblique line (ob-**leek**)   Crest on the lateral side of the mandible, where the ramus joins the body.

Extrinsic tongue muscles (eks-**trin**-sik)   Tongue muscles with different origins outside the tongue.

Eyelids   Movable upper and lower tissues that cover and protect each eyeball.

F

Facial (**fay**-shal)   Structures closest to the facial surface.

Facial artery   Anterior arterial branch from the external carotid artery with a complicated path as it gives off the ascending palatine, submental, inferior and superior labial, and angular arteries.

Facial bones   Skull bones that create the face and include the lacrimal bone, nasal bone, vomer, inferior nasal concha, zygomatic bone, maxilla, and mandible.

Facial lymph nodes   Superficial nodes located along the facial vein that include the malar, nasolabial, buccal, and mandibular nodes.

Facial nerve   Seventh cranial nerve (VII) that serves the muscles of facial expression, posterior suprahyoid muscles, lacrimal gland, sublingual and submandibular salivary glands, tongue portion, and portion of skin through its greater petrosal, chorda tympani, and posterior auricular nerves and muscular branches.

Facial paralysis (pay-**ral**-i-sis)   Loss of action of the facial muscles.

Facial vein   Vein that drains into the internal jugular vein after draining the facial areas.

Fascia, fasciae (**fash**-e-ah, **fash**-e-ay)   Layers of fibrous connective tissue that underlie the skin and also surround the muscles, bones, vessels, nerves, organs, and other structures of the body.

Fascial spaces (**fash**-e-al)   Potential spaces between the layers of fascia in the body.

Fauces (**faw**-seez)   Faucial isthmus or junction between the oral region and oropharynx.

Filiform lingual papillae (**fil**-i-form)   Papillae that give the tongue its velvety texture.

Fissure (**fish**-er)   Opening in bone that is narrow and cleftlike.

Fistula, fistulae (**fis**-chool-ah, **fis**-chool-ay)   Passageway in the skin, mucosa, or even bone allowing drainage of an abscess at the surface.

Foliate lingual papillae (**fo**-le-ate)   Ridges of papillae on lateral tongue surface.

Foramen, foramina (for-**ay**-men, for-**am**-i-nah)   Short windowlike opening in bone.

Foramen cecum (for-**ay**-men **se**-kum)   Depression on the dorsal surface of the tongue where the sulcus terminalis points backward toward the pharynx.

Foramen lacerum (lah-**ser**-um)   Foramen between the sphenoid, occipital, and temporal bones that is filled with cartilage.

Foramen magnum (**mag**-num)   Foramen in the occipital bone that carries the spinal cord, vertebral arteries, and eleventh cranial nerve.

Foramen ovale (**ova**-lee)   Foramen in the sphenoid bone for the mandibular division of the trigeminal or fifth cranial nerve.

Foramen rotundum (row-**tun**-dum)   Foramen in the sphenoid bone that carries the trigeminal or fifth cranial nerve.

Foramen spinosum (**spine**-o-sum)   Foramen in the sphenoid bone for the middle meningeal artery.

Fossa, fossae (**fos**-ah, **fos**-ay)   Depression on a bony surface.

Frontal bone (**frunt**-il)   Single cranial bone that forms the forehead and a portion of the orbits.

Frontal eminence (**frunt**-il **em**-i-nins)   Prominence of the forehead.

Frontal nerve (**frunt**-il)   Nerve from the merger of the supraorbital and supratrochlear nerves that continues into the ophthalmic nerve when joined by the lacrimal and nasociliary nerves.

Frontal plane (**frunt**-il) Plane created by an imaginary line that divides the body at any level into anterior and posterior parts.

Frontal process of the maxilla (**frunt**-il) Process that forms a portion of the orbital rim.

Frontal process of the zygomatic bone (**frunt**-il) Process that forms a portion of the orbital wall.

Frontal region (**frunt**-il) Region of the head that includes the forehead and supraorbital area.

Frontal section (**frunt**-il) Section of the body through any frontal plane.

Frontal sinuses (**frunt**-il **sy**-nuses) Paired paranasal sinuses located internally in the frontal bone.

Frontonasal duct (frunt-o-**na**-zil dukt) Drainage canal of each frontal sinus to the nasal cavity.

Fungiform lingual papillae (**fung**-i-form) Papillae with a mushroom-shaped appearance.

G

Ganglion, ganglia (**gang**-gle-on, **gang**-gle-ah) Accumulation of neuron cell bodies outside the central nervous system.

Genial tubercles (ji-**ni**-il) Midline bony projections or the mental spines on the inner aspect of the mandible.

Genioglossus muscle (ji-nee-o-**gloss**-us) Extrinsic tongue muscle that arises from the genial tubercles.

Geniohyoid muscle (ji-nee-o-**hi**-oid) Anterior suprahyoid muscle that is deep to the mylohyoid muscle.

Gingiva, gingivae (jin-**ji**-vah, jin-**ji**-vay) Mucosa surrounding the maxillary and mandibular teeth.

Glabella (glah-**bell**-ah) Smooth elevated area on the frontal bone between the supraorbital ridges.

Gland (gland) Structure that produces a chemical secretion necessary for normal body functioning.

Glossopharyngeal nerve (**gloss**-oh-fah-**rin**-je-al) Ninth cranial nerve that serves the parotid salivary gland, a pharyngeal muscle, and a tongue portion.

Goiter (**goit**-er) Enlarged thyroid gland due to a disease process.

Gow-Gates mandibular nerve block Block that anesthetizes the inferior alveolar, mental, incisive, lingual, mylohyoid, auriculotemporal, and buccal (long) nerves.

Greater cornu Pair of projections from the sides of the body of the hyoid bone.

Greater palatine artery (**pal**-ah-tine) Arterial branch from the maxillary artery that travels to the palate.

Greater palatine (GP) block (**pal**-ah-tine) Local anesthetic block that achieves anesthesia for the lingual tissues of the maxillary posterior teeth and posterior palatal tissues.

Greater palatine (GP) foramen (**pal**-ah-tine) Foramen in the palatine bone that carries the greater palatine nerve and blood vessels.

Greater palatine (GP) nerve (**pal**-ah-tine) Nerve that serves the posterior hard palate and posterior lingual gingiva and then joins the maxillary nerve.

Greater petrosal nerve (peh-**troh**-sil) Branch of the facial nerve that serves the lacrimal gland, nasal cavity, and minor salivary glands of the hard and soft palates.

Greater wing of the sphenoid bone (**sfe**-noid) Posterolateral process of the body of the sphenoid bone.

H

Hamulus (**ha**-mu-lis) Process of the medial pterygoid plate of the sphenoid bone.

Hard palate (**pal**-it) Anterior portion of the palate formed by the palatine processes of the maxilla and the horizontal plates of the palatine bones.

Head (hed) Rounded surface projecting from a bone by a neck.

Helix (**heel**-iks) The superior and posterior free margin of the auricle.

Hematoma (hee-mah-**toe**-mah) Bruise that results when a blood vessel is injured and a small amount of blood escapes into the surrounding tissue and clots.

Hemorrhage (**hem**-ah-rij) Large amounts of blood that escape into the surrounding tissue without clotting when a blood vessel is seriously injured.

Hilus (**hi**-lus) Depression on one side of a lymph node where lymph flows out by way of an efferent lymphatic vessel.

Horizontal plane (hor-i-**zon**-tal) Plane created by an imaginary line that divides the body at any level into superior and inferior parts.

Horizontal plates of the palatine bones Plates that form the posterior portion of the hard palate.

Hyoglossus muscle (hi-o-**gloss**-us) Extrinsic tongue muscle that originates from the hyoid bone.

Hyoid bone (**hi**-oid) Bone suspended in the neck that allows the attachment of many muscles.

Hyoid muscles (**hi**-oid) Muscles that attach to the hyoid bone and can be classified by whether they are superior or inferior to the hyoid bone.

Hypoglossal canal (hi-poh-**gloss**-al) Canal in the occipital bone that carries the twelfth cranial nerve.

Hypoglossal nerve (hi-poh-**gloss**-al) Twelfth cranial nerve (XII) that serves the muscles of the tongue.

Hypothalamus (**hi**-po-**thal**-a-mus) Portion of the diencephalus that regulates homeostasis.

I

Incisive artery (in-**sy**-ziv) Arterial branch from the inferior alveolar artery that divides into dental and alveolar branches to supply the pulp tissue and periodontium of the mandibular anterior teeth.

Incisive block (in-**sy**-ziv) Local anesthetic block that achieves anesthesia of the pulp and facial tissues of the mandibular anterior and premolar teeth.

Incisive foramen (in-**sy**-ziv) Foramen in the maxilla that carries branches of the right and left nasopalatine nerves and blood vessels and is marked by the incisive papilla.

Incisive nerve (in-**sy**-ziv) Nerve that is formed from dental and interdental branches of the mandibular anterior teeth and merges with the mental nerve to form the inferior alveolar nerve.

Incisive papilla (in-**sy**-ziv pah-**pil**-ah) Bulge of tissue on the hard palate over the incisive foramen.

Incisura (in-si-**su**-rah) Indentation or notch at the edge of the bone.

Inferior (in-**fere**-ee-or) Area that faces away from the head and toward the feet of the body.

Inferior alveolar artery (al-**ve**-o-lar) Arterial branch from the maxillary artery that supplies the mandibular posterior teeth and branches into the mental and incisive arteries.

Inferior alveolar (IA) block (al-**ve**-o-lar) Local anesthetic block that achieves anesthesia of the pulp and lingual tissues of the mandibular teeth, as well as facial tissues of the mandibular anterior and premolar teeth.

Inferior alveolar (IA) nerve (al-**ve**-o-lar) Nerve formed from the merger of the incisive and mental nerves that serves the tissues of the chin, lower lip, and labial mucosa of the mandibular anterior and premolar teeth and later joins the posterior trunk of the mandibular division of the trigeminal nerve.

Inferior alveolar vein (al-**ve**-o-lar) Vein formed by the merger of the dental, alveolar, and mental branches that drains the pulp tissue and periodontium of the mandibular teeth, as well as the tissues of the chin.

Inferior articular processes (ar-**tik**-you-lar) Processes of the first and second cervical vertebrae that allow articulation with the vertebrae below.

Inferior labial artery Arterial branch from the facial artery that supplies the lower lip tissues.

Inferior labial vein Vein that drains the lower lip and then drains into the facial vein.

Inferior nasal conchae (**nay**-zil **kong**-kay) Paired facial bones that project inwardly from the maxilla to form walls of the nasal cavity.

Inferior orbital fissure (**or**-bit-al) Fissure between the greater wing of the sphenoid bone and maxilla that carries the infraorbital and zygomatic nerves, as well as the infraorbital artery and inferior ophthalmic vein.

Infrahyoid muscles (in-frah-**hi**-oid) Hyoid muscles that are inferior to the hyoid bone.

Infraorbital artery (in-frah-**or**-bit-al) Arterial branch from the maxillary artery that gives off the anterior superior alveolar artery and branches to the orbit.

Infraorbital (IO) block (in-frah-**or**-bit-al) Local anesthetic block that achieves anesthesia in the tissues supplied by the middle and anterior superior alveolar nerves, including the pulp and facial tissues of the maxillary anterior and premolar teeth.

Infraorbital canal (in-frah-**or**-bit-al) Canal off the infraorbital sulcus that terminates on the surface of the maxilla as the infraorbital foramen.

Infraorbital foramen (in-frah-**or**-bit-al) Foramen of the maxilla that transmits the infraorbital nerve and blood vessels.

Infraorbital (IO) nerve (in-frah-**or**-bit-al) Nerve that is involved in forming the maxillary nerve and is formed from branches of the upper lip, cheek portion, lower eyelid, and side of the nose.

Infraorbital region (in-frah-**or**-bit-al) Region of the head that is located below the orbital region and lateral to the nasal region.

Infraorbital rim (in-frah-**or**-bit-al) Inferior rim of the orbit.

Infraorbital sulcus (in-frah-**or**-bit-al) Groove in the floor of the orbital surface.

Infratemporal crest (in-frah-**tem**-poh-ral) Crest that divides each greater wing of the sphenoid bone into temporal and infratemporal surfaces.

Infratemporal fossa (in-frah-**tem**-poh-ral) Fossa inferior to the temporal fossa and infratemporal crest on the greater wing of the sphenoid bone.

Infratemporal space (in-frah-**tem**-poh-ral) Space that occupies the infratemporal fossa.

Infratrochlear nerve (in-frah-**trok**-lere) Nerve from the medial eyelid and side of the nose that converges with other branches to form the nasociliary nerve.

Innervation (in-er-**vay**-shin) Supply of nerves to tissues or organs.

Insertion (in-**sir**-shun) End of the muscle that is attached to the more movable structure.

Interdental gingiva (in-ter-**den**-tal) Attached gingiva between the teeth.

Intermediate tendon (in-ter-**me**-dee-it **ten**-don) Tendon between two muscle bellies, such as the anterior and posterior bellies of the digastric muscle.

Internal (in-**tern**-il) Inner side of the wall of a hollow structure.

Internal acoustic meatus (ah-**koos**-tik) Bony meatus in the temporal bone that carries the seventh and eighth cranial nerves.

Internal carotid artery (kah-**rot**-id) Artery off the common carotid artery that gives rise to the ophthalmic artery and also supplies intracranial structures.

Internal jugular vein (**jug**-you-lar) Vein that travels in the carotid sheath from the jugular foramen and drains the tissues of the head and neck.

Internal nasal nerves (**nay**-zil) Nerves from the nasal cavity that converge with other branches to form the nasociliary nerve.

Intertragic Notch (in-ter-**tra**-gic) Deep notch between the tragus and antitragus on the surface of the ear.

Intrinsic tongue muscles (in-**trin**-sik) Muscles located entirely inside the tongue.

Investing fascia (in-**vest**-ing) Most external layer of the deep cervical fascia.

Ipsilateral (ip-see-**lat**-er-il) Structures on the same side of the body.

Iris (**eye**-ris) Central area of coloration of the eyeball.

J

Joint (joint) Site of a junction or union between two or more bones.

Joint capsule of the temporomandibular joint Fibrous capsule that encloses the temporomandibular joint.

Jugular foramen (**jug**-you-lar) Foramen between the occipital and temporal bones that carries the internal jugular vein and ninth, tenth, and eleventh cranial nerves.

Jugular notch of the occipital bone (**jug**-you-lar) Occipital or medial portion of the jugular foramen.

Jugular notch of the temporal bone (**jug**-you-lar) Temporal or lateral portion of the jugular foramen.

Jugular trunk (**jug**-you-lar trungk) Lymphatic vessel that drains one side of the head and neck and then empties into that side's lymphatic duct.

Jugulodigastric lymph node (jug-you-lo-di-**gas**-trik) Superior deep cervical node located below the posterior belly of the digastric muscle.

Jugulo-omohyoid lymph node (jug-you-lo-o-mo-**hi**-oid) Inferior deep cervical node located at the crossing of the omohyoid muscle and internal jugular vein.

L

Labial (**lay**-be-al) Structures closest to the lips.

Labial commissure (**kom**-i-shoor) Corner of the mouth where the upper and lower lips meet.

Labial frenum (**free**-num) Fold of tissue or frenulum located at the midline between the labial mucosa and alveolar mucosa of the maxilla and mandible.

Labial mucosa Lining of the inner portions of the lips.

Labiomental groove (lay-bee-o-**ment**-il) A groove that separates the lower lip from the chin.

Lacrimal bones (**lak**-ri-mal) Paired facial bones that help form the medial wall of the orbit.

Lacrimal fluid (**lak**-ri-mal) Tears or watery fluid excreted by the lacrimal gland.

Lacrimal fossa (**lak**-ri-mal) Fossa of the frontal bone that contains the lacrimal gland.

Lacrimal gland (**lak**-ri-mal) Gland in the lacrimal fossa of the frontal bone that produces lacrimal fluid or tears.

Lacrimal nerve (**lak**-ri-mal) Nerve that serves the lateral part of the eyelid and other eye tissues and joins the frontal and nasociliary nerves to form the ophthalmic nerve.

Lambdoidal suture (lam-**doid**-al) Suture between the occipital bone and both parietal bones.

Laryngopharynx (lah-ring-gah-**far**-inks) Inferior portion of pharynx close to the laryngeal opening.

Lateral (**lat**-er-il) Area that is farther away from the median plane of the body or structure.

Lateral canthus, canthi (**kan**-this, **kan**-thy) Outer corner of the eye or outer canthus where the upper and lower eyelids meet.

Lateral deviation of the mandible (de-vee-**ay**-shun) Shifting of the lower jaw to one side.

Lateral masses (**mass**-ez) Lateral portions of the first cervical vertebra where it articulates with the occipital bone above and the axis below.

Lateral pterygoid muscle (**teh**-ri-goid) Muscle of mastication that lies in the infratemporal fossa.

Lateral pterygoid nerve (**teh**-ri-goid) Muscular branch from the anterior trunk of the mandibular division of the trigeminal nerve that serves the lateral pterygoid muscle.

Lateral pterygoid plate (**teh**-ri-goid) Portion of the pterygoid process.

Lateral surface of the tongue Side of the tongue.

Lesser cornu Pair of projections of the hyoid bone.

Lesser palatine artery (**pal**-ah-tine) Arterial branch from the maxillary artery that travels to the soft palate.

Lesser palatine foramen (**pal**-ah-tine) Foramen in the palatine bone that transmits the lesser palatine nerve and blood vessels.

Lesser palatine nerve (**pal**-ah-tine) Nerve that serves the soft palate and palatine tonsillar tissues along with the posterior nasal cavity and then joins the maxillary nerve.

Lesser petrosal nerve (peh-**troh**-sil) Parasympathetic fibers from the ninth cranial nerve that exit the skull through the foramen ovale of the sphenoid bone.

Lesser wing of the sphenoid bone (**sfe**-noid) Anterior process of the body of the sphenoid bone.

Levator anguli oris muscle (le-**vate**-er **an**-gu-lie **or**-is) Muscle of facial expression in the mouth region that elevates the angle of the mouth.

Levator labii superioris alaeque nasi muscle (le-**vate**-er **lay**-be-eye soo-per-ee-**or**-is a-lah-cue **naz**-eye) Muscle of facial expression in the mouth region that elevates the upper lip and ala of the nose.

Levator labii superioris muscle (le-**vate**-er **lay**-be-eye soo-per-ee-**or**-is) Muscle of facial expression in the mouth region that elevates the upper lip.

Levator veli palatini muscle (le-**vate**-er **vee**-lie pal-ah-**teen**-ee) Muscle of the soft palate that raises the soft palate to close off the nasopharynx.

Ligament (**lig**-ah-mint) Band of fibrous tissue connecting bones.

Line (line) Straight small ridge of bone.

Lingual (**ling**-gwal) Structures closest to the tongue.

Lingual artery Anterior arterial branch from the external carotid artery that supplies tissues superior to the hyoid bone, as well as the tongue and floor of the mouth.

Lingual frenum (**free**-num) Midline fold of tissue or frenulum between the ventral surface of the tongue and floor of the mouth.

Lingual nerve Nerve that serves the tongue, floor of the mouth, and lingual gingiva of the mandibular teeth and joins the posterior trunk of the mandibular division of the trigeminal nerve.

Lingual papillae (pah-**pil**-ay) Small elevated structures covering the dorsal surface of the body of the tongue.

Lingual tonsil (**ton**-sil) Indistinct layer of lymphoid tissue located on the dorsal surface of the tongue's base.

Lingual veins Veins that include the deep lingual, dorsal lingual, and sublingual veins.

Lingula (**ling**-gul-ah) Bony spine overhanging the mandibular foramen.

Lobule (**lob**-yule) Inferior fleshy protuberance from the helix of the auricle.

Local infiltration (lo-kal in-fil-**tray**-shun) Type of injection that anesthetizes a small area, one or two teeth and associated structures when the anesthetic solution is deposited near terminal nerve endings.

Ludwig's angina (**lood**-vigz an-**ji**-nah) Serious infection of the submandibular space, with a risk of spread to the neck and chest.

Lymph (limf) Tissue fluid that drains from the surrounding region and into the lymphatic vessels.

Lymphadenopathy (lim-fad-in-**op**-ah-thee) Process in which there is an increase in the size and a change in the consistency of lymphoid tissue.

Lymphatic ducts (lim-**fat**-ik dukts) Larger lymphatic vessels that drain smaller vessels and then empty into the venous system.

Lymphatics (lim-**fat**-iks) Part of the immune system.

Lymphatic vessels (lim-**fat**-ik **ves**-els) System of channels that drain tissue fluid from the surrounding regions.

Lymph nodes (limf nodes) Organized bean-shaped lymphoid tissue that filters the lymph by way of lymphocytes to fight disease and is grouped into clusters along the connecting lymphatic vessels.

M

Major salivary glands Large, paired glands with associated named ducts that include the parotid, submandibular, and sublingual glands.

Malar lymph nodes (**may**-lar) Superficial nodes of the face located in the infraorbital region.

Mandible (**man**-di-bl) Single facial bone that articulates bilaterally with the temporal bones at the temporomandibular joints.

Mandibular canal (man-**dib**-you-lar) Canal in the mandible where the inferior alveolar nerve and blood vessels travel.

Mandibular foramen (man-**dib**-you-lar) Foramen of the mandible that allows the inferior alveolar nerve and blood vessels to exit or enter the mandibular canal.

Mandibular lymph nodes (man-**dib**-you-lar) Superficial nodes of the face located over the surface of the mandible.

Mandibular nerve (man-**dib**-you-lar) Mandibular division of the trigeminal nerve that is formed by the merger of posterior and anterior trunks and joins with the ophthalmic and maxillary nerves to form the trigeminal ganglion of the trigeminal nerve.

Mandibular notch (man-**dib**-you-lar) Notch located on the mandible between the condyle and coronoid process.

Mandibular teeth (man-**dib**-you-lar) Teeth of the mandible.

Marginal gingiva (**mar**-ji-nal) Nonattached gingiva at the gingival margin of each tooth.

Masseter muscle (**mass**-et-er **mus**-il) Most obvious and strongest muscle of mastication.

Masseteric artery (mass-et-**tehr**-ik) Arterial branch from the maxillary artery that supplies the masseter muscle.

Masseteric nerve (mass-et-**tehr**-ik) Muscular nerve branch from the anterior trunk of the mandibular division of the trigeminal nerve

that serves the masseter muscle and temporomandibular joint.

Masseteric-parotid fascia (mass-et-**tehr**-ik-pah-**rot**-id) Deep fascia that is located inferior to the zygomatic arch and over the masseter muscle.

Masticator space (mass-ti-**kay**-tor) Space that includes the entire area of the mandible and muscles of mastication.

Mastoid air cells (**mass**-toid) Air spaces in the mastoid process of the temporal bone that communicate with the middle ear cavity.

Mastoid notch (**mass**-toid) Notch on the mastoid process of the temporal bone.

Mastoid process (**mass**-toid) Area on the petrous portion of the temporal bone that contains the air cells and on which the cervical muscles attach.

Maxilla, maxillae (mak-**sil**-ah, mak-**sil**-lay) Upper jaw that consists of two maxillary bones.

Maxillary artery (**mak**-sil-lare-ee) Terminal arterial branch from the external carotid artery.

Maxillary nerve (**mak**-sil-ar-ee) Second division of the sensory root of the trigeminal nerve that is formed by the convergence of many nerves, including the infraorbital nerve, and serves many maxillary tissues, such as the maxillary sinus, palate, nasopharynx, and overlying skin.

Maxillary process of the zygomatic bone (**mak**-sil-lare-ee) Process that forms a portion of the infraorbital rim and orbital wall.

Maxillary sinuses (**mak**-sil-lare-ee **sy**-nuses) Paranasal sinuses in each body of the maxilla.

Maxillary sinusitis (**si**-nu-**si**-tis) Infection of the maxillary sinus.

Maxillary teeth (**mak**-sil-lare-ee) Teeth of the maxilla.

Maxillary tuberosity (**mak**-sil-lare-ee too-beh-**ros**-i-tee) Elevation on the posterior aspect of the maxilla that is perforated by the posterior superior alveolar foramina.

Maxillary vein (**mak**-sil-lare-ee) Vein that after collecting from the pterygoid plexus merges with the superficial temporal vein to form the retromandibular vein.

Meatus (me-**ate**-us) Opening or canal in the bone.

Medial (**me**-dee-il) Area that is closer to the median plane of the body or structure.

Medial canthus, canthi (**kan**-this, **kan**-thy) Inner angle or canthus of the eye.

Medial pterygoid muscle (**teh**-ri-goid) Muscle of mastication that inserts on the medial surface of the mandible.

Medial pterygoid plate (**teh**-ri-goid) Portion of the pterygoid process.

Median (**me**-dee-an) Structure at the median plane.

Median lingual sulcus (**ling**-wal **sul**-kus) Midline depression on the dorsal surface of the tongue that corresponds to the deeper median septum.

Median palatine raphe (**pal**-ah-tine **ra**-fe) Midline fibrous band of the palate.

Median palatine suture (**pal**-ah-tine) Midline suture between the palatine processes of the maxillae and between the horizontal plates of the palatine bones.

Median pharyngeal raphe (fah-**rin**-je-al **ra**-fe) Midline fibrous band on the posterior wall of the pharynx.

Median plane (**me**-dee-an) Plane created by an imaginary line dividing the body into right and left halves.

Median septum (**sep**-tum) Midline fibrous structure that divides the tongue and corresponds to a midline depression, the median lingual sulcus, on the dorsal surface of the tongue.

Medulla (me-**dul**-ah) Portion of the brainstem that is involved with the regulation of heartbeat, breathing, vasoconstriction, and reflex centers.

Meningitis (men-in-**jite**-is) Inflammation of the meninges of the brain or spinal cord.

Mental artery (**ment**-il) Arterial branch from the inferior alveolar artery that exits the mental foramen and supplies the tissues of the chin.

Mental block (**ment**-il) Local anesthetic block that achieves anesthesia of the facial tissues of the mandibular premolars and anterior teeth.

Mental foramen (**ment**-il) Foramen between the apices of the mandibular first and second premolars that transmits the mental nerve and blood vessels.

Mental nerve (**ment**-il) Nerve that joins the incisive nerve to form the inferior alveolar nerve and serves the tissues of the chin and lower lip and the labial mucosa of the mandibular anterior teeth.

Mental protuberance (**ment**-il pro-**too**-ber-ins) Mandibular bony prominence of the chin.

Mental region (**ment**-il) Region of the head where the major feature is the chin.

Mentalis muscle (ment-**ta**-lis) Muscle of facial expression in the mouth region that raises the chin.

Metastasis (meh-**tas**-tah-sis) Spread of cancer from the original or primary site to another or secondary site.

Midbrain Portion of the brainstem that includes relay stations for hearing, vision, and motor pathways.

Middle meningeal artery (meh-**nin**-je-al) Arterial branch from the maxillary artery that supplies the meninges of the brain by the way of the foramen spinosum.

Middle meningeal vein (meh-**nin**-je-al) Vein that drains blood from the meninges of the brain into the pterygoid plexus of veins.

Middle nasal conchae (**nay**-zil **kong**-kay) Lateral portions of the ethmoid bone in the nasal cavity.

Middle superior alveolar (MSA) block (al-**ve**-o-lar) Local anesthetic block that achieves anesthesia of the pulp and buccal tissues of the maxillary premolars and the mesiobuccal root of the maxillary first molar.

Middle superior alveolar (MSA) nerve (al-**ve**-o-lar) Nerve that serves the maxillary premolar teeth and tissues, as well as the mesiobuccal root of the maxillary first molar, is formed from dental, interdental, and interradicular branches, and later joins the infraorbital nerve.

Middle temporal artery (**tem**-poh-ral) Arterial branch from the superficial temporal artery that supplies the temporalis muscle.

Midsagittal section (mid-**saj**-i-tl) Section of the body through the median plane.

Minor salivary glands Small glands scattered in the tissues of the buccal, labial, and lingual mucosa; soft and hard palates; and floor of the mouth, as well as associated with the circum-vallate lingual papillae.

Motor root of the trigeminal nerve Root of the trigeminal nerve.

Mucobuccal fold (mu-ko-**buk**-al) Fold in the vestibule where the labial or buccal mucosa meets the alveolar mucosa.

Mucogingival junction (mu-ko-**jin**-ji-val). Border between the alveolar mucosa and attached gingiva.

Mucosa (mu-**ko**-sah) Mucous membrane, such as that lining the oral cavity.

Muscle (**mus**-il) Type of body tissue that short-ens under neural control, causing soft tissue and bony structures to move.

Muscle of the uvula (**u**-vu-lah) Muscle of the soft palate that is within the uvula.

Muscles of facial expression Paired muscles that give the face expression and are located in the superficial fascia of the facial tissues.

Muscles of mastication (mass-ti-**kay**-shun) Pairs of muscles attached to and moving the mandible, including the temporalis, masseter, and medial and lateral pterygoid muscles.

Muscles of the pharynx (**far**-inks) Muscles that include the stylopharyngeus, pharyngeal constrictor, and soft palate muscles.

Muscles of the soft palate (**pal**-it) Muscles that include the palatoglossal, palatopharyn-geus, levator veli palatini, and tensor veli pala-tini muscles and muscle of the uvula.

Muscles of the tongue Muscles of the tongue that can be further grouped according to whether they are intrinsic or extrinsic.

Mylohyoid artery (my-lo-**hi**-oid) Arterial branch from the inferior alveolar artery that supplies the floor of the mouth and the mylohyoid muscle.

Mylohyoid groove (my-lo-**hi**-oid) Groove on the mandible where the mylohyoid nerve and blood vessels travel.

Mylohyoid line (my-lo-**hi**-oid) Line on the inner aspect of the mandible.

Mylohyoid muscle (my-lo-**hi**-oid) Anterior suprahyoid muscle that forms the floor of the mouth.

Mylohyoid nerve (my-lo-**hi**-oid) Nerve branch from the inferior alveolar nerve that serves the mylohyoid muscle and the anterior belly of the digastric muscle.

N

Naris, nares (**nay**-ris, **nay**-rees) Nostril of the nose.

Nasal bones (**nay**-zil) Paired facial bones that form the bridge of the nose.

Nasal cavity (**nay**-zil **kav**-it-ee) Cavity of the nose.

Nasal conchae (**nay**-zil **kong**-kay) Projecting structures that extend inward from the lateral walls of the nasal cavity.

Nasal meatus (**nay**-zil) Groove beneath each nasal concha that contains openings for com-munication with the paranasal sinuses or naso-lacrimal duct.

Nasal region (**nay**-zil) Region of the head where the main feature is the external nose.

Nasal septum (**nay**-zil **sep**-tum) Vertical parti-tion of the nasal cavity.

Nasion (**nay**-ze-on) Midline junction between the nasal and frontal bones.

Nasociliary nerve (nay-zo-**sil**-ee-a-re) Nerve that joins the frontal and lacrimal nerves to form the ophthalmic nerve.

Nasolabial lymph nodes (nay-zo-**lay**-be-al) Superficial nodes of the face located near the nose.

Nasolabial sulcus (nay-zo-**lay**-be-al **sul**-kus) Groove running upward between the labial commissure and ala of the nose.

Nasolacrimal duct (nay-zo-**lak**-rim-al **dukt**) Duct formed at the junction of the lacrimal and maxillary bones that drains the lacrimal fluid or tears.

Nasopalatine (NP) block (nay-zo-**pal**-ah-tine) Local anesthetic block that achieves anesthesia of the anterior portion of the hard palate.

Nasopalatine (NP) nerve (nay-zo-**pal**-ah-tine) Nerve that serves the anterior hard palate and lingual gingiva of the maxillary anterior teeth and then joins the maxillary nerve.

Nasopharynx (nay-zo-**far**-inks) Portion of the pharynx that is superior to the level of soft palate.

Nerve (nurv) Bundle of neural processes outside the central nervous system, part of the peripheral nervous system.

Nerve block (nurv) Type of injection that anesthetizes a larger area than the local infiltration because the anesthetic solution is deposited near large nerve trunks.

Neuron (**noor**-on) Cellular component of the nervous system that is individually composed of a cell body and neural processes.

Neurotransmitter (**nu**-ro-**tranz**-mitt-er) Chemical agent of the neuron that is discharged with the arrival of the action potential, diffuses across the synapse, and binds to receptors on the other cell's membrane.

Normal flora (**flor**-ah) Resident microorganisms that usually do not cause infections.

Notch (noch) Indentation at the edge of a bone.

O

Occipital artery (ok-**sip**-it-tal) Posterior arterial branch from the external carotid artery that supplies the suprahyoid and sternocleidomastoid muscles and posterior scalp tissues.

Occipital bone (ok-**sip**-it-al) Single cranial bone in the most posterior portion of the skull.

Occipital condyles (ok-**sip**-it-al) Projections of the occipital bone that articulate with lateral masses of the first cervical vertebra.

Occipital lymph nodes (ok-**sip**-it-al) Superficial nodes located on the posterior base of the head.

Occipital region (ok-**sip**-it-al) Region of the head overlying the occipital bone and covered by the scalp.

Oculomotor nerve (ok-yule-oh-**mote**-er) Third cranial nerve (III) that serves some of the eye muscles.

Olfactory nerve (ol-**fak**-ter-ee) First cranial nerve (I) that transmits smell from the nose to the brain.

Omohyoid muscle (o-mo-**hi**-oid) Infrahyoid muscle with superior and inferior bellies.

Ophthalmic artery (of-**thal**-mic) Arterial branch that supplies the eye, orbit, and lacrimal gland.

Ophthalmic nerve (of-**thal**-mic) First division of the sensory root of the trigeminal nerve that arises from the frontal, lacrimal, and nasociliary nerves.

Ophthalmic veins (of-**thal**-mic) Veins that drain the tissues of the orbit.

Opportunistic infections (op-or-tu-**nis**-tik) Normal flora creating an infectious process because the body's defenses are compromised.

Optic canal (**op**-tik) Canal in the orbital apex between the roots of the lesser wing of the sphenoid bone.

Optic nerve (**op**-tik) Second cranial nerve (II) that transmits sight from the eye to the brain.

Oral cavity Inside of the mouth.

Oral region Region of the head that contains the lips, oral cavity, palate, tongue, and floor of the mouth and portions of the pharynx.

Orbicularis oculi muscle (or-bik-you-**laa**-ris **oc**-yule-eye) Muscle of facial expression that encircles the eye.

Orbicularis oris muscle (or-bik-you-**laa**-ris **or**-is) Muscle of facial expression that encircles the mouth.

Orbit (**or**-bit) Eye cavity that contains the eyeballs.

Orbital apex (**or**-bit-al) Deepest portion of the orbit composed of portions of the sphenoid and palatine bones.

Orbital plate of the ethmoid bone (**or**-bit-al) Plate that forms most of the medial orbital wall.

Orbital region (**or**-bit-al) Region of the head with the eyeball and all its supporting structures.

Orbital walls (**or**-bit-al) Walls of the orbit composed of portions of the frontal, ethmoid, lacrimal, maxillary, zygomatic, and sphenoid bones.

Origin (**or**-i-jin) End of the muscle that is attached to the least movable structure.

Oropharynx (or-o-**far**-inks) Portion of the pharynx that is between the soft palate and opening of the larynx.

Osteomyelitis (os-tee-o-my-il-**ite**-is) Inflammation of bone marrow.

Ostium, ostia (**os**-tee-um, **os**-tee-ah) Small opening in bone.

Otic ganglion (**ot**-ik) Ganglion associated with the lesser petrosal nerve and branches of the mandibular nerve.

P

Palatal (**pal**-ah-tal) Structures closest to the palate.

Palate (**pal**-it) Roof of the mouth.

Palatine bones (**pal**-ah-tine) Paired bones of the skull that consist of two plates, a vertical and a horizontal plate.

Palatine process of the maxilla (**pal**-ah-tine) Paired processes that articulate with each other and form the anterior portion of the hard palate.

Palatine rugae (**pal**-ah-tine **ru**-gay) Irregular ridges of tissues surrounding the incisive papilla on the hard palate.

Palatine tonsils (**pal**-ah-tine) Tonsils located between the anterior and posterior faucial pillars.

Palatoglossal muscle (pal-ah-to-**gloss**-el) Muscle of the soft palate that forms the anterior faucial pillar.

Palatopharyngeus muscle (pal-ah-to-fah-**rin**-je-us) Muscle of the soft palate that forms the posterior faucial pillar.

Paranasal sinuses (pare-ah-**na**-zil **sy**-nuses) Paired air-filled cavities in bone that include the frontal, sphenoid, ethmoid, and maxillary sinuses.

Parapharyngeal space (pare-ah-fah-**rin**-je-al) Space located lateral to the pharynx.

Parasympathetic nervous system (pare-ah-sim-pah-**thet**-ik) Portion of the autonomic nervous system that is involved in 'rest or digest.'

Parathyroid glands (par-ah-**thy**-roid) Small endocrine glands located close to or even inside the thyroid gland.

Parathyroid hormone (par-ah-**thy**-roid) Hormone produced and secreted by the parathyroid glands directly into the blood to regulate calcium and phosphorus levels.

Paresthesia (par-es-**the**-ze-ah) Abnormal sensation from an area, such as burning or prickling.

Parietal bones (pah-**ri**-it-al) Paired cranial bones of the skull that articulate with each other and other skull bones.

Parietal region (pah-**ri**-it-al) Region of the head that overlies the parietal bones and is covered by the scalp.

Parotid duct (pah-**rot**-id) Duct associated with the parotid salivary gland that opens into the oral cavity at the parotid papilla.

Parotid fascia (pah-**rot**-id) Space created inside the investing fascia as it envelops the parotid salivary gland.

Parotid papilla (pah-**rot**-id pah-**pil**-ah) Small elevation of tissue that marks the opening of the parotid salivary gland and is located opposite the second maxillary molar on the inner cheek.

Parotid salivary gland (pah-**rot**-id) Major gland located over the mandibular ramus that is divided into superficial and deep lobes.

Parotid space (pah-**rot**-id) Space enveloping parotid gland.

Pathogens (**path**-ah-jens) Flora that are not normal body residents and can cause an infection.

Perforation (per-fo-**ray**-shun) Abnormal hole in a hollow organ, such as in the wall of a sinus.

Peripheral nervous system (PNS) (per-**if**-er-al) Portion of the nervous system that consists of the afferent and efferent nervous systems.

Perpendicular plate (per-pen-**dik**-you-lar) Midline vertical plate of the ethmoid bone.

Petrotympanic fissure (pe-troh-tim-**pan**-ik) Fissure between the tympanic and petrosal portions of the temporal bone, just posterior to the articular fossa, through which the chorda tympani nerve emerges.

Petrous portion of the temporal bone (**pet**-rus) Inferior portion of the bone that contains the mastoid process and air cells.

Pharyngeal constrictor muscles (fah-**rin**-je-il kon-**strik**-tor) Three paired muscles that form the lateral and posterior walls of the pharynx.

Pharyngeal tonsil (fah-**rin**-je-il) Tonsil located on the posterior wall of the nasopharynx.

Pharynx (**far**-inks) Portion of both the respiratory and digestive tracts that is divided into the nasopharynx, oropharynx, and laryngopharynx.

Philtrum (**fil**-trum) Vertical groove in the midline of the upper lip.

Piriform aperture (**pir**-i-form) Anterior opening of the nasal cavity.

Plate (plate) Flat structure of bone.

Platysma muscle (plah-**tiz**-mah) Muscle of facial expression that runs from the neck to the mouth.

Plexus (**plek**-sis) Network of blood vessels, usually veins.

Plica fimbriata, plicae fimbriatae (**pli**-kah fim-bree-**ay**-tah, **pli**-kay fim-bree-**ay**-tay) Fold with fringelike projections on the ventral surface of the tongue.

Pons (ponz) Portion of the brainstem that connects the medulla with the cerebellum.

Posterior (pos-**tere**-ee-or) Back of an area of the body.

Posterior arch Arch on the first cervical vertebra.

Posterior auricular artery (aw-**rik**-yule-lar) Posterior arterial branch from the external carotid artery that supplies the tissues around the ear.

Posterior auricular nerve (aw-**rik**-yule-lar) Branch of the facial nerve that serves the occipital belly of the epicranial muscle, the stylohyoid muscle, and the posterior belly of the digastric muscle.

Posterior cervical triangle (**ser**-vi-kal) Lateral region of the neck.

Posterior digastric nerve (di-**gas**-trik) Nerve that supplies the posterior belly of the digastric muscle.

Posterior nasal apertures (**nay**-zil) Posterior openings of the nasal cavity.

Posterior superior alveolar artery (al-**ve**-o-lar) Arterial branches from the maxillary artery that supply the pulp tissue and periodontium of the maxillary posterior teeth and maxillary sinus.

Posterior superior alveolar (PSA) block (al-**ve**-o-lar) Local anesthetic block that is used to achieve pulpal and buccal tissue anesthesia of the maxillary molars.

Posterior superior alveolar foramina (al-**ve**-o-lar) Foramina on the maxillary tuberosity that carry the posterior superior alveolar nerve and blood vessels.

Posterior superior alveolar (PSA) nerve (al-**ve**-o-lar) Nerve that directly joins the maxillary nerve after serving maxillary molars and tissues.

Posterior superior alveolar vein (al-**ve**-o-lar) Vein that is formed from the merger of dental and alveolar branches that drain the pulp tissue and periodontium of the maxillary teeth.

Posterior suprahyoid muscle group (soo-prah-**hi**-oid) Suprahyoid muscles posterior to the hyoid bone that include the posterior belly of the digastric and stylohyoid muscles.

Posterior faucial pillar (**faw**-shawl **pil**-er) Vertical fold posterior to each palatine tonsil created by the palatopharyngeus muscle.

Postglenoid process (post-**gle**-noid) Process of the temporal bone.

Previsceral space (pre-**vis**-er-al) Space located between the visceral and investing fasciae.

Primary node Lymph node that drains lymph from a particular region.

Primary sinusitis (sy-nu-**si**-tis) Inflammation of the sinus.

Process (**pros**-es) General term for any prominence on a bony surface.

Protrusion of the mandible (pro-**troo**-shun) Bringing of the lower jaw forward.

Proximal (**prok**-si-mil) Area closer to the median plane of the body.

Pterygoid arteries (**teh**-ri-goid) Arterial branches from the maxillary artery that supply the pterygoid muscles.

Pterygoid canal (**teh**-ri-goid) Small canal at the superior border of each posterior nasal aperture.

Pterygoid fascia (**teh**-ri-goid) Deep fascia located on the medial surface of the media pterygoid muscle.

Pterygoid fossa (**teh**-ri-goid) Fossa between the medial and lateral pterygoid plates of the sphenoid bone.

Pterygoid fovea (**teh**-ri-goid **fo**-vee-ah) Depression on the anterior surface of the condyle of the mandible.

Pterygoid plexus of veins (**teh**-ri-goid) Collection of veins around the pterygoid muscles and maxillary arteries that drain the deep face and alveolar veins into the maxillary vein.

Pterygoid process (**teh**-ri-goid) Portion of the sphenoid bone that forms the lateral borders of the posterior nasal apertures.

Pterygomandibular fold (teh-ri-go-man-**dib**-yule-lar) Fold of tissue in the oral cavity that covers the pterygomandibular raphe.

Pterygomandibular raphe (teh-ri-go-man-**dib**-yule-lar **ra**-fe) Fibrous structure that extends from the hamulus to the posterior end of the mylohyoid line.

Pterygomandibular space (teh-ri-go-man-**dib**-yule-lar) Space that is a portion of the infratemporal space.

Pterygopalatine fossa (teh-ri-go-**pal**-ah-tine) Fossa deep to the infratemporal fossa and between the pterygoid process and maxillary tuberosity.

Pterygopalatine ganglion (teh-ri-go-**pal**-ah-tine) Ganglion associated with the greater petrosal nerve and branches of the maxillary nerve.

Pupil (**pew**-pil) Area in the center of the iris that responds to changing light conditions.

Pustule (**pus**-tule) Small, elevated, circumscribed suppuration-containing lesion of either the skin or the oral mucosa.

R

Ramus (**ray**-mus) Plate of the mandible that extends superiorly from the body of the mandible.

Regions of the head Regions that include the frontal, parietal, occipital, temporal, orbital, nasal, infraorbital, zygomatic, buccal, oral, and mental regions.

Regions of the neck Regions that include the anterior and posterior cervical triangles.

Resting potential (po-**ten**-shal) Charge difference between the fluid outside and inside a cell that results in differences in the distribution of ions.

Retraction of the mandible (re-**trak**-shun) Bringing of the lower jaw backward.

Retroauricular lymph nodes (reh-tro-aw-**rik**-you-lar) Superficial nodes located posterior to the ear.

Retromandibular vein (reh-tro-man-**dib**-you-lar) Vein that is formed by the merger of the superficial temporal and maxillary veins and divides into anterior and posterior divisions below the parotid salivary gland.

Retromolar pad (re-tro-**moh**-lar) Dense pad of tissue distal to the last tooth of the mandible that covers the retromolar triangle.

Retromolar triangle (re-tro-**moh**-lar) Portion of the mandibular alveolar process just posterior to the most distal mandibular molar that is covered by the retromolar pad.

Retropharyngeal lymph nodes (ret-ro-far-**rin**-je-al) Deep nodes located near the deep parotid nodes and at the level of the first cervical vertebra.

Retropharyngeal space (ret-ro-far-**rin**-je-al) Fascial space located immediately posterior to the pharynx.

Right lymphatic duct Duct formed from the convergence of the lymphatics of the right arm and thorax and the right jugular trunk that drains this side of the head and neck.

Risorius muscle (ri-**soh**-ree-us) Muscle of facial expression in the mouth region that is used when smiling widely.

Root of the nose Area of the nasal region between the eyes.

S

Sagittal plane (**saj**-i-tel) Any plane of the body created by an imaginary plane parallel to the median plane.

Sagittal suture (**saj**-i-tel) Suture between the paired parietal bones.

Saliva (sah-**li**-vah) Product produced by the salivary glands.

Salivary gland (**sal**-i-ver-ee) Gland that produces saliva that lubricates and cleanses the oral cavity and helps in digestion.

Scalp (skalp) Layers of soft tissue overlying the bones of the cranium.

Sclera (**skler**-ah) White area of the eyeball.

Secondary node Lymph node that drains lymph from a primary node.

Secondary sinusitis (sy-nu-**si**-tis) Inflammation of the sinus related to another source.

Sensory root of the trigeminal nerve Root of the trigeminal nerve that has ophthalmic, maxillary, and mandibular divisions.

Skull (skul) Structure composed of both the cranial bones or cranium and facial bones.

Soft palate (**pal**-it) Posterior nonbony portion of the palate.

Somatic nervous system (SNS) Portion of the peripheral nervous system that includes all nerves controlling the muscular system and external sensory receptors.

Space of the body of the mandible (**man**-di-bl) Space formed by the periosteum covering the body of the mandible.

Spinal cord (**spi**-nal) Runs along the dorsal side of the body and links the brain to the rest of the body.

Sphenoid bone (**sfe**-noid) Single midline cranial bone with a body and several pairs of processes.

Sphenoid sinuses (**sfe**-noid **sy**-nuses) Paired sinuses located in the body of the sphenoid bone.

Sphenomandibular ligament (**sfe**-no-man-**dib**-you-lar) Ligament that connects the spine of the sphenoid bone with the lingula of the mandible.

Sphenopalatine artery (sfe-no-**pal**-ah-tine) Terminal arterial branch from the maxillary artery that supplies the nose, including a branch through the incisive foramen.

Spine (spine) Abrupt small prominence of bone.

Spine of the sphenoid bone Spine located at the posterior extremity of the sphenoid bone.

Squamosal suture (**skway**-mus-al) Suture between the temporal and parietal bones.

Squamous portion of the temporal bone (**skway**-mus) Portion that forms the braincase and portions of the zygomatic arch and temporomandibular joint.

Sternocleidomastoid muscle (SCM) (stir-no-klii-do-**mass**-toid **mus**-il) Paired cervical muscle that serves as a primary landmark of the neck.

Sternohyoid muscle (ster-no-**hi**-oid) Infrahyoid muscle that is located superficial to the thyroid gland and cartilage.

Sternothyroid muscle (ster-no-**thy**-roid) Infrahyoid muscle that inserts on the thyroid cartilage.

Stoma (**stow**-mah) Opening, such as a fistula.

Styloglossus muscle (sty-lo-**gloss**-us) Extrinsic tongue muscle that originates from the styloid process of the temporal bone.

Stylohyoid muscle (sty-lo-**hi**-oid) Posterior suprahyoid muscle that originates from the styloid process of the temporal bone.

Stylohyoid nerve (sty-lo-**hi**-oid) Branch of the facial nerve that supplies the stylohyoid muscle.

Styloid process (**sty**-loid) Bony projection of the temporal bone that serves as an attachment for muscles and ligaments.

Stylomandibular ligament (sty-lo-man-**dib**-you-lar) Ligament that connects the styloid process with the angle of the mandible.

Stylomastoid artery (sty-lo-**mass**-toid) Artery that is a branch from the posterior auricular artery and supplies the mastoid air cells.

Stylomastoid foramen (sty-lo-**mass**-toid) Foramen in the temporal bone that carries the facial or seventh cranial nerve.

Stylopharyngeus muscle (sty-lo-fah-**rin**-je-us) Paired longitudinal muscle of the pharynx arising from the styloid process.

Subclavian artery (sub-**klay**-vee-an) Artery that arises from the aorta on the left and the brachiocephalic artery on the right and gives off branches to supply both intracranial and extracranial structures, as well as the arm.

Subclavian vein (sub-**klay**-vee-an) Vein from the arm that drains the external jugular vein and then joins with the internal jugular vein to form the brachiocephalic vein.

Sublingual artery (sub-**ling**-gwal) Arterial branch from the lingual artery that supplies the sublingual salivary gland, floor of the mouth, and mylohyoid muscle.

Sublingual caruncle (sub-**ling**-gwal **kar**-unk-el) Papilla near the midline of the floor of the mouth where the sublingual and submandibular ducts open into the oral cavity.

Sublingual duct (sub-**ling**-gwal) Duct associated with the sublingual salivary gland that opens at the sublingual caruncle.

Sublingual fold (sub-**ling**-gwal) Fold of tissue on the floor of the mouth where other smaller ducts of the sublingual salivary gland open into the oral cavity.

Sublingual fossa (sub-**ling**-gwal) Fossa on the medial surface of the mandible, above the mylohyoid line, that contains the sublingual salivary gland.

Sublingual salivary gland (sub-**ling**-gwal) Major gland located in the sublingual fossa.

Sublingual space (sub-**ling**-gwal) Space located below the oral mucosa, thus making this tissue its roof.

Subluxation (sub-luk-**ay**-shun) Acute episode of temporomandibular joint disorder in which both joints become dislocated, often due to excessive mandibular protrusion and depression.

Submandibular fossa (sub-man-**dib**-you-lar) Fossa on the medial surface of the mandible, below the mylohyoid line, that contains the submandibular salivary gland.

Submandibular ganglion (sub-man-**dib**-you-lar) Ganglion superior to the deep lobe of the submandibular salivary gland that communicates with the chorda tympani and lingual nerves.

Submandibular lymph nodes (sub-man-**dib**-you-lar) Superficial cervical nodes located at the inferior border of the ramus of the mandible.

Submandibular salivary gland (sub-man-**dib**-you-lar) Major gland that is located in the submandibular fossa.

Submandibular space (sub-man-**dib**-you-lar) Space located lateral and posterior to the submental space on each side of the jaws.

Submandibular triangle (sub-man-**dib**-you-lar) Portion of the anterior cervical triangle formed by the mandible and anterior and posterior bellies of the digastric muscle.

Submasseteric space (sub-mas-et-**tehr**-ik) Space located between the masseter muscle and external surface of the vertical ramus.

Submental artery (sub-**men**-tal) Arterial branch from the facial artery that supplies the submandibular lymph nodes, submandibular salivary glands, and mylohyoid and digastric muscles.

Submental lymph nodes (sub-**men**-tal) Superficial cervical nodes located inferior to the chin.

Submental space (sub-**men**-tal) Space located midline between the symphysis and hyoid bone.

Submental triangle (sub-**men**-tal) Unpaired midline portion of the anterior cervical triangle created by the right and left anterior bellies of the digastric muscle and the hyoid bone.

Submental vein (sub-**men**-tal) Vein that drains the tissues of the chin and then drains into the facial vein.

Sulcus, sulci (**sul**-kus, **sul**-ky) Shallow depression or groove, such as that on a bony surface or between a tooth and the inner surface of the marginal gingiva.

Sulcus terminalis (**sul**-kus ter-mi-**nal**-is) V-shaped groove on the dorsal surface of the tongue.

Superficial (soo-per-**fish**-al) Structures located toward the surface of the body.

Superficial parotid lymph nodes (pah-**rot**-id) Nodes located just superficial to the parotid salivary gland.

Superficial temporal artery (**tem**-poh-ral) Terminal arterial branch from the external carotid artery that arises in the parotid salivary gland and gives off the transverse facial and middle temporal arteries, as well as frontal and parietal branches.

Superficial temporal vein (**tem**-poh-ral) Vein that drains the side of the scalp and goes on to form the retromandibular vein along with the maxillary vein.

Superior (soo-**pere**-ee-or) Area that faces toward the head of the body, away from the feet.

Superior articular processes (ar-**tik**-you-lar) Processes from a vertebra that allow articulation with the vertebra above.

Superior labial artery Arterial branch from the facial artery that supplies the upper lip tissues.

Superior labial vein Vein that drains the upper lip and then drains into the facial vein.

Superior nasal conchae (**nay**-zil **kong**-kay) Lateral portions of the ethmoid bone in the nasal cavity.

Superior orbital fissure (**or**-bit-al) Fissure between the greater and lesser wings of the sphenoid bone that transmits structures from the cranial cavity to the orbit.

Superior thyroid artery (**thy**-roid) Anterior arterial branch from the external carotid artery that supplies the tissues inferior to the hyoid bone, including the thyroid gland.

Superior vena cava (**vee**-na **kay**-va) Vein formed from the union of the brachiocephalic veins that empties into the heart.

Suppuration (sup-u-**ray**-shun) Pus containing pathogenic bacteria, white blood cells, tissue fluid, and debris.

Supraclavicular lymph nodes (soo-prah-klah-**vik**-you-ler) Deep cervical nodes located along the clavicle.

Suprahyoid muscles (soo-prah-**hi**-oid) Hyoid muscles located superior to the hyoid bone that can be further divided by their anterior or posterior relationship to the hyoid bone.

Supraorbital nerve (soo-prah-**or**-bit-al) Nerve from the forehead and anterior scalp that merges with the supratrochlear nerve to form the frontal nerve.

Supraorbital notch (soo-prah-**or**-bit-al) Notch on the frontal bone located on the supraorbital ridge.

Supraorbital ridge (soo-prah-**or**-bit-al) Ridge on the frontal bone located over the orbit.

Supraorbital vein (soo-prah-**or**-bit-al) Vein that joins the supratrochlear vein to form the facial vein in the frontal region.

Supratrochlear nerve (soo-prah-**trok**-lere) Nerve from the nose bridge and medial parts of the upper eyelid and forehead that merges with the supraorbital nerve to form the frontal nerve.

Supratrochlear vein (soo-prah-**trok**-lere) Vein that joins the supraorbital vein to form the facial vein in the frontal region.

Suture (**su**-cher) Generally immovable articulation in which bones are joined by fibrous tissue.

Sympathetic nervous system (sim-pah-**thet**-ik) Portion of the autonomic nervous system that is involved in 'fight or flight.'

Symphysis (**sim**-fi-sis) Midline articulation where bones are joined by fibrocartilage, such as the midline ridge on the mandible that fuses together in early childhood.

Synapse (**sin**-aps) Junction between two neurons or between a neuron and an effector organ where neural impulses are transmitted by electrical or chemical means.

Synovial cavities of the temporomandibular joint (sy-**no**-vee-al **kav**-i-tees) Upper and lower spaces created by the division of the joint by the disc.

Synovial fluid of the temporomandibular joint (sy-**no**-vee-al) Fluid secreted by the membranes lining the synovial cavities.

T

T-cell lymphocytes (**lim**-fo-sites) White blood cells of the immune system that mature in the thymus gland in response to stimulation by thymus hormones.

Temporal bones (tem-poh-ral) Paired cranial bones that form the lateral walls and articulate with the mandible at the temporomandibular joint.

Temporal fascia (tem-poh-ral) Deep fascia covering the temporalis muscle down to the zygomatic arch.

Temporal fossa (tem-poh-ral) Fossa on the lateral surface of the skull that contains the body of the temporalis muscle.

Temporalis muscle (tem-poh-**ral**-is) Muscle of mastication that fills the temporal fossa.

Temporal lines (tem-poh-ral) Two separate parallel ridges, superior and inferior, on the lateral surface of the skull.

Temporal process of the zygomatic bone (**tem**-poh-ral) Process that forms part of the zygomatic arch.

Temporal region (tem-poh-ral) Region of the head where the external ear is a prominent feature.

Temporal space (**tem**-poh-ral) Space formed by the temporal fascia covering the temporalis muscle.

Temporomandibular disorder (TMD) (tem-poh-ro-man-**dib**-you-lar) Disorder involving one or both temporomandibular joints.

Temporomandibular joint (TMJ) (tem-poh-ro-man-**dib**-you-lar) Articulation between the temporal bone and mandible that allows for movement of the mandible.

Temporomandibular joint ligament (tem-poh-ro-man-**dib**-you-lar) Ligament associated with the temporomandibular joint.

Temporozygomatic suture (tem-por-oh-zi-go-**mat**-ik) Suture between the temporal and zygomatic bones.

Tensor veli palatini muscle (**ten**-ser **vee**-lie pal-ah-**teen**-ee) Muscle of the soft palate that stiffens it.

Thalamus (**thal**-a-mus) Portion of the diencephalon that serves as a central relay point for incoming nervous impulses.

Thoracic duct (tho-**ras**-ik) Lymphatic duct draining the lower half of the body and left side of the thorax and draining the left side of the head and neck through the left jugular trunk.

Thrombus, thrombi (**throm**-bus, **throm**-by) Clot that forms on the inner blood vessel wall.

Thymus gland (**thy**-mus) Endocrine gland located inferior to the thyroid gland and deep to the sternum.

Thyrohyoid muscle (thy-ro-**hi**-oid) Infrahyoid muscle that appears as a continuation of the sternothyroid muscle.

Thyroid gland (**thy**-roid) Endocrine gland having two lobes and located inferior to the thyroid cartilage.

Thyroxine (thy-**rok**-sin) Hormone produced and secreted by the thyroid gland directly into the blood.

Tonsillar tissue (**ton**-sil-lar) Masses of lymphoid tissue located in the oral cavity and pharynx to protect the body against disease processes.

Tonsils (**ton**-sils) Tonsillar tissue that includes the palatine, lingual, pharyngeal, and tubal tonsils.

Tragus (**tra**-gus) Flap of tissue that is part of the auricle and anterior to the external acoustic meatus.

Transverse facial artery Arterial branch from the superficial temporal artery that supplies the parotid salivary gland.

Transverse foramen Foramen on the transverse processes of each cervical vertebra that carries the vertebral artery.

Transverse palatine suture (**pal**-ah-tine) Suture between the palatine processes of the maxillae and horizontal plates of the palatine bones.

Transverse process Lateral projections of the cervical vertebrae.

Transverse section (**trans**-vers) Section of the body through any horizontal plane.

Trapezius muscle (trah-**pee**-zee-us) Cervical muscle that covers the lateral and posterior surfaces of the neck.

Trigeminal ganglion (try-**jem**-i-nal **gang**-gle-on) Sensory ganglion located intracranially on the petrous portion of the temporal bone.

Trigeminal nerve (try-**jem**-i-nal) Fifth cranial nerve (V) that serves the muscles of mastication and cranial muscles through its motor root and serves the teeth, tongue, and oral cavity and most of the facial skin through its sensory root.

Trigeminal neuralgia (try-**jem**-i-nal noor-**al**-je-ah) Type of lesion of the trigeminal nerve involving facial pain.

Trochlear nerve (**trok**-lere) Fourth cranial nerve (IV) that serves an eye muscle.

Tubal tonsil (**tube**-al) Tonsil located in the nasopharynx near the auditory tube.

Tubercle (**too**-ber-kl) Eminence or small rounded elevation on the bony surface.

Tubercle of the upper lip (**too**-ber-kl) Thicker area in the upper lip where the philtrum terminates.

Tuberosity (too-beh-**ros**-i-tee) Large, often rough, prominence on the surface of bone.

Tympanic portion of the temporal bone (tim-**pan**-ik) Portion that forms most of the external acoustic meatus.

U

Uvula of the palate (**u**-vu-lah) Midline muscular structure that hangs from the posterior margin of the soft palate.

V

Vagus nerve (**vay**-gus) Tenth cranial nerve (X) that serves the muscles of the soft palate, pharynx, and larynx, a portion of the ear skin, and many organs of the thorax and abdomen.

Vein (vane) Type of blood vessel that travels to the heart carrying blood.

Venous sinus (**vee**-nus **sy**-nus) Blood-filled space between two layers of tissue.

Ventral (**ven**-tral) Front of an area of the body.

Ventral surface of the tongue Underside of the tongue.

Venule (**ven**-yule) Smaller vein that drains the capillaries of the tissue area and then joins larger veins.

Vermilion border (ver-**mil**-yon) Outline of the entire lip from the surrounding skin.

Vermilion zone (ver-**mil**-yon) Darker appearance of the lips.

Vertebral fascia (**ver**-teh-brahl) Deep cervical fascia that covers the vertebrae, spinal column, and associated muscles.

Vertebral foramen (**ver**-teh-brahl) Central foramen in the vertebrae for the spinal cord and associated tissues.

Vertical plates of the palatine bones Plates that form part of the lateral wall of the nasal cavity and orbital apex.

Vestibular space of the mandible (**man**-di-bl) Space of the lower jaw.

Vestibular space of the maxilla (mak-**sil**-ah) Space of the upper jaw.

Vestibules (**ves**-ti-bules) Upper and lower spaces between the cheeks, lips, and gingival tissues in the oral region.

Vestibulocochlear nerve (ves-tib-you-lo-**kok**-lear) Eighth cranial nerve (VIII) that serves to convey signals from the inner ear to the brain.

Visceral fascia (**vis**-er-al) Deep cervical fascia that is a single midline tube running down the neck.

Vomer (**vo**-mer) Single facial bone that forms the posterior portion of the nasal septum.

von Ebner's glands (**eeb**-ners) Minor salivary glands associated with the circumvallate lingual papilla.

Z

Zygomatic arch (zy-go-**mat**-ik) Arch formed by the union of the temporal process of the zygomatic bone and zygomatic process of the temporal bone.

Zygomatic bones (zy-go-**mat**-ik) Paired facial bones that form the cheek bones.

Zygomatic nerve (zy-go-**mat**-ik) Nerve that is formed from the merger of the zygomaticofa-cial and zygomaticotemporal nerves and joins the maxillary nerve.

Zygomatic process of the frontal bone (zy-go-**mat**-ik) Process lateral to the orbit.

Zygomatic process of the maxilla (zy-go-**mat**-ik) Process that forms a portion of the infra-orbital rim.

Zygomatic region (zy-go-**mat**-ik) Region of the head that overlies the cheek bone.

Zygomaticofacial nerve (zy-go-**mat**-i-ko-**fay**-shal) Nerve that serves the skin of the cheek and joins with the zygomaticotemporal nerve to form the zygomatic nerve.

Zygomaticotemporal nerve (zy-go-**mat**-i-ko-**tem**-poh-ral) Nerve that serves the skin of the temporal region and joins with the zygomaticofacial nerve to form the zygomatic nerve.

Zygomaticus major muscle (zy-go-**mat**-i-kus **may**-jer) Muscle of facial expression in the mouth region that is used when smiling.

Zygomaticus minor muscle (zy-go-**mat**-i-kus **my**-ner) Muscle of facial expression in the mouth region that elevates the upper lip.

APPENDICES

Extraoral and Intraoral Clinical Assessment

PROCEDURES FOR PERFORMING EXTRAORAL AND INTRAORAL EXAMINATIONS

EXTRAORAL REGIONS	STEPS
Overall evaluation of the face, head, and neck including skin	With patient sitting upright and relaxed, visually observe symmetry and coloration.
Parietal and Occipital Regions including scalp, hair, and occipital nodes	Standing near the patient, visually inspect the entire scalp by moving the hair, especially around the hairline, starting from one ear and proceeding to the other ear. Standing behind the patient, have the patient lean the head forward to allow bilateral palpation of the occipital nodes located at the base of the head.
Temporal Region including auricular nodes and ears	Standing near the patient, visually inspect and bilaterally palpate the auricular nodes and scalp and face around each ear. Visually inspect and palpate each ear.
Frontal Region including forehead and frontal sinuses	Standing near the patient, visually inspect and bilaterally palpate the forehead, including the frontal sinuses.
Orbital Region including the eyes	Standing near the patient, visually inspect the eyes and their movements and responses.
Nasal Region including the nose	Standing near the patient, visually inspect and bilaterally palpate the nasal region, starting at the root of the nose and proceeding to its apex.
Infraorbital and Zygomatic Regions including the muscles of facial expression, facial nodes, maxillary sinuses and bone, and temporomandibular joint	Standing near the patient, visually inspect the infraorbital and zygomatic regions, especially noting the use of the muscles of facial expression. Visually inspect and bilaterally palpate the facial nodes by moving from the infraorbital region to the labial commissure and then to the surface of the mandible. Visually inspect and bilaterally palpate the maxillary sinuses. To examine the entire joint and its associated muscles effectively, use bilateral palpation and ask the patient to open and close the mouth several times. Then ask the patient to move the opened jaw to the left, then the right, and then forward. Or using digital palpation of the mandible's movement at the temporomandibular joint,

EXTRAORAL REGIONS	STEPS
	gently place a finger into the outer portion of the external acoustic meatus. Auscultate the joint.
Buccal Region including the masseter muscle, parotid salivary gland, and mandible	Standing near the patient, visually inspect and bilaterally palpate the masseter muscle and parotid gland by starting in front of each ear and moving to the cheek area and down to the angle of the mandible. Place the fingers of each hand over the masseter muscle and ask the patient to clench the teeth together several times.
Oral and Mental Region including the chin	Standing near the patient, bilaterally palpate and visually inspect the chin.
Anterior and Posterior Cervical Triangle Regions including sternocleidomastoid muscle and associated nodes	Have the patient look straight ahead and then have the patient turn the head to the side to make the sternocleidomastoid muscle more prominent. Using two hands first on one side of the neck, then on the other, manually palpate the superficial cervical nodes, starting below the ear and continuing the whole length of the muscle surface to the clavicles. Then have the patient turn the head and palpate the deep cervical nodes on the underside of the anterior and posterior aspects of the muscle. To examine the nodes in the most inferior portion of the neck, in the area of the clavicles, have the patient raise the shoulders up and forward. Then manually palpate the nodes using one hand on each side.
Submandibular and Submental Triangle Regions including submandibular and sublingual salivary glands and associated nodes	Standing slightly behind the patient first on one side, then on the other, have the patient lower the chin and manually palpate the submental and submandibular triangular region, with its nodes and submandibular gland. Push the tissue in the area over the bony edge, where it is grasped and rolled over the angle of the mandible. The opposite side is examined in the same way.
Anterior Midline Cervical Region including hyoid bone, thyroid gland, and cartilage	Standing near the patient, place one hand on each side of the trachea. Then gently displace the thyroid tissue to the other side of the neck while the other hand manually palpates the displaced glandular tissue. Compare the two lobes of the thyroid using bimanual or manual palpation and visual inspection. Ask the patient to swallow to check for mobility of the gland by visually inspecting it while it moves superiorly.
Oral Cavity including lips, buccal and labial mucosa, parotid glands and ducts, alveolar ridges, and attached gingiva	Visually inspect the lips, including the labial frena and commissures. Bidigitally palpate the lower lip in a systematic manner from one commissure of the mouth to the other. Use the same technique for the upper lip. Have the

INTRAORAL REGIONS	STEPS
	patient open the mouth slightly and gently pull the lower lip away from the teeth to observe the labial mucosa. Use the same technique for the upper lip. Then gently pull the buccal mucosa slightly away from the teeth to palpate bidigitally, using circular compression. Dry the area and observe the flow of saliva from each duct. Retract the labial and buccal mucosa enough to visually inspect the vestibular area. Visually examine and palpate, using digital compression, the alveolar ridges, attached gingiva, maxillary tuberosity, and retromolar area. Perform olfaction of the breath.
Palate and Pharynx including the hard and soft palates, tonsillar pillars, uvula, and portions of the oropharynx and nasopharynx	Use a mouth mirror to intensify the light source and view the palatal and pharyngeal regions. Have the patient extend the tongue and observe the soft palate. Gently place the mouth mirror (mirror side down) on the middle of the tongue and ask the patient to say "aah." As this is done, visually observe the uvula and the visible portions of the pharynx. Compress the hard and soft palates with the first or second finger of one hand. Avoid circular compression on the soft palate to avoid initiating the gag reflex.
Tongue including all surfaces and swallowing pattern	To examine the dorsal and lateral surfaces of the tongue, wrap a gauze square around the anterior one third of the tongue to obtain a firm grasp while the patient gently extends it. If the patient is forced to extend the tongue too far, the gag reflex is triggered. Palpate the dorsal surface digitally. Turn the tongue slightly on its side and inspect its base and lateral borders. Bidigitally palpate the lateral surfaces of the tongue. To examine the ventral surface, have the patient lift the tongue; inspect and digitally palpate the surface. While holding the lips apart, ask the patient to swallow and observe the swallowing pattern.
Floor of the Mouth including the submandibular and sublingual salivary glands and ducts	Use the mouth mirror to facilitate lighting and direct observation. While the patient lifts the tongue to the palate, observe the mucosa of the floor of the mouth. Check the lingual frenum. Wipe the sublingual caruncle with gauze and observe the saliva flow from the duct. Bimanually palpate the sublingual area by placing the right index finger intraorally and the fingertips of the left hand extraorally under the chin to feel the tissue between the two hands. Bidigitally palpate the sublingual gland on the floor of the mouth, behind each mandibular canine, by placing the index finger of one hand intraorally and one finger extraorally and compressing the gland between the fingers.

Head and Neck Anatomy Review Cases

CASE STUDY 1

Patient Profile: Male, age 48

Chief Complaint: Floor of mouth that bleeds and burning sensation in entire lower lip

Medical History: Radiation treatment to anterior floor of mouth due to presence of squamous cell carcinoma; smoker and tobacco chewer.

Dental History: Poor prognosis for mandibular teeth

Supplemental History: Intraoral examination shows bone damage of mandibular alveolar process with hemorrhaging (Figure B–1) and paresthesia of entire lower lip.

CASE STUDY 1 QUESTIONS

1. Why does bone damage of this kind happen mainly in the mandible?
   A. Thicker cortical plates and increased vascularization
   B. Thinner cortical plates and reduced vascularization
   C. Thicker cortical plates and reduced vascularization

FIGURE B–1

D. Thinner cortical plates and increased vascularization

2. What term is used to describe the infection of the bone?
   A. Cellulitis
   B. Abscess
   C. Pericoronitis
   D. Osteomyelitis
   E. Ludwig's angina

3. Which lymph nodes are the primary nodes for the site of this lesion?
   A. Submental nodes only
   B. Submandibular nodes only
   C. Submental and submandibular nodes
   D. Deep cervical nodes only

4. Which muscle creates the patient's floor of the mouth?
   A. Zygomaticus major muscle
   B. Mylohyoid muscle
   C. Omohyoid muscle
   D. Superior pharyngeal constrictor muscle

5. Which arteries are most likely to supply the site of infection?
   A. Inferior labial artery
   B. Submental artery
   C. Occipital artery
   D. Middle meningeal artery

CASE STUDY 2

Patient Profile: Female, age 72

Chief Complaint: Dry mouth, achy jaws, and dark front tooth

Medical History: Arthritis and antidepressant medication

Dental History: Dry mouth due to medication; nightly clenching of teeth, jaws ache in the morning; and the permanent maxillary right central incisor has had root canal treatment.

Supplemental History: Extraoral examination shows firmly enlarged cheeks (Figure B–2), and intraoral examination shows a darkened permanent maxillary right central incisor.

CASE STUDY 2 QUESTIONS

1. Which areas of the mouth would need to be palpated to evaluate salivary gland function?
   A. Only the parotid duct on each side of the buccal mucosa
   B. The parotid duct on the buccal mucosa and the submandibular duct on the floor of the mouth
   C. Only the submandibular duct in the mandibular vestibule of the buccal mucosa
   D. The parotid duct on the buccal mucosa, as well as the submandibular and sublingual ducts on the floor of the mouth

2. Which gland normally produces the most saliva for this patient?
   A. Parotid gland
   B. Submandibular gland
   C. von Ebner's glands
   D. Sublingual gland

FIGURE B–2

3. What is the efferent nerve supply for the submandibular gland?
   A. Glossopharyngeal nerve
   B. Facial nerve
   C. Cervical ganglion
   D. Trigeminal nerve

4. Which bones form a joint that may be affected by arthritis?
   A. Parietal and occipital bones
   B. Maxillary and palatine bones
   C. Temporal bone and mandible
   D. Occipital bone and mandible
   E. Maxillary bone and mandible

5. What nerves may be involved in the ache she feels in her jaw?
   A. Chorda tympani
   B. Buccal branch of the facial nerve
   C. Maxillary division of the trigeminal nerve
   D. Mandibular division of the trigeminal nerve

6. What has caused the patient's firmly enlarged cheeks?
   A. Overuse of the masseter muscle
   B. Underuse of the temporomandibular ligament
   C. Excess fluid in the synovial cavities
   D. Excess blood in the disc of the joint

7. Which lymph nodes drain the periodontium associated with the darkened tooth?
   A. Buccal nodes
   B. Submandibular nodes
   C. Submental nodes
   D. Deep parotid nodes

8. Which veins drain the periodontium associated with the darkened tooth?
   A. Superficial temporal vein
   B. Posterior superior alveolar vein
   C. Incisive vein
   D. Mylohyoid vein

9. If the dentist wants to perform further treatment on the darkened tooth, which nerve must be anesthetized?
   A. Inferior alveolar nerve
   B. Posterior superior alveolar nerve
   C. Mental nerve
   D. Anterior superior alveolar nerve

10. Which local anesthetic blocks could be used to anesthetize the darkened tooth if further dental work were expected?
    A. Posterior superior alveolar block
    B. Middle superior alveolar block
    C. Infraorbital block
    D. Greater palatine block

▓ CASE STUDY 3

Patient Profile: Male, age 7

Chief Concern: Burn on front roof of mouth from hot pizza

Medical History: None

Dental History: Missed previous 6-month appointment

Supplemental History: Intraoral examination shows enlarged bilateral tonsils near the fauces (Figure B–3) and a small area of superficial ulceration on the anterior hard palate.

CASE STUDY 3 QUESTIONS

1. Which nerves are involved in the discomfort possibly felt by the patient due to the thermal burn?
   A. Posterior superior alveolar nerve
   B. Lesser palatine nerve
   C. Incisive nerve
   D. Nasopalatine nerves
   E. Anterior superior alveolar nerve

2. Which bone(s) underlie(s) the thermal burn when gently palpated during the intraoral examination?
   A. Palatine bones
   B. Zygomatic bone
   C. Maxillary bone
   D. Maxillary and palatine bones

3. Which unique intraoral landmark is nearby or within the thermal burn area?
   A. Parotid papilla
   B. Incisive papilla
   C. Retromolar pad
   D. Maxillary tuberosity

FIGURE B–3

4. Which tonsils are involved in the enlargement seen on examination?
   A. Lingual tonsil
   B. Palatine tonsils
   C. Pharyngeal tonsil
   D. Tubal tonsil

5. Which group of lymph nodes may be palpable during the extraoral examination because the patient has enlarged tonsils?
   A. Superior deep cervical nodes
   B. Submandibular nodes
   C. Submental nodes
   D. Mandibular nodes

6. Which specific lymph nodes may be palpable due to the enlarged tonsils?
   A. Jugulo-omohyoid nodes
   B. Occipital nodes
   C. Jugulodigastric nodes
   D. Auricular nodes

7. When the patient tried to chew the pizza, which of the muscles were used primarily?
   A. Temporalis muscle
   B. Epicranial muscle
   C. Mentalis muscle
   D. Risorius muscle
   E. Platysma muscle

8. Which muscle helps keep the pizza in the "correct" position during chewing?
   A. Masseter muscle
   B. Buccinator muscle
   C. Risorius muscle
   D. Medial pterygoid muscle

9. Which nerve innervates the muscles mainly involved in chewing the hot pizza?
   A. Facial nerve
   B. Glossopharyngeal nerve
   C. Trigeminal nerve
   D. Abducens nerve

10. Pressure upon examination of the ulcerated area causes the patient to frown, contracting which muscles?
    A. Zygomaticus minor muscle
    B. Corrugator supercilii muscle
    C. Risorius muscle
    D. Zygomaticus major muscle

▓ CASE STUDY 4

Patient Profile: Male, age 32

Chief concern: Bad breath and soreness in lower left jaw area

Medical history: Smoker

Dental history: Last appointment 5 years ago

Supplemental History: Intraoral examination shows pericoronal inflammation around a partially erupted permanent mandibular left third molar (Figure B–4), and the patient presents with halitosis and coated tongue.

CASE STUDY 4 QUESTIONS

1. Which lymph nodes drain the site of the oral infection?
   A. Submandibular nodes
   B. Mandibular nodes
   C. Buccal nodes
   D. Malar nodes

2. Which arteries provide the blood supply to the site of the oral infection?
   A. Inferior labial artery
   B. Inferior alveolar artery
   C. Posterior superior alveolar artery
   D. Retromandibular artery

FIGURE B–4

3. Which nerves could be involved in the discomfort at the site of the oral infection?
   A. Mental nerve
   B. Long buccal nerve
   C. Incisive nerve
   D. Posterior superior alveolar nerve

4. Which muscle is contracted when the patient sticks out his tongue during the examination?
   A. Pharyngeal constrictor muscles
   B. Hyoglossus muscle
   C. Genioglossus muscle
   D. Styloglossus muscle

5. When the patient brushes his tongue, as directed later during an oral hygiene care discussion, which nerve feels the sensation?
   A. Posterior superior alveolar nerve
   B. Lingual nerve
   C. Mental nerve
   D. Inferior alveolar nerve

6. Which nerve would need to be anesthetized to extract the involved tooth?
   A. Posterior superior alveolar nerve
   B. Middle superior alveolar nerve
   C. Greater palatine nerve
   D. Inferior alveolar nerve

7. If the involved tooth is extracted, from which bone and its process would the extraction take place?
   A. Maxillary bone and zygomatic process
   B. Mandible and coronoid process
   C. Zygomatic bone and maxillary process
   D. Mandible and alveolar process

8. If the infection progresses, which of the following locations of an abscess presentation would be most likely?
   A. Palate
   B. Buccal space
   C. Submental space
   D. Sublingual space
   E. Submandibular space

9. If the spaces associated with the involved tooth were to undergo cellulitis, into which location could the infection travel?
   A. Unilateral zygomatic region
   B. Cavernous sinus
   C. Retropharyngeal space
   D. Maxillary sinus

10. If the patient needs to take pain medication, which muscle will help close off the nasopharynx when he swallows it?
    A. Genioglossus muscle
    B. Inferior pharyngeal constrictor muscle
    C. Hyoglossus muscle
    D. Muscle of the uvula

Answers to Case Study Questions

CASE STUDY 1

1. C
2. D
3. C
4. B
5. B

CASE STUDY 2

1. D
2. B
3. B
4. C
5. D
6. A
7. B
8. B
9. D
10. C

CASE STUDY 3

1. D
2. C
3. B
4. B

5. A
6. C
7. A
8. B
9. C
10. B

CASE STUDY 4

1. A
2. B
3. B
4. C
5. B
6. D
7. D
8. E
9. C
10. D

Index

Note: Page numbers followed by f indicate figures; those followed by t indicate tables.